Practical Musculoskeletal Ultrasound

Eugene G McNally FRCR FRCPI

Consultant Musculoskeletal Radiologist
Nuffield Orthopaedic Centre
and John Radcliffe Hospitals
Oxford
UK

ELSEVIER
CHURCHILL
LIVINGSTONE

PHILADELPHIA • EDINBURGH • LONDON • NEW YORK • OXFORD • ST LOUIS • SYDNEY • TORONTO • 2005

CHURCHILL LIVINGSTONE
An imprint of Elsevier Limited

First published 2005
   Reprinted 2005

ISBN 0 443 07350 3

BRITISH LIBRARY CATALOGUING IN PUBLICATION DATA
A catalogue record for this book is available from the British
Library

LIBRARY OF CONGRESS CATALOGUING IN PUBLICATION
DATA
A catalogue record for this book is available from the Library of
Congress

NOTICE
Medical knowledge is constantly changing. Standard safety
precautions must be followed, but as new research and clinical
experience broaden our knowledge, changes in treatment and
drug therapy may become necessary or appropriate. Readers are
advised to check the most current product information provided
by the manufacturer of each drug to be administered to verify
there commended dose, the method and duration of
administration, and contraindications. It is the responsibility of the
practitioner, relying on experience and knowledge of the patient,
to determine dosages and the best treatment for each individual
patient. Neither the Publisher nor the authors assumes any
liability for any injury and/or damage to persons or property
arising from this publication.

The Publisher

ELSEVIER your source for books,
journals and multimedia
in the health sciences
www.elsevierhealth.com

Working together to grow
libraries in developing countries
www.elsevier.com | www.bookaid.org | www.sabre.org
ELSEVIER BOOK AID International Sabre Foundation

The
publisher's
policy is to use
**paper manufactured
from sustainable forests**

Printed in China
Last digit is the print number: 9 8 7 6 5 4 3 2

Contents

Contributors

Ian Beggs FRCR
Consultant Musculoskeletal Radiologist
Department of Radiology
Royal Infirmary
Edinburgh
UK

Stefano Bianchi MD PD
Consultant Musculoskeletal Radiologist
Fondation et Clinique des Grangettes
Geneva
SWITZERLAND

Nathalie Boutry MD
Consultant Musculoskeletal Radiologist
Musculoskeletal Radiology Department
Roger Salengro Hospital
Lille
FRANCE

Rethy K Chhem MD PhD FRCPC
Professor of Radiology
Chief, Department of Radiology and
    Nuclear Medicine
University of Western Ontario
London Health Sciences Centre
London, Ontario
CANADA

Michael Cohen MD
Consultant Radiologist
Medical Imaging Centre
Marseilles
FRANCE

Lawrence Friedman MBBCh FFRAD DJSA
    FRCPC FACR
Associate Professor of Radiology
Department of Radiology
Hamilton Health Sciences, Henderson Division
Hamilton, Ontario
CANADA

Wayne Gibbon FRCS FRCR
Consultant Musculoskeletal Radiologist
Department of Medical Imaging
Royal Brisbane and Women's Hospital
Brisbane, Queensland
AUSTRALIA

Andrew J Grainger MRCP FRCR
Consultant Musculoskeletal Radiologist
Department of Radiology
Leeds General Infirmary
Leeds
UK

Carlo Martinoli MD
Associate Professor of Radiology
Department of Radiology
University of Genoa
Genoa
ITALY

Eugene G McNally FRCR FRCPI
Consultant Musculoskeletal Radiologist
Nuffield Orthopaedic Centre
and John Radcliffe Hospitals
Oxford
UK

Simon J Ostlere FRCP FRCR
Consultant Musculoskeletal Radiologist
Nuffield Orthopaedic Centre
and John Radcliffe Hospitals
Oxford
UK

Philip J O'Connor MRCP FRCR
Consultant Musculoskeletal Radiologist
Department Of Radiology
Leeds General Infirmary
Leeds
UK

Philip Robinson MRCP FRCR
Consultant Musculoskeletal Radiologist
Honorary Senior Lecturer
St James's University Hospital
Leeds
UK

James L Teh MBBS BSc FRCP FRCR
Consultant Musculoskeletal Radiologist
Department of Radiology
Nuffield Orthopaedic Centre
and John Radcliffe Hospitals
Oxford
UK

David J Wilson MBBs BSc FRCP FRCR
Consultant Musculoskeletal Radiologist
Nuffield Orthopaedic Centre
and John Radcliffe Hospitals
Oxford
UK

Jane Wolstencroft BA (Hons) DCR
Senior Radiographer
Nuffield Orthopaedic Centre
Oxford
UK

Contributors

Preface

Ultrasound is the most rapidly developing technique in musculoskeletal imaging. Continuing advances in technology have broadened its application, such that it now replaces MRI in many specific clinical settings and serves as an important adjunct in others. This book owes much to the contributors who work at the forefront of these developments. The majority are dedicated musculoskeletal radiologists, who have access to the full range of imaging techniques and are therefore best placed to recommend where ultrasound is most useful and to understand its limitations. The purpose of this book is to bring this expertise together in one place, in a format designed to make this information easily accessible. With colour-coded chapters, anatomical positioning diagrams and highlighted key points and practical tips, I hope it will earn its place on the busy benches of the ultrasound department.

Eugene G McNally
Oxford 2004

To Cath, Cian, Lise and Rebecca – the real loves of my life.

Upper limb: anatomy and technique

1

Eugene G McNally

SHOULDER

Pain is the most frequent presenting complaint in patients with injuries to the rotator cuff occurring particularly during arm abduction. It is not uncommon for pain to be referred either to the posterior aspect of the shoulder or to the lateral aspect of the upper arm close to the deltoid insertion. The differential diagnosis of shoulder pain is wide and involves not only injuries related to the shoulder but also the conditions affecting the cervical spine. As a general rule, pain that is felt medial to the shoulder, particularly medial to the supraclavicular fossa, is felt to arise from the cervical spine rather than the shoulder.

The complete ultrasound examination of the shoulder involves eight standard sections. In the majority of patients these can be easily achieved with the patient seated. The examiner can be either seated or standing, in front of or behind the patient. The author's preference is to examine the patient from behind. This allows the supraspinatus to be inspected for muscle wasting and allows the patient to view the screen and become involved in their examination.

Transverse bicipital groove view

With the patient seated, the hand of the shoulder to be examined is placed on the knee, palm upwards in order to rotate the bicipital groove anteriorly. Placing the probe transversely anteriorly should easily locate the bicipital groove as a smooth defect on the anterior aspect of the humeral head. The transverse ligament, which maintains the biceps tendon within its groove, can also be depicted on high-resolution equipment as a thin hypo-reflective structure that resembles ligaments elsewhere in the body (Fig. 1.1). The normal tendon on ultrasound has a very characteristic appearance of low reflective tendon fibrils surrounded by reflective collective tissue matrix. Overall the tendon will appear bright on ultrasound provided it is interrogated with the direction of the ultrasound beam perpendicular to the tendon. If the tendon runs obliquely to the direction of the ultrasound beam then reflectivity is reduced and

Transverse bicipital
  groove view
Longitudinal biceps view
Transverse subscapularis view
Transverse free edge view
Transverse midsection view
Posterior joint, infraspinatus and
  teres view
Coronal view supraspinatus
Coronal infraspinatus view

**Ligaments around
the shoulder**

Dynamic shoulder examination

The arm

The elbow joint

Lateral coronal
Medial coronal
Anterior biceps view
Sagittal posterior

The forearm

Wrist

Volar aspect wrist
Transverse section palm
Transverse dorsal aspect
Sagittal fingers
Nerves at the wrist

Practical musculoskeletal ultrasound**1**

this can simulate tendon disease. This is termed "anisotropy".

> **Key point**
>
> A tendon running obliquely to the direction of an ultrasound beam will cause reduced reflectivity, which can simulate tendon disease.

A small quantity of fluid is frequently detected within the biceps tendon sheath. This is best appreciated in the lower part of the bicipital groove just above the musculo-tendinous junction. Alternating internal and external rotation and keeping the probe in the axial position overlying the bicipital groove is a technique used to detect dynamic biceps tendon subluxation. Patients with subluxation of biceps tendon will often complain of a painful click. The biceps tendon is kept in its groove by the transverse ligament. Rupture of this ligament can occur as an isolated injury although biceps tendon subluxation is more usually seen as a consequence of subscapularis muscle, itself most commonly the consequences of advanced rotator cuff disease. If the biceps tendon subluxes, it is important to identify whether this is superficial to, or deep to, the subscapularis tendon as this will differentiate between simple

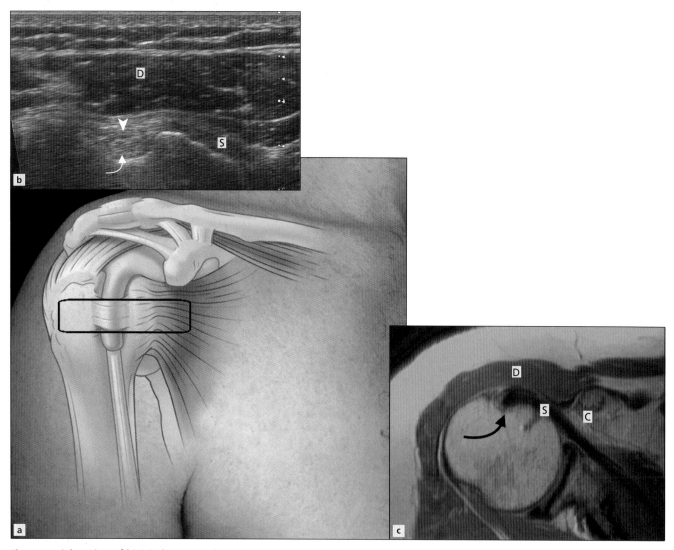

Fig. 1.1 Axial section of bicipital groove. The patient is seated with the back of the hand placed on the ipsilateral knee of the side being examined. (b) An axial plane initially demonstrates the bicipital groove on the anterior aspect of the humerus. The oval-shaped reflective biceps tendon is just visible within its groove (curved arrow), which is covered by the transverse ligament (arrowhead). The overlying muscle is the deltoid (D) and medially the subscapularis tendon (S) is just visible. The position of the probe is shown figuratively as a rectangle in (a). The overlying deltoid muscle has been removed. (c) The equivalent MRI position with the groove demonstrate (black curved arrow) and deltoid (D), subscapularis (S) and coracoid (C) is depicted.

intertransverse ligament rupture and more complex rupture of the subscapularis from its insertion.

Longitudinal biceps view

From the transverse position as described above, the probe can easily be turned 90° to demonstrate the biceps tendon in longitudinal section. It is often helpful to apply a little pressure with the distal end of the probe in order to bring the biceps tendon into a more longitudinal plane (Fig. 1.2). If there are difficulties in identifying the biceps tendon it is helpful to scan from medial to lateral and notice how the reflective leading edge of the humerus falls away as the probe overlies the bicipital groove. With a little practice it is not difficult to easily and readily achieve this position.

> **Practical tip**
>
> Applying a little pressure with the distal end of the probe helps to bring the biceps tendon into a more longitudinal plane.

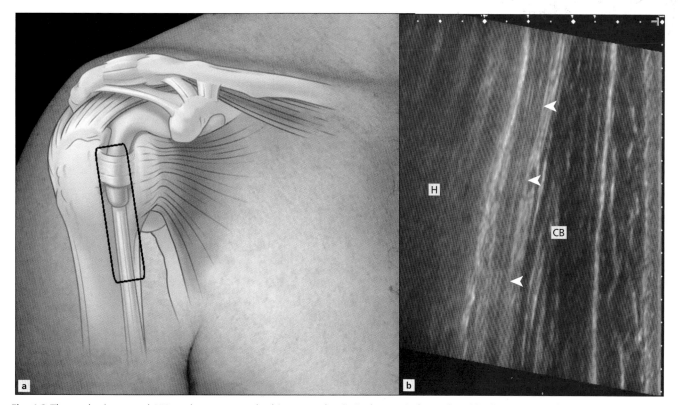

Fig. 1.2 The probe is rotated 90° to demonstrate the biceps tendon in its long axis (arrowheads). The position of the probe is shown figuratively as a rectangle in (a). The biceps tendon in its upper two-thirds is held tightly bound to the underlying humerus (H). A little pressure on the distal end of the probe helps to improve consipiquity of the tendon that can be easily traced to the musculotendinous junction. CB = coracobrachialis.

Transverse subscapularis view

This image is obtained by returning the probe in the axial plane and externally rotating the shoulder. This manoeuvre brings the subscapularis tendon out from under the coracoid and into fuller view. The insertion of the subscapularis along the medial margin of the bicipital groove, just medial to the biceps tendon, is easily recognised (Fig. 1.3). If desired, the probe can be rotated 90° to demonstrate the multipennate muscle in sagittal cross section. This is a useful image for detecting early subscapularis tendinopathy, which often begins in the superior part of the tendon. Isolated subscapularis rupture is uncommon but can occur in the absence of transverse ligament rupture.

Transverse free edge view

The supraspinatus is examined in two planes, transverse and coronal. It is the author's preference to begin with a transverse plane as the majority of rotator cuff tears can be detected on this projection. The supraspinatus tendon is best examined with the shoulder adducted with full internal rotation (Fig. 1.4). There are a variety of ways in which this can be achieved; the simplest is to ask the patient to place the back of their hand against the small of their back. Most patients can achieve this position with a minimum of discomfort. Patients with severe pain or restricted motion, such as a frozen shoulder, may have some difficulty. An alternative position is to ask the patient to place the palm of the hand as though they were

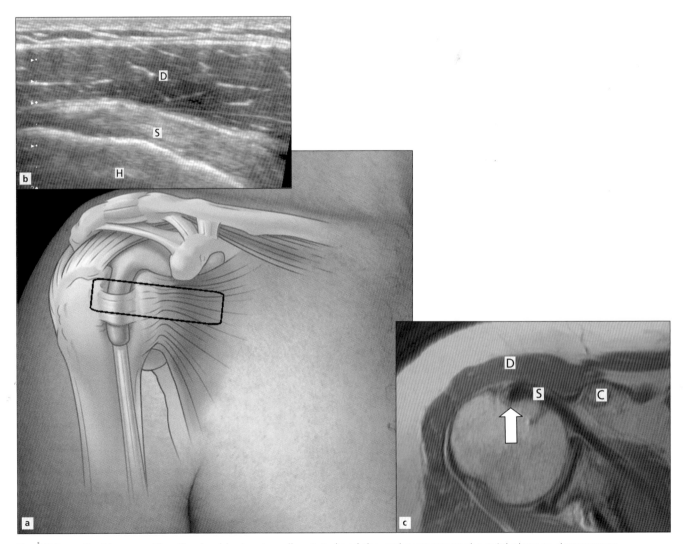

Fig. 1.3 From the biceps position the shoulder is externally rotated and the probe returns to the axial plane to demonstrate subscapularis muscle (a). The position of the probe is shown figuratively as a rectangle in (a). External rotation exposes the distal portion of subscapularis (S), which can be traced to the bicipital groove (arrow). The deltoid (D) overlies the coracoid (C) and subscapularis. H = Humerus.

putting it into their back pocket. Patients with more severe restriction of motion, e.g., those in a wheelchair or bed-bound patients, can be examined by hanging their arms at their sides and internally rotating by pointing the palm backwards.

The axial section is the position used to examine the anterior free edge of the tendon. The probe is placed transversely and anteriorly so that the image includes the reflective leading edge of the coracoid process and humeral head (Fig. 1.4). In this position the intra-articular portion of the biceps tendon can usually be identified as a reflective oval structure (Fig. 1.4b). Some patients with an excellent range of motion may internally rotate sufficient to completely

obscure the biceps tendon. In these cases the hand on pocket position should be employed. Immediately lateral to the biceps tendon is the anterior free edge of the supraspinatus tendon. The supraspinatus tendon itself is seen as a tongue of tendinous tissue lying between the humerus and the deltoid muscle. The most medial portion of it represents the free or leading edge.

> **Practical tip**
>
> Examine the supraspinatus in the transverse plane first as most rotator cuff tears can be detected there.

> **Practical tip**
>
> To diagnose a rotator-cuff tear in the axial plane, find the free edge of supraspinatus and determine whether there is a gap between it and the biceps tendon. If so, this is a free-edge tear. If not, move the probe laterally to detect a mid-substance tear.

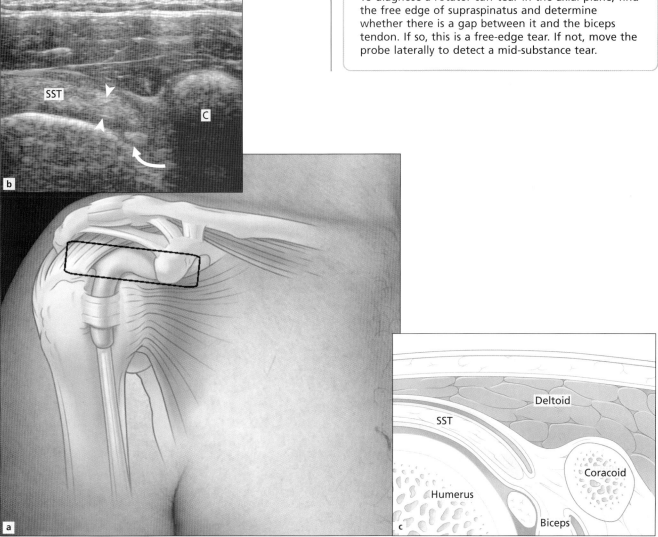

Fig. 1.4 From the subscapularis position the shoulder is internally rotated and adducted. Subscapularis disappears beneath the coracoid (C) and the intra-articular portion of the biceps tendon (curved arrow) demarcates the anterior free edge of the supraspinatus tendon (SST), which is depicted in (b) between the arrowheads. This is one of the most important sections for evaluating the supraspinatus tendon and is depicted anatomically in (a) and schematically in (c). The position of the probe is shown figuratively as a rectangle in (a).

Transverse midsection view

From the above position the probe is kept in the transverse plane and moved laterally around the curvature of the shoulder to demonstrate the mid-substance region (Fig. 1.5). The key feature to recognise is the reflective supraspinatus tendon lying between the humerus and deltoid. Supraspinatus can be followed posteriorly to a point where the posterior supraspinatus meets the anterior infraspinatus. The junctional area is visualised as the interdigitation of dark and reflective tendon slips. These poorly reflective slips may arise as a consequence of differences in the direction of tendon fibril orientation within infraspinatus, creating an anisotropic affect or differences in the degree of tendon muscle interdigitation between the two muscles. In either case the junctional area between supraspinatus and infraspinatus is difficult to appreciate with most other imaging techniques and on arthroscopy. At arthroscopy, the supraspinatus is said to attach to articular cartilage directly and the infraspinatus does not. This point is used to discriminate between the two tendons.

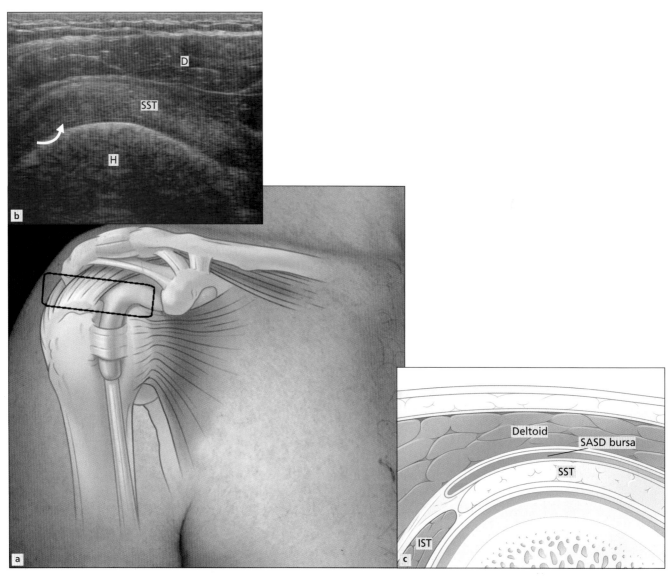

Fig. 1.5 From the free edge position the probe is moved laterally but its axial orientation is preserved. The position of the probe is shown figuratively as a rectangle in (a). The supraspinatus tendon (SST) represents the middle layer between the overlying deltoid muscle (D) on the underlying humerus (H). Posteriorly, the more poorly reflective slips of infraspinatus tendon (curved arrow) are becoming just visible. IST = infraspinatus tendon.

Posterior joint, infraspinatus and teres view

Continuing with the circular motion posteriorly and keeping the probe in the transverse plane, the posterior margin of the glenohumeral joint will be encountered (Fig. 1.6). In thin patients the posterior labrum is visualised. The overlying muscle is the infraspinatus muscle superiorly and the teres major muscle inferiorly. This is also a useful position for detecting glenohumeral effusion. Fluid in the glenohumeral joint can be seen as an area of decreased reflectivity in the region of the glenoid margin and posterior labrum and deep to the infraspinatus. This is also the position for guided aspirations and injections of the shoulder joint (see chapter 15).

Coronal view supraspinatus

Although this is referred to as the coronal view, the probe is held in the anatomical sagittal plane. A coronal view of the tendon is seen as a consequence of shoulder internal rotation. It also equates with the appearance of the supraspinatus as seen on coronally orientated MR images

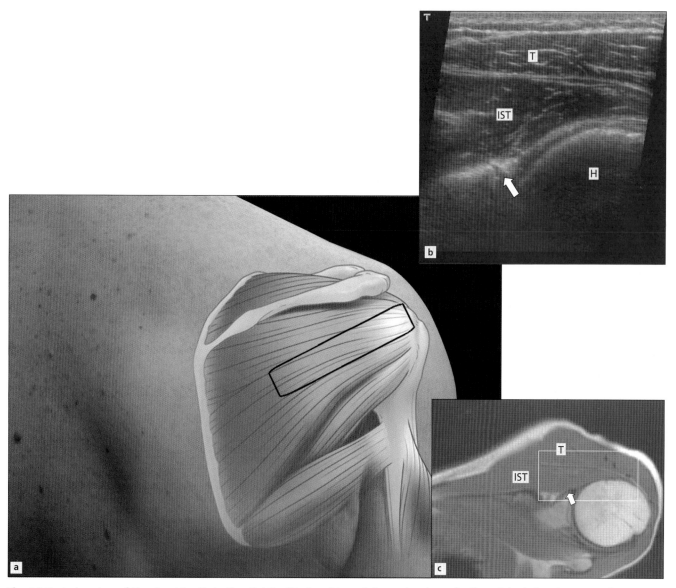

Fig. 1.6 Posterior view of the shoulder. Note the slightly tilted position of the probe along the line of the infraspinatus tendon (represented figuratively as a rectangle). (b) The infraspinatus tendon (IST) is shown between the trapezius (T) and humerus (H). The MRI equivalent position is shown in (c). The posterior labrum (arrow) is just visible.

(Fig. 1.7). The classic appearance of the supraspinatus tendon in this position is of a triangular-shaped hyper-reflective structure deep to the deltoid muscle, which is itself deep to skin subcutaneous fat. The apex of the triangle is lateral and the base is formed by acoustic shadowing from the lateral margin of the acromium. Separating the deltoid muscle from the supraspinatus tendon is the subacromial subdeltoid bursa. On good resolution equipment this is depicted as two bands of increased reflectivity representing a small quantity of fat that surrounds the bursal lining. This demarcates the bursal surface of the infraspinatus tendon, which should have a smooth convex superior surface. On the deeper joint surface of the supraspinatus the tendon can be seen to insert into the greater tuberosity. Separating the humeral head from the joint surface of the supraspinatus medial to its insertion is the humeral head articular cartilage. Occasionally areas of decreased reflectivity can be identified within the supraspinatus insertion caused by anisotropic artefact. Moving the probe more laterally and tilting it across the insertion can help to increase reflectivity and confirm this finding as artefact.

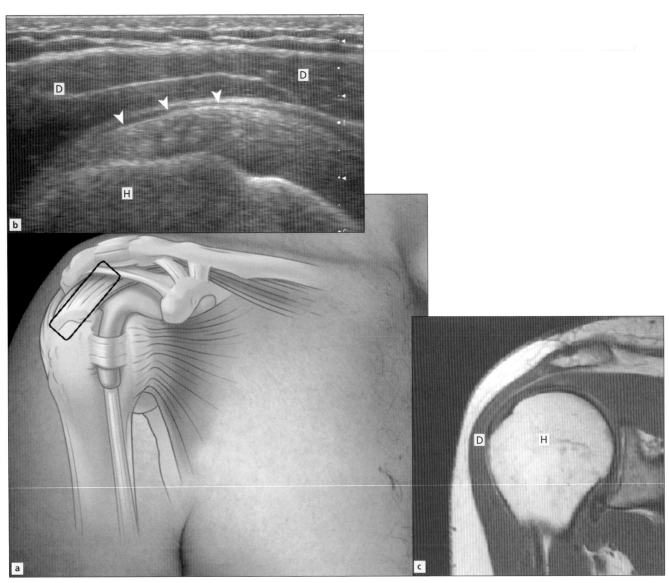

Fig. 1.7 The patient is seated with the shoulder interiorly rotated and abducted. The probe is orientated along the long axis of the supraspinatus tendon [the position of the probe is represented figuratively as a rectangle in (a)]. This is termed the "coronal view" as it is equivalent to the coronal MR image (c). (b) The ultrasound image shows the typical triangular shape to the reflective supraspinatus tendon. There is clear demarcation between the supraspinatus tendon and the overlying more poorly reflective deltoid muscle (D). The fatty tissue planes demarcating the subacromial subdeltoid bursa are seen (arrowheads). The spatial resolution as depicted by ultrasound is considerably superior to the MR equivalent (c), although the field of view and ability to demonstrate intra-articular structures and to more easily demonstrate supraspinatus muscle belly is clearly superior on the MR image. H = Humerus.

Coronal infraspinatus view

From the above position the probe is moved laterally and somewhat posteriorly to demonstrate the normal coronal appearance to infraspinatus. This is of slightly decreased reflectivity and usually a slightly thinner tendon than supraspinatus (Fig. 1.6). This can be augmented by the axial supraspinatus image which is obtained by asking the patient to place their hand on the opposite shoulder and rotating the probe until it is parallel to the infraspinatus tendon.

LIGAMENTS AROUND THE SHOULDER

Apart from the transverse ligament overlying the bicipital groove, a number of other important ligamentous structures can be identified during the routine shoulder examination. The most important of these is the coraco-acromial ligament. This is best identified by initially placing the probe in the transverse plane used to show the free edge of the supraspinatus (Fig. 1.4). The probe is then moved laterally until its most medial edge overlies the coracoid and the lateral edge of the probe is rotated upwards towards the acromium (Fig. 1.8). This reveals the

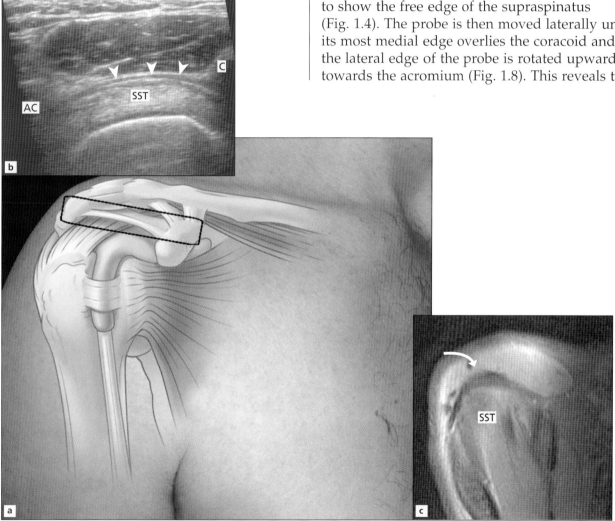

Fig. 1.8 The coraco-acromial ligament (arrowheads) is most easily seen by moving the probe medially until the reflective surface of the coracoid (C) is just visible on the medial side of the picture. The approximate orientation for the probe is shown as a rectangle in (a). (b) The ultrasound appearance of the coraco-acromial ligament (arrowheads) is shown. The supraspinatus muscle is deep. The reflective free edge of the coracoid (C) makes a useful landmark. (c) The equivalent MR image is not a conventional plane: an axial image has been used to show a near equivalent appearance with the coraco-acromial ligament seen as a low attenuation structure (curved arrow) in this T1-weighted image. The supraspinatus tendon (SST) can be seen to pass beneath the coraco-acromial ligament on both ultrasound and MR images. AC = acromium

coraco-acromial ligament, which has the characteristic appearance typical of ligaments elsewhere in the body. With a little practice the ligament can be identified relatively quickly in the majority of patients. Other ligaments include the coraco-humeral ligament, which lies in a more axial plane and blends with the transverse ligament. The glenohumeral ligaments are seen variably on ultrasound examinations; injuries are usually the consequence of recurrent dislocation and assessing the full extent of ligament and labral injuries requires MR arthrography.

> **Key point**
>
> In practice, a shoulder examination is a dynamic interaction between the positioning of the probe over the various anatomical areas and the appropriate arm and shoulder movements of the patient to bring the relevant tendons into view.

Dynamic shoulder examination

Although the examination described above has been in terms of a series of static images, in practice it is a dynamic interaction between the probe moving over the various anatomical areas in turn, in concert with the appropriate arm and shoulder movements of the patient needed to bring the relevant tendons to the field of view. It is the dynamic aspect of the examination that offers considerable advantages over other imaging techniques, particularly MRI. When fluid is present the dynamic examination can be augmented by the gentle application and release of pressure with the probe. This can be sufficient to force fluid into small tendon defects and render them more clearly visible. Information can also be gleaned from the manner in which tissue responds to this pressure and to normal patient movement. Although three possible arm positions for examining the supraspinatus tendon have been described above, none are either correct or incorrect. Indeed there are advantages in using several in any given patient, to either increase or decrease the degree of internal rotation or add or remove tension from the cuff and bursa (Figs 1.9a and 1.9b). If a small defect is suspected in the position you use as standard but you are uncertain, move the arm to another of the positions, for example, from the "arm-lock" position to the "hand in back pocket" position. The manner in which the tendon responds and or the movement of small amounts of free fluid can help to add to your suspicions or show the tendon to be normal.

> **Practical tip**
>
> In a shoulder examination, varying the degree of rotation and amount of tension on the cuff and bursa by using more than one arm position with a patient is advantageous.

A dynamic examination with more gross movement of the shoulder is necessary to detect impingement or to assess the integrity of a cuff repair. Impingement can be detected by the movement of small quantities of fluid out of the subacromial portion of the SASD bursa on abduction, or by the bunching up of thickened bursa against the acromium or coraco-acromial ligament. The latter is thought to be the more important area, and it is the coraco-acromial ligament that is divided during arthroscopic

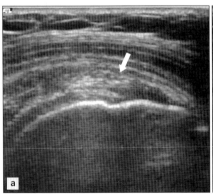 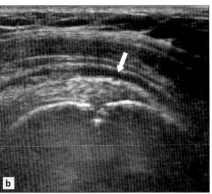

Fig. 1.9 (a) Coronal image of the supraspinatus tendon obtained with the arm fully abducted and internally rotated (arm-lock position). There is minimal separation of the SASD bursa (arrow). (b) The arm has been moved to a more moderate degree of internal rotation (hand in back pocket) and the SASD bursa opens (arrow).

subacromial decompression. The best probe position to detect these often subtle findings is one oriented 90° to the coraco-acromial ligament. The abnormal fluid and bursal movement can be seen against the coraco-acromial ligament seen in cross section. The full technique, indication and relevance of the dynamic technique in this assessment and that of the post repair cuff are discussed in chapter 4.

THE ARM

The anatomy of the arm is relatively straightforward. There are two compartments, anterior and posterior (Fig. 1.10). The anterior compartment is occupied by three muscles, the biceps forming the anterior muscle bulk with the brachialis lying posterior and posterolateral. The coraco-brachialis lies posterior and medial, deep

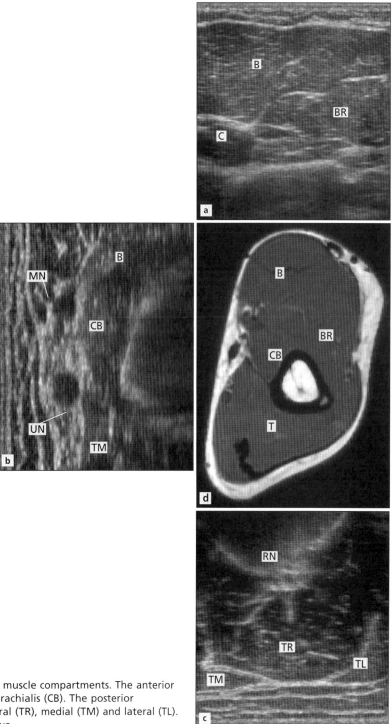

Fig. 1.10 Axial images through the arm. There are two muscle compartments. The anterior contains the biceps (B), brachialis (BR) and the coracobrachialis (CB). The posterior compartment contains the three heads of triceps, central (TR), medial (TM) and lateral (TL). MN = median nerve, UN = ulnar nerve, RN = radial nerve.

to the major neurovascular bundle that comprises the brachial artery, vein and median and ulnar nerves. The posterior compartment is occupied by one muscle, the triceps. As its name implies, there are three heads, medial, lateral (deep abutting the humerus) and the more superficial long head. In the distal arm the radial nerve and profunda brachii artery and veins lie between the brachialis and the lateral head of the triceps.

THE ELBOW JOINT

Due to its complex anatomy, the elbow joint is one of the more difficult joints to examine comprehensively with ultrasound. Once again standard sections are described, which fit well with the common clinical presentations.

Lateral coronal

The lateral coronal position is the standard position for the examination of the common extensor origin (CEO), the radiocapitellar joint

and the lateral collateral ligament. This position is best achieved with the patient sitting opposite the operator with both arms extended on the examination table into a position that mimics the hands in prayer (Fig. 1.11). It is useful to have the contralateral asymptomatic side for comparison. The common extensor origin is identified as a triangular-shaped, hyper-reflective structure comprising four superficial extensor

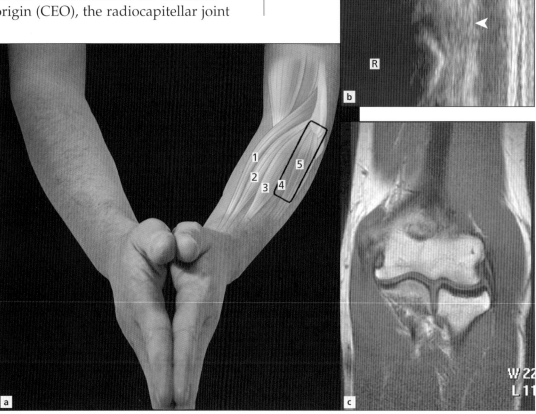

Fig. 1.11 (a) The so-called praying position exposes both elbows, particularly the lateral aspects for examination, and has the advantage of allowing immediate side-by-side comparison. The position of the probe for examination of the common extensor origin is shown figuratively as a rectangle in (a). (b) The coronal ultrasound image depicts the common extensor origin demarcated superficially by the arrowheads overlying the bony reflective interfaces for the humerus (H) and radius (R). The common extensor origin is made up of a series of muscle slips, although these cannot always be reliably separated. The lateral oblique anatomical diagram demonstrates from anterior to posterior the extensor carpi radialis longus (1), the extensor carpi radialis brevis (2), the extensor digitorum (3), the extensor carpi ulnaris (4) and the anconeus (5).

muscles (extensor carpi ulnaris, extensor digiti minimi, extensor digitorum, and extensor carpi radialis brevis). The latter is felt to be the most important in epicondylitis. The radial collateral ligament can be seen as a more organised ligament deep to the CEO. This position is also useful in the assessment of the radiocapitellar joint, particularly in children, looking for proximal radial subluxation or pulled elbow.

> **Practical tip**
>
> Placing the patient's arms in the so-called praying position allows for immediate side-by-side comparison of the elbow joints.

Medial coronal

In the same way as the common extensor origin can be examined in the lateral coronal position, the common flexor origin and ulnar collateral ligament can be examined by placing the probe in the coronal position in the medial aspect of the elbow (Fig. 1.12). The common flexor origin has a similar reflective appearance as the common extensor origin. The ulnar collateral ligament attaches to the coronoid process, provides the main resistance to valgus stress, and is therefore of particular importance in the throwing athlete. The ulnar collateral ligament comprises three bands; the anterior, posterior and transverse, of which the anterior is the largest and most important. Examining the ligament during active valgus stress has been shown by De Smet (personal communication) to improve the detection of ligament injury.

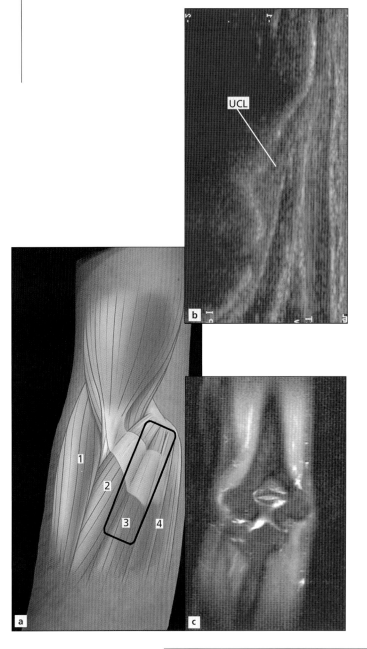

Fig. 1.12 The common flexor origin has a similar appearance to the CEO. (b) In the ultrasound image the ulnar collateral ligament (UCL) is seen. (c) The flexor muscles are (1) the prontor teres, (2) the flexor carpi radialis, (3) the flexor digitorum superficialis and (4) the flexor carpi ulnaris.

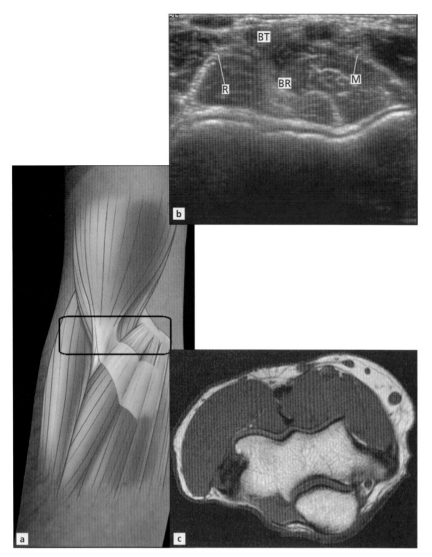

Fig. 1.13 Anterior elbow axial section. The position of the probe is shown figuratively in (a). (b) This is the easiest plane to follow the biceps tendon (BT) as it rests on brachialis (BR). The radial (R) and median (M) nerves are identified.

Anterior biceps view

By keeping the patient's arm in the same position, a transverse view of the anterior elbow can be obtained (Fig. 1.13). This is useful for examining the biceps tendon, which lies between the common flexor and extensor muscle groups. The biceps tendon is a difficult structure to examine because of anisotropy and because of its close proximity to the medial nerve and antecubital vessels. Obtaining a good sagittal view is especially challenging. Ostlere has described an alternative long-axis (coronal) view obtained by moving the probe medially and angling it laterally (Fig. 1.14). The anatomy of the anterior elbow is straightforward. Muscles are divided into three groups, medial, lateral and central. The central group comprises the brachialis muscle predominantly, with the tendon of the biceps overlying it. The medial group is the pronator teres and the common flexors; the

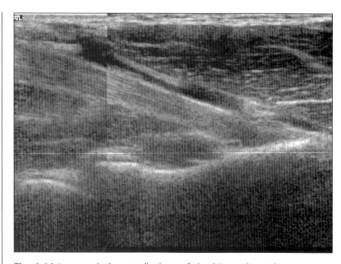

Fig. 1.14 Long-axis (coronal) view of the biceps insertion obtained by moving the probe from the central sagittal position medially, then angled laterally. Tilting the probe to follow the course of the biceps tendon as it heads towards its insertion improves visualisation.

lateral group is the brachio-radialis superficially with the common extensors.

The neural pathways across the elbow joint are important as several nerve compression syndromes can occur. The median nerve lies between the medial and central muscle groups and is least often compressed. Should compression occur, it is usually in the distal arm where a bony supracondylar process may combine with the ligament of Struthers to compress the nerve. If compression is not detected here, the nerve should be followed distally to the proximal margin of the pronator teres muscle where compression may also occur. The radial nerve lies between the central and lateral groups and may be compressed in its course from the anterior capsule of the elbow joint proximally to the arcade of Frohse at the level of the upper margin of supinator. A careful examination of the nerve and its posterior interosseus division in the axial plane is necessary to detect compression. Symptoms of radial compression may mimic lateral epicondylitis. The ulnar nerve is the most frequently compressed. Examination in the axial plane should cover from 10 cm proximal to 5 cm distal to the joint, though the commonest site of compression is within the cubital tunnel itself.

Sagittal posterior

The sagittal posterior view is ideal for the assessment of the triceps muscle, tendon, the olecranon fossa, posterior joint space and for the assessment of effusion (Fig. 1.15). There are several methods for achieving this image. When the patient is sitting opposite the examiner, a simple manoeuvre is for the patient to place their hand flat on the examination couch, then rotate it inwards whilst the elbow flexes. This is the so-called crab position and it presents the

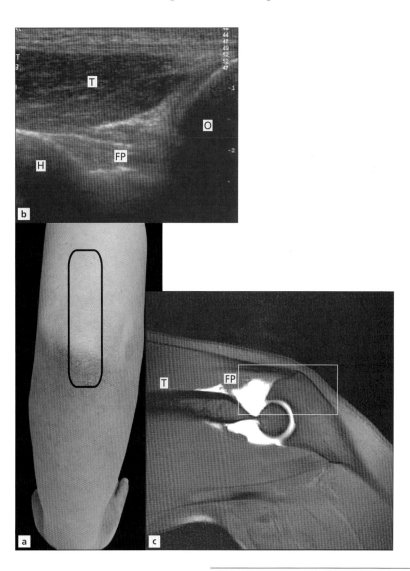

Fig. 1.15 An image through the dorsal aspect of the elbow can be achieved in a number of ways. If there is reasonably good elbow movement, the crab position is relatively easy to achieve. The arm and probe position is demonstrated as a rectangle in (a). This yields an excellent view of the olecranon fossa and is therefore particularly good for assessing elbow effusion. Its superficial muscle bulk is the triceps (T), whose tendon can be traced to its insertion into the olecranon (O). The deep bony landmark of the distal humerus (H) and trochlea. The reflective posterior fat pad (FP) separates the triceps from the joint space. If fluid is present it will be identified separating the fat pad from the humerus. If necessary, the elbow can be rotated so that a small quantity of joint fluid gravitates posteriorly and is more easily seen. The MRI equivalent is demonstrated in (c), where the fat-saturated, T1-weighted MR arthrogram shows the fat pad to be posteriorly displaced.

posterior joint for easy examination. The triangular-shaped reflective posterior fat pad is easily identified. Intra-articular fluid, if present, can be identified lying between the posterior aspect of the distal humerus and the posterior fat pad. This position is also useful for the assessment of loose bodies. A variation on this position is to externally rotate the shoulder 90° to create a mirror image of the crab position. This facilitates the detection of small amounts of intra-articular fluid as gravity brings fluid to the posterior joint space. Not all patients can manage these manoeuvres, especially if the elbow is painful or stiff, so an alternative is to have the patient sit with their back to the examiner, as in a shoulder examination, and place the affected-side hand across the chest. This presents the elbow to the seated ultrasonologist. Whilst examining the posterior elbow, the probe can be turned to the axial plane to look at the ulnar groove (Fig. 1.16).

THE FOREARM

In the forearm, muscle anatomy is best divided into three groups, anterior, posterior and lateral (Fig. 1.17). The anterior group comprises the main flexors of which there are five, three superficial and two deep. The three superficial muscles are, from medial to lateral, flexor carpi ulnaris, flexor digitorum superficialis and flexor carpi radialis. In some individuals a fourth muscle is seen anteriorly representing palmaris longus. The deep group comprise two muscles, the bulk of which is formed by the flexor digitorum profundus with the smaller flexor pollicis longus overlying the radius.

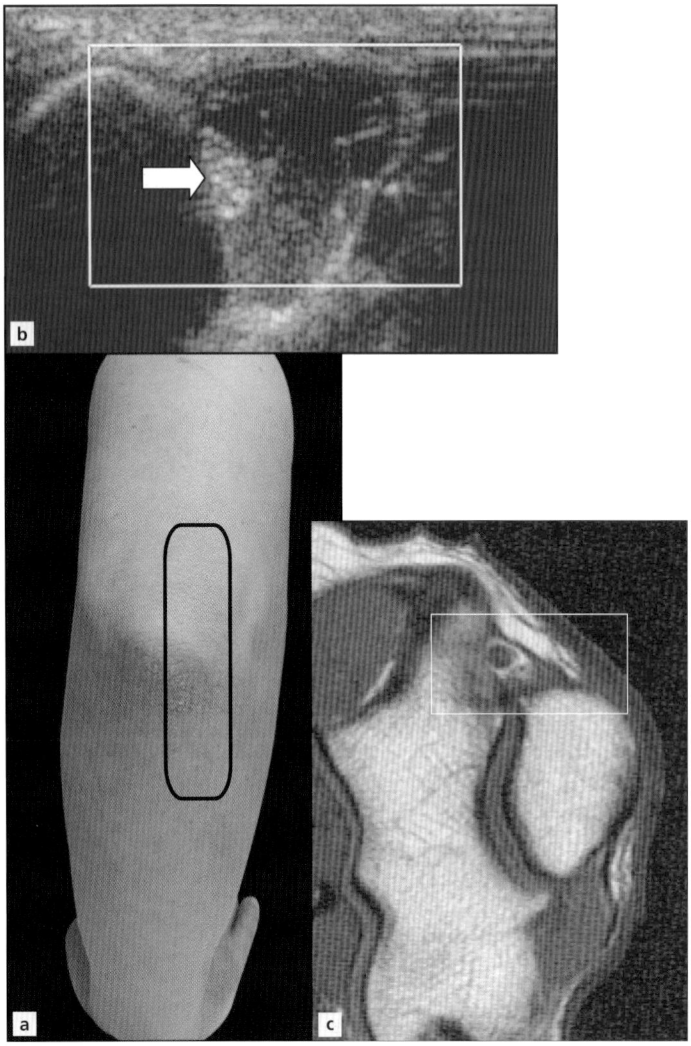

Fig. 1.16 Axial section through the ulnar groove showing the oval-shaped speckle but predominantly reflective ulnar nerve (arrow).

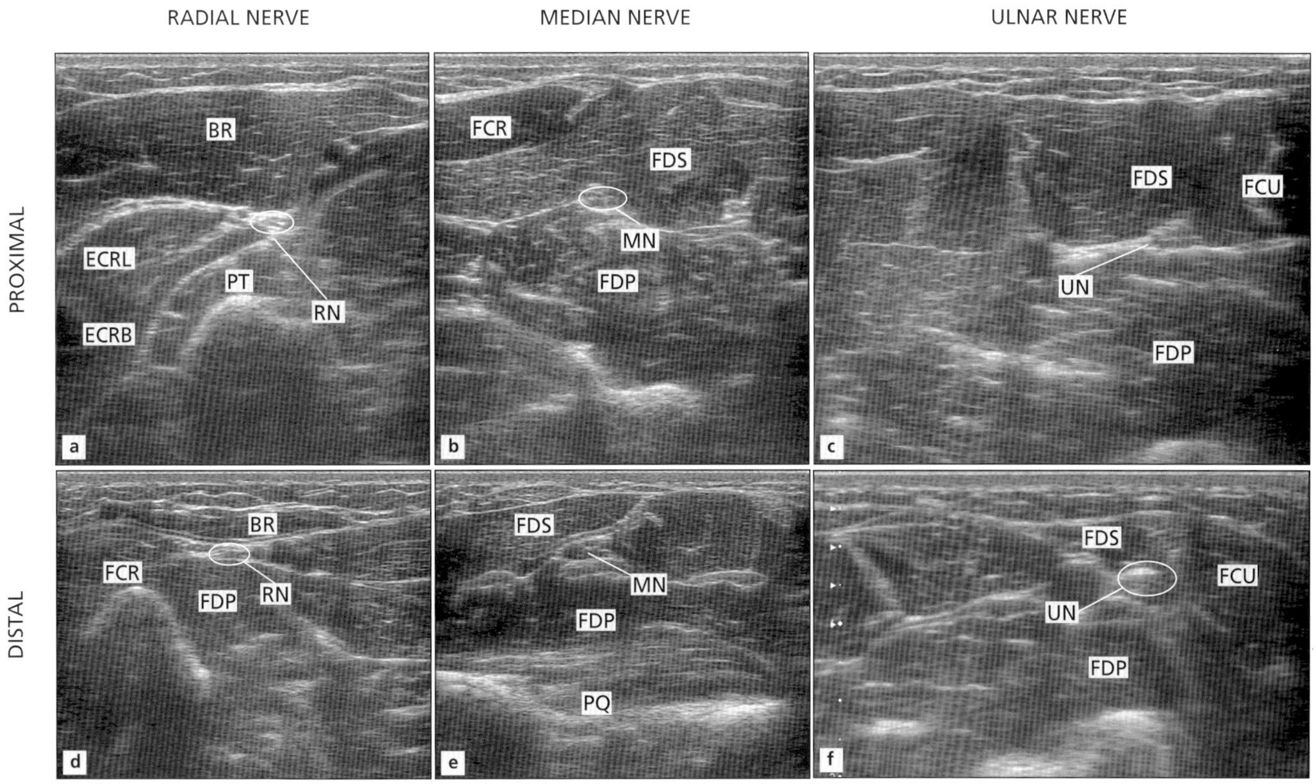

| RADIAL NERVE | MEDIAN NERVE | ULNAR NERVE |

Fig. 1.17 Transverse sections showing the course of the major nerves of the forearm, radial (a, proximal and d, distal), median (b and e) and radial (c and f). Brachioradialis (BR), extensor carpi radialis longus (ECRL) and Brevis (ECRB), pronator teres (PT), flexor carpi radialis (FCR), flexor digitorum superficialis (FDS) and profundus (FDP), flexor carpi ulnaris (FCU) and pronator quadratus (PQ). RN = radial nerve, MN = median nerve, UN = Ulnar nerve.

The dorsal group are the extensors, comprising six muscles, three superficial and three deep. The three superficial muscles from medial to lateral are extensor carpi ulnaris, extensor digiti minimi and extensor digitorum. The three deep muscles, which are in general smaller, are extensor pollicis longus, abductor pollicis longus and the supinator.

The lateral group are also predominantly extensors and comprises four muscles that are essentially parallel. From superficial to deep they are brachio-radialis, extensor carpi radialis longus, extensor carpi radialis brevis and pronator teres.

WRIST

As per the elbow, the examiner is best seated opposite the patient with the hands placed on a table. Plenty of coupling jelly is required due to the varied contours of the hand; consequently an absorbent pad placed beneath the hand is essential. The complex anatomy of the wrist and hand requires that many different techniques be used, and these are described in Chapter 6. Despite this, transverse sections at the level of

the wrist and sagittal sections at the level of the fingers are robust in providing an initial assessment (Fig. 1.18).

Volar aspect wrist

Three standard sections will be described, through the level of the distal radius, the carpal tunnel and the palm.

There are four groups of tendons on the flexor aspect of the distal wrist and these should be examined separately. The largest group comprises those tendons contained within the carpal tunnel, which is one of the fibro-osseus tunnels that transmit tendons and neurovascular structures on the volar aspect of the wrist. Its medial bony boundary is made up of the hamate and the triquetral; the lateral bony boundary is the scaphoid. A thin fibrous band, the flexor retinaculum, which can usually be depicted on good quality equipment, forms its roof (Fig. 1.18). Its main contents are the flexor tendons, but it is best known for transmission of the median nerve. The precise technique for examining the medial

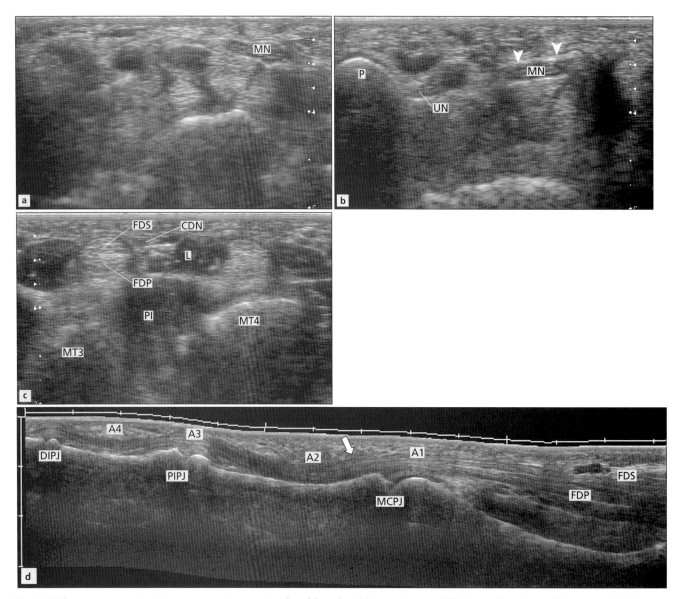

Fig. 1.18 Flexor aspect wrist. Transverse sections proximal to (a) and within carpal tunnel (b). Note that the median nerve (MN) is darker than the adjacent tendons. The ligamentous retinaculum is just visible (arrowheads). Guyon's canal on the ulnar aspect of the wrist, adjacent to the pisiform (P) transmits the ulnar nerve (UN). (c) Transverse section distal to the carpal tunnel. The lumbricals (L) lie adjacent to the superficial (FDS) and deep (FDP) flexor tendons, which lie in close proximity to the common digital nerve (CDN). The deeper muscles are the palmar interosseii (PI). (d) Sagittal panorama of the flexor tendons, showing the position of the four A pulleys. The most prominent of these, the A2 is just visible (arrow).

nerve will be described in a later section. The second and smaller tunnel is Guyon's canal, which lies to the ulnar side of the carpal tunnel and transmits the ulnar neurovascular bundle.

Outside the tunnel there is one tendon group on the ulnar side of the carpus and two on the radial. The ulnar side tendon is the flexor carpi ulnaris, which overlies the ulnar nerve at the wrist. The flexor carpi ulnaris is easily identified as it is traced to its insertion first in the pisiform and then into the hook of the hamate and base of the fifth metacarpal. The latter two insertions are sometimes termed the "pisohamate ligament" and the "pisometacarpal ligament". This is one of the more easily palpated tendons; a useful landmark is the ulnar artery, which lies just on its radial aspect.

The more ulnar of the two tendon groups on the radial aspect of the carpal tunnel is the flexor pollicis longus tendon, which inserts at the base of the distal phalanx of the thumb. It has its own synovial sheath but does pass through the flexor retinaculum. This can then be tested clinically by asking the patient to flex the thumb against resistance. Clinically this tendon can be tested by radial deviation of the wrist and thumb.

Transverse section palm

This is a complex section comprising many small muscles. Recognising each individual one and remembering their names is difficult and fortunately rarely necessary in practice. The majority of deeply placed muscles are interosseii. It is helpful to remember that the dorsal interosseii lie between the metacarpals, and that there are four, one for each interspace and numbered accordingly. The palmar interosseii, of which there are three, are more superficial. A more bulky band-like muscle, more superficial again and on the radial side, is the adductor pollicis. Most superficial of all are the flexor tendons. There are two additional muscles each for the thumb and little finger, which lie anterior and lateral to their respective fingers. For the thumb they are abductor and flexor pollicis brevis and for the little finger they are abductor and opponens digiti minimi.

Transverse dorsal aspect

Although the extensor tendons at the level of the wrist can be assessed in this position, it is most useful for the diagnosis of occult ganglia. The majority of wrist ganglia arise from the dorsal aspect of the scapholunate ligament. This ligament is best located in the axial plane. The probe is first positioned in the distal forearm so that the two-bone (radius and ulna) image is obtained. It can then be moved slowly, distally across the radio-carpal joint, to a point where the two bones become three. This is the proximal carpal row comprising the triquetral, lunate and scaphoid. Keeping in the axial plane, the probe is then moved in a radial direction (i.e., towards the thumb) to help identify the scaphoid and lunate. On good quality images the scapholunate ligament can be identified running between them. It is not absolutely necessary to identify the scapholunate ligament per se, but merely to use this as an anatomical reference point. If there is a dorsal ganglion it should be seen as a poorly reflective fluid collection arising in this region. Occasionally recesses of the wrist joint filled with synovial fluid can mimic a ganglia but these are not usually in this location and if present are easily compressible, unlike a more tense ganglion cyst.

There are six separate extensor compartments numbered 1–6 beginning on the radial aspect of the wrist (Fig. 1.19). Extensor compartment 1 contains two tendons, extensor pollicis brevis and abductor pollicis longus. Abductor pollicis longus can be traced to its insertion on the base of the thumb whereas the extensor pollicis brevis can be traced more distally to its insertion at the base of the proximal phalanx of the thumb. The two tendons together form the palmar boundary of the anatomical snuff box. Pathologically they are most commonly encountered in patients with de Quervain's tenosynovitis. This has to be distinguished from intersection syndrome, which is a tendinopathy ocurring more proximally where the first and second extensor compartments cross over each other.

Extensor compartment 2 comprises two tendons, the extensor carpi radialis longus and brevis. The brevis tendon is the more ulnar of the two inserting into the base of the third metacarpal whereas the longus inserts into the base of the second. They form the dorsal aspect of the anatomical snuff box.

The second extensor compartment is separated from the third extensor compartment by Lister's tubercle, which is a prominent anatomical landmark on the dorsal aspect of the radius.

The third compartment comprises the extensor pollicis longus as the sole tendon. It passes through its own retinaculum where it forms the dorsal aspect of the anatomical snuff box. It is easily recognised by the sharp radial deviation that it takes around Lister's tubercle as it heads towards its insertion in the base of the distal phalanx of the thumb. It is one of the more common extensor tendon ruptures in patients with rheumatoid arthritis due to this relationship with Lister's tubercle.

The fourth compartment comprises five tendons, four of which are extensor tendons to the four fingers while the fifth, which lies deep to the other four, is the extensor indices.

The fifth compartment is the extensor digiti minimi, which inserts in the extensor apparatus of the little finger. This may be a paired tendon or become a paired tendon as it moves distally. It is joined by the extensor digitorum tendon to the little finger just proximal to the metacarpal phalangeal joint.

The sixth compartment is most easily identified lying within the groove on the medial aspect of the distal ulna. It contains the extensor carpi ulnaris tendon, which inserts in the base of the fifth metacarpal.

The first and sixth compartments are the most frequently involved by tenosynovitis.

Sagittal fingers

Sagittal sections are most useful in the assessment of flexor and extensor tendons. These are best examined in long axis with the probe placed along the tendon. The flexor tendons are easier to examine, being considerably larger and more rounded structures than the more band-like extensor tendons. The superficial and deep tendons are easily separated in the distal palm but this differentiation becomes more difficult once they enter the flexor tendon sheath. Turning the probe axially is the best means of demonstrating the insertion of the superficialis tendon as it splits into two slips, one of which passes medially while the other passes laterally to the profundus tendon before recombining to insert in the base of the middle phalanx. The profundus tendon can then be traced, the sole occupant of the flexor sheath, to its insertion in the base of the distal phalanx. In this position, the metacarpal phalangeal and interphalangeal joints can also be assessed.

Several small structures can be identified in the

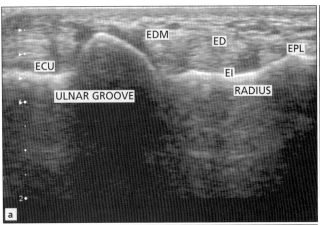

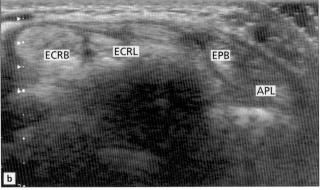

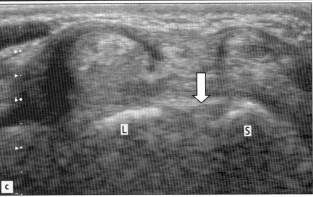

Fig. 1.19 Extensor aspect wrist. (a) Ulnar side with extensor compartments 6 (extensor carpi ulnaris, ECU) easily identified within the ulnar groove, 5 (extensor digiti minimi, EDM) and 4 (extensor digiti, ED; and extensor indicis, EI). Extensor compartment 3 (extensor pollicis longis, EPL) is just visible recognised by its proximity to Listers tubercle. (b) Extensor compartments 2 (extensor carpi radialis longus, ECRL; and brevis, ECRB) and 1 (extensor pollicis brevis, EPB; and abductor pollicis longus, APL). (c) More distal transverse section at level of first carpal row showing the scapholunate ligament (arrow) linking the scaphoid (S) and lunate (L).

fingers on good quality equipment. The A pulleys are seen as a thin hyporeflective band parallel to the proximal phalanx (A2) and middle phalanx (A3). The C pulleys are more difficult to clearly define but the collateral ligaments and volar plate are easily identified at each joint. Injuries to these structures will be discussed in more detail in Chapter 6.

Nerves at the wrist

Median nerve

The medial nerve is usually examined in patients suspected of having carpal tunnel syndrome. The important anatomical point therefore is that portion of the nerve just proximal to and within the carpal tunnel. At this level the nerve can be difficult to differentiate from adjacent tendons although it is usually of relatively lower reflectivity and does not move in the same manner as the flexor tendons. For this reason it is easier to identify the nerve in the mid-forearm on axial section. The nerve is located centrally between the muscle bellies of the superficial and deep flexor groups. It can then be traced more distally, keeping the probe in the axial plane as it migrates around the superficial tendon group before it drops down into the flexor retinaculum. At this point the probe can be rotated 90° and an excellent image of the long axis of the medial nerve identified. Carpal tunnel syndrome will be discussed elsewhere.

> ### Practical tip
>
> One of the easier places to identify the median nerve is in the mid-forearm on axial section where it will have a reflectivity lower than that of the flexor tendons and not move as they do.

Just beyond the carpal tunnel, the median nerve can be seen to divide into the recurrent motor and the common palmar digital nerves. The common nerves then divide again into the proper palmar digital branches. These smaller nerves are best detected by locating the palmar digital arteries and locating the adjacent nerve. The fasicular structure of the nerve even at this distal level is still preserved, though the tubular structure and absence of vascular flow are sufficient to identify them.

Ulnar nerve

Guyon's canal is a smaller fibro-osseus on the volar medial aspect of the wrist. Its floor is formed by the transverse carpal ligament its medial wall by the pisiform and its roof by an extension from the flexor retinaculum. In the proximal tunnel the nerve lies between the ulnar artery and the pisiform. In the distal tunnel, the ulnar nerve divides into a superficial sensory branch and a deep motor branch, which separate on either side of flexor digiti minimi brevis. The deep branch lies adjacent to the hook of the hamate where it may be injured by compression against the hook along with injury to the adjacent ulnar artery (hammer hand syndrome).

Radial Nerve

The radial nerve at the wrist is a small structure on the volar radial aspect. It reaches clinical significance if inflamed as it crosses the first extensor compartment to reach the dorsal aspect of the wrist. This is termed Wartenbergs syndrome and comes into the differential diagnosis of De Quervains tenosynovitis and intersection syndrome.

Lower limb: anatomy and technique

2

Eugene G McNally

THE ADULT HIP

Anterior hip

Initial orientation is best achieved with the probe in the axial position. The femoral vessels are easily identified and are a useful landmark from which to start. The femoral nerve is lateral and the vein medial to the artery with the lymphatic channel, through which femoral hernias pass, the most medial (think NAVeL: Nerve, Artery, Vein, Lymphatic). The femoral vessels lie in a bed of two muscles, the smaller more medial one is the pectineus (Fig. 2.1) and the latter larger muscle bulk represents the conjoint psoas and iliacus. The space between these two muscles represents a potential area for expansion of the iliopsoas bursa should it distend. The normal iliopsoas bursa lies deep to the iliopsoas muscle group and is usually not visualised unless it contains fluid.

The iliopsoas muscle is roughly triangular in shape, which also helps with its identification. Its base lies along the iliopsoas bursa and capsule, and its anteromedial border faces the femoral vessels. Two other muscles abut the anterolateral border; the more anterior of these is the sartorius and the deeper is the rectus femoris. Rotating the probe to the long axis over the sartorius will allow the muscle to be traced to its origin from the anterior superior iliac spine. It can be traced distally to a combined insertion with the gracilis and semitendinosus, termed the "pes anserinus" in the medial aspect of the tibia. The rectus femoris has its origin on the anterior inferior iliac spine and can be traced distally to where it forms the quadriceps group and the quadriceps tendon.

When the probe is moved more laterally but kept in the axial plane, the next column of three muscles is encountered. The most anterior of these is the tensor fascia lata, which arises from the iliac crest anteriorly. Distally this muscle forms the fibrous iliotibial tract that can be traced to the knee. Deep to this muscle and running perpendicular to it are the gluteus minimis and medius (Fig. 2.2). These are an important and often underdiagnosed source of groin pain, particularly in older individuals. The minimis is the more medial of the two muscles

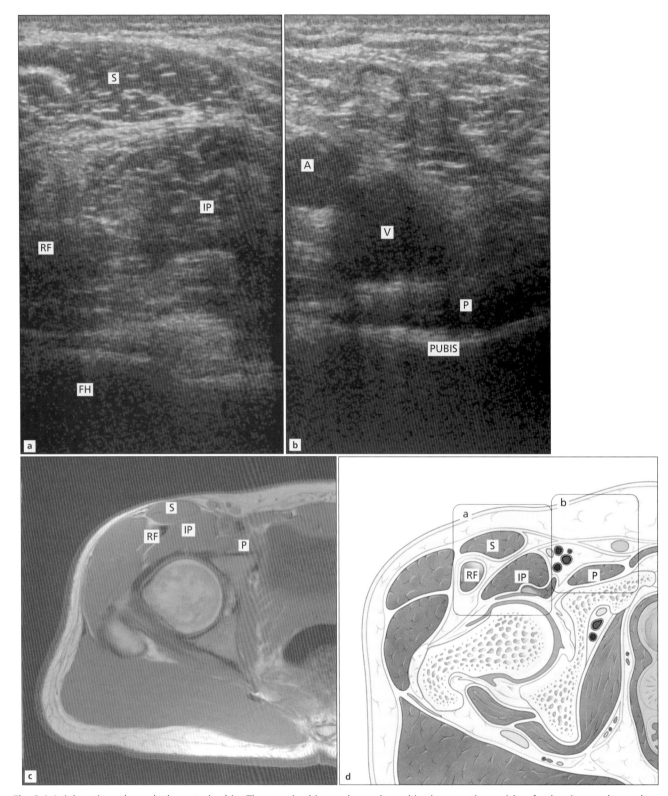

Fig. 2.1 Axial sections through the anterior hip. The anterior hip can be evaluated in three sections with a further image devoted to the adductor origin (Figs 2.4, 2.5). (a) The middle section with the prominent iliopsoas muscle (IP) lying centrally. Against the lateral aspect of this structure are two easily identified muscles with sartorius (S) anteriorly and rectus femoris (RF) laterally. The bony structure deep to the muscle groups is the femoral head (FH). (b) A more medial axial section showing pectineus (P) deep to the femoral artery (A) and vein (V). (c, d) MR correlation and Axial anatomy.

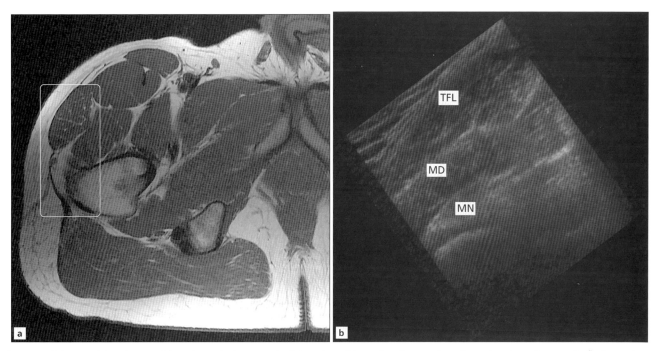

Fig. 2.2 Axial T1-weighted MRI with enlarged ultrasound of the gluteal insertional area; the triangular-shaped anterolateral muscle, tensor fasciae latae (TFL) is a useful landmark. The gluteal insertion is complex with the gluteus minimus (MN) inserting on the more anterior aspect of the greater trochanter with the gluteus medius (MD) inserting laterally.

separated by a small bursa termed the "subgluteus medius bursa". The gluteus minimis can be traced to its insertion on the anterior aspect of the greater trochanter and the gluteus medius to its insertion more laterally. Continuing in the axial plane now, moving over the lateral aspect of the hip to the posterolateral position, the largest muscle bulk is the gluteus maximus. This inserts on the dorsal aspect of the greater trochanter, with more anterior fibres contributing to the ilio-tibial tract. On the dorsal aspect of the trochanter separating it from the gluteus maximus is the trochanteric bursa.

Sciatic Nerve

The axial anatomy on the dorsal aspect of the hip joint can be difficult to discriminate on ultrasound due predominantly to its depth. A good knowledge of the anatomy in this region is needed if ischial bursal injections or sciatic blocks are being considered. In thin individuals the

ischial tuberosity provides a useful landmark from which to identify the other structures in this area (Fig. 2.3). The precise anatomy depends on the level scanned. At upper levels close to the superior margin of the femoral head, the sciatic nerve and adjacent vessels lie directly on the bony posterior column of the acetabulum. They are separated from the gluteus maximus by the piriformis muscle. At the level of the femoral neck the sciatic nerve is separated from the bony acetabulum by the gemelli. From there it passes on to lie on the quadratus femoris, which itself lies superficial to the obturator externus. In this position the sciatic nerve lies in a fatty triangle bordered superficially by the gluteus maximus, deeply by the quadratus femoris and medially by the ischial tuberosity from which the semimembranosis and long head of the biceps femoris arise. A small bursa is normally present adjacent to the ischium though usually not normally seen unless distended. When inflamed as ischial bursitis, sciatic symptoms can result.

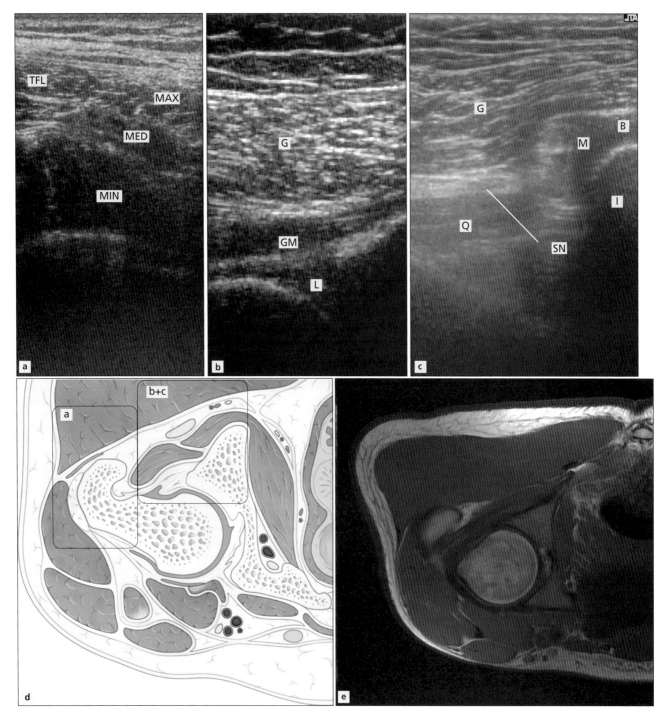

Fig. 2.3 Muscles on the posterior aspect of the hip joint. Axial diagrams and T1-weighted MR have been reversed so that ultrasound images can be positioned as they would be seen during an examination. The most medial section is adjacent to the bony line mark of the ischial tuberosity (I). This gives rise to the hamstrings. The conjoint tendon of the semitendinosus and the long head of the biceps femoris is more superficial with the tendinous origin of the semimembranosus being deeper. Immediately lateral to these is the sciatic nerve (SN), which rests at this level on the quadratus femoris (Q) and the overlying muscle bulk is of course the gluteus maximus (G). More lateral to this is a section taken over the posterior joint itself and in this figure is at a slightly higher level, showing the posterior labrum (L). At this level the traversing muscles are the gemellii (GM). If the axial section is taken at a higher level in through the upper aspect of the joint then the traversing muscle is the piriformis, which runs in a parallel plane above the gemellii. More laterally still the insertion of the gluteus maximus (G) can be seen deep to which lies the trochanteric bursa.

THE THIGH

The muscles of the thigh are divided into three compartments.

Adductor compartment

Returning to the axial position overlying the femoral neurovascular bundle and moving the probe medially the two most superficial muscles are the adductor longus and gracilis with the latter being the more medial. Both of these arise from the pubic bone adjacent to the symphysis. Deep to this muscle pair are the adductor brevis and then the larger adductor magnus (Figs 2.4, 2.5). The area is examined with the hip adducted and externally rotated with knee flexion. This is similar to the frog position of paediatric radiography. The adductor longus is the prominent and most easily recognised muscle. It has both muscular and tendinous components close to its origin.

The longus and gracilis arise from the body of the symphysis itself and can be traced distally. This pattern is preserved throughout the adductor compartment with the three adductor muscles (from anterior longus, brevis and magnus) descending into the thigh capped by the more medially placed and perpendicularly lying gracilis muscle.

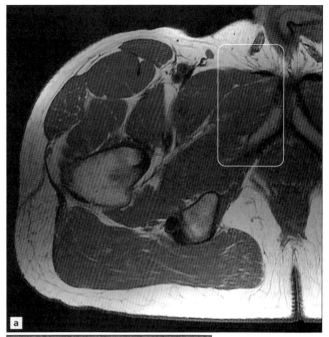

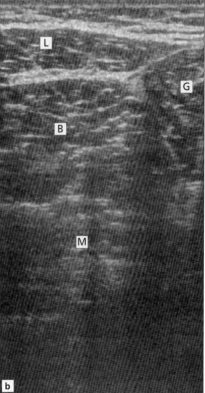

Fig. 2.4 Axial T1-weighted MRI with axial ultrasound enlargement of the adductor origin area. With the hip abducted and externally rotated (frog position) the prominent superficial muscle is the gracilis. This can be confirmed by tracing it distally to its insertion in the medial aspect of the knee. Deep to the gracilis muscle (G) are the three adductors. Their configuration, with longus (L) most anterior, brevis (B) centrally and magnus (M) most posterior, is preserved throughout their length.

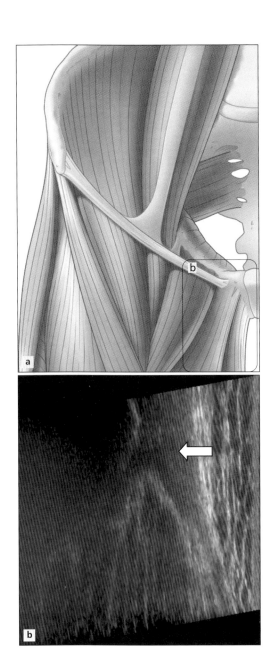

Fig. 2.5 Longitudinal view of the adductor origin showing the adductor group sweeping towards the reflective conjoint tendon origin (arrow).

Hamstring compartment

The hamstrings comprise the semimembranosis, semitendinosus and biceps femoris (Fig. 2.6). Their origins have already been mentioned in relation to the posterior hip described earlier. The former two have distal insertions that are *medially* located and in the distal thigh run in close proximity to the sartorius and gracilis muscles. The biceps femoris inserts *laterally* into the lateral surface of the fibula head along with the fibular collateral ligament with which it sometimes forms a conjoint tendon. This separation gives rise to the terms medial and lateral hamstrings. The principal clinical importance of these muscles is the identification of proximal avulsions and insertional tendinopathy. These will be discussed in the relevant chapters. As the muscle groups diverge, the sciatic nerve comes between them. Identification of the sciatic nerve in this region is the first step in locating the common peroneal nerve. The sciatic nerve divides into the posterior tibial and common peroneal nerves roughly at the upper border of the popliteal fossa.

The quadriceps compartment

The anterior compartment of the knee is filled with five muscles, four of which make up the quadriceps group (Fig. 2.6); the fifth is the sartorious. The quadriceps comprise the vastus intermedius, which lies between the vastus medialis and vastus lateralis, and rectus femoris, which fills the anterior space between the medialis and lateralis. These four muscles form a conjoint insertion as the quadriceps tendon into the upper pole of the patella. Four distinct layers can be identified within the quadriceps tendon separated by fibrofatty tissue. Deep to the quadriceps tendon lies the suprapatellar fat triangle, the suprapatellar bursa and the prefemoral fat. Separation between the suprapatellar fat triangle and the prefemoral fat of more than 5 mm indicates an effusion that is easily detectable. The medial adductor group is separated from the medial components of the quadriceps group by the saphenous nerve.

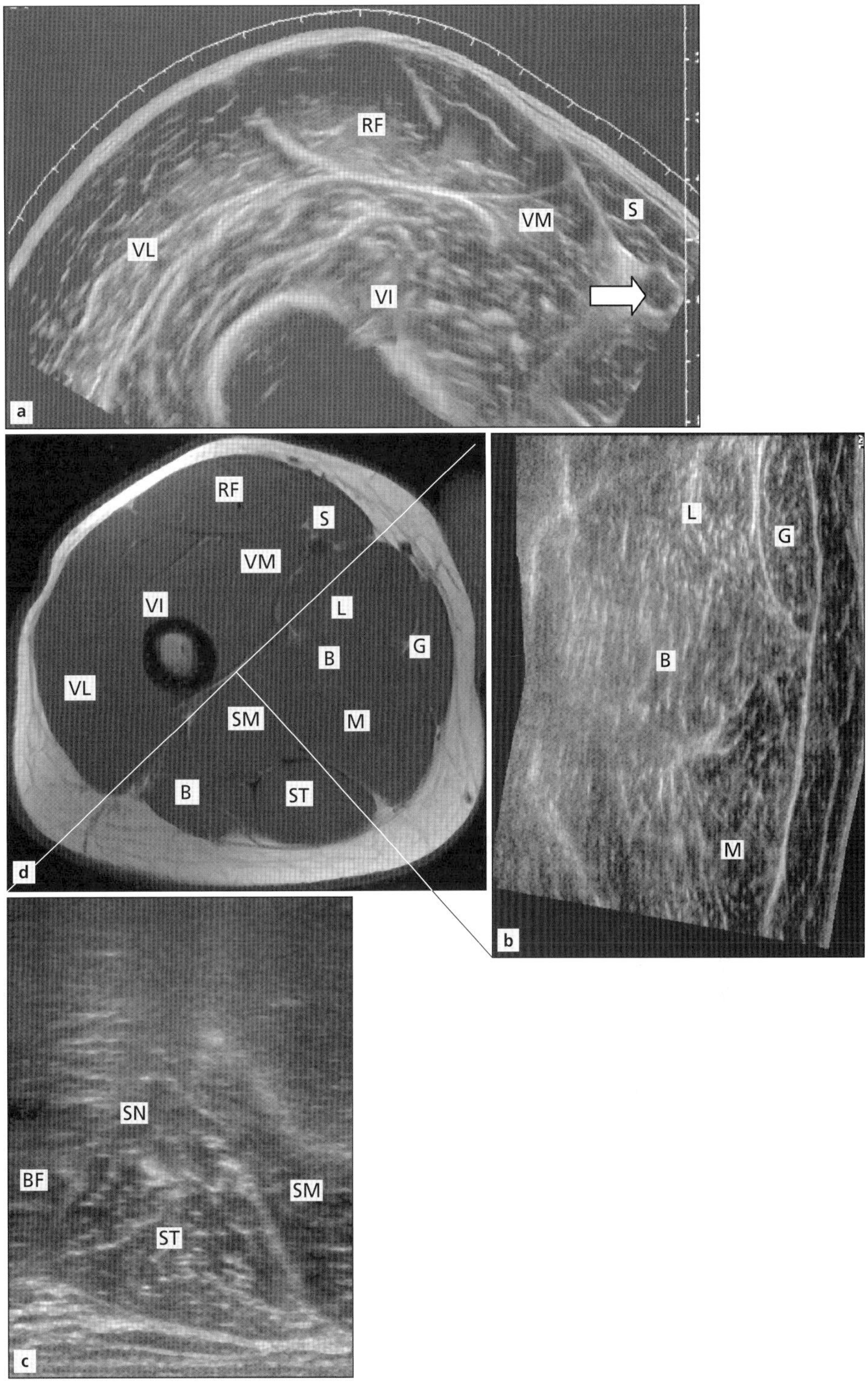

Fig. 2.6 The muscle anatomy of the thigh is divided into three compartments anteriorly. There are five muscles, representing the quadriceps and sartorius (S). The sartorius is a strap-like muscle that overlies the femoral vessels, which can be used as a useful landmark. The quadriceps group is made up of the rectus femoris (RF) anteriorally. Deep to this lies the vastus intermedius (VI) and on either side the vastus medialis (VM) and vastus lateralis (VL). On the medial aspect of the thigh is the adductor group with a similar configuration between the overlying gracilis (G) and deep adductolongus (L), brevis (B), and magnus (M). Posteriorly is the hamstring compartment and again there is some variation in muscle contact and configuration, depending on the level scanned. At the upper levels some fibres of the gluteus maximus may still be visible on the lateral aspect of this compartment. The compartment is mainly occupied by the hamstrings from medial to lateral, semimembranosus (SM), semitendinosus (ST) and biceps femoris. At upper levels the biceps femoris (BF) may be seen as two separate muscle bulks representing the two heads. The relationship of the semimembranosus and semitendinosus is curious in that the semitendinosus starts as the bulkier of the two structures lying lateral and deep to the semimembranosus but in the distal thigh becomes very much the smaller and more tendinous structure and lies superficial to the bulkier semimembranosus. The principle nerve in this compartment is the sciatic nerve (SN) and would be identified on the deep surface of the biceps.

THE KNEE

With the patient in the supine position and the knee slightly flexed, the anterior aspect of the knee can be examined from the medial collateral ligament to the iliotibial tract laterally.

Medial structures

On the medial aspect of the knee with the probe held in the coronal plane, the medial collateral ligament can be identified extending from its superior attachment of the medial femoral condyle to the tibia (Figs 2.7a, 2.7b). The most

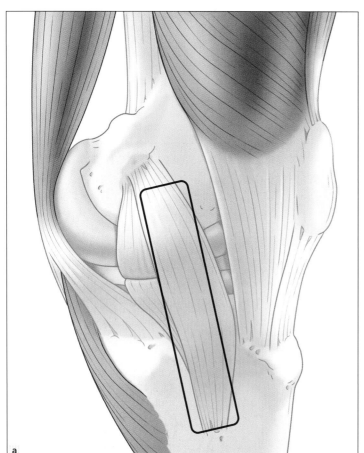

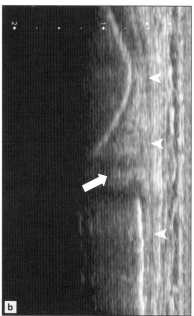

Fig. 2.7 (a, b) Long-axis section through medial collateral ligament. The position of the ultrasound probe is shown figuratively as a rectangle in (a). The medial collateral ligament is identified as a typical ligament-like structure crossing the joint line (arrowheads). The medial meniscus is just visible (arrow). (c, d) Sagittal section through the extensor mechanism showing the quadriceps insertion, patella and patellar tendon.

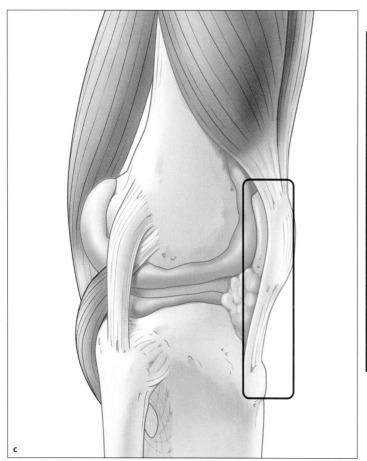

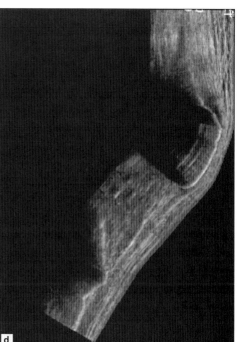

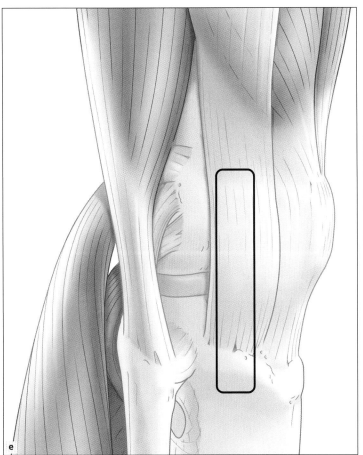

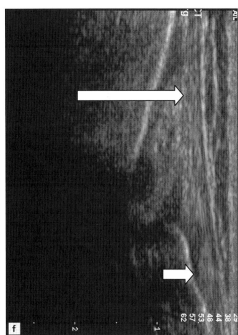

(e, f) Coronal section through the lateral knee anterior aspect. The iliotibial tract (long arrow) is easily recognised as it is traced to Gerdy's tubercle (arrow). (g, h) Coronal view lateral knee posterior aspect. Note the tilt of the probe is needed to demonstrate the fibular collateral ligament (curved arrow). At its distal portion a conjoint insertion with the biceps femoris can be seen.

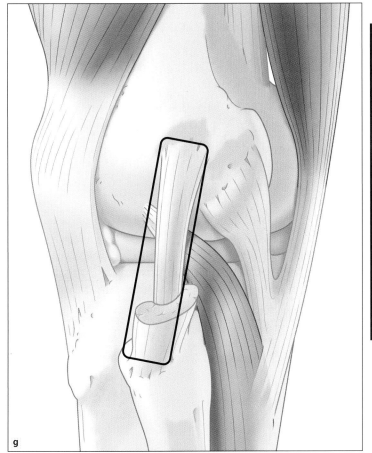

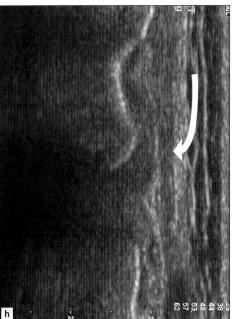

common site of injury of this collateral ligament is proximal, close to the femoral condylar origin. When viewed axially, the medial collateral ligament is seen to be larger inferiorly than it is superiorly. On its deep surface, fibrous bands extend to the medial meniscus. These are called the medial meniscofemoral ligament and the medial meniscotibial ligament. Occasionally a bursa can be seen separating the superficial from the deep portions of the ligament.

When the probe is kept in the coronal plane and moved posteriorly and with slight clockwise rotation the group of three muscles comprising the pes anserinus is encountered (Fig. 2.8). The most anterior of these is the sartorius followed by, in sequence, the gracilis and the

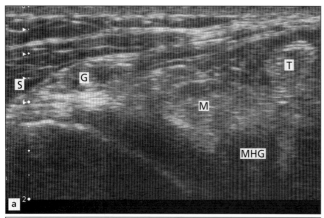

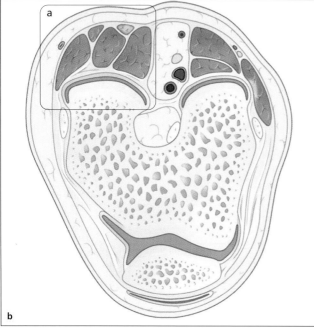

Fig. 2.8 Posteriomedial aspect of the knee axial section in the dorsal aspect of the medial femoral condyle shows four muscles, sartorius (S), gracilis (G), semimembranosus (M) and semitendinosus (T). The medial head of gastrocnemius (MHG) is just visible. There are no significant nerves.

semitendinosus. All three insert as a conjoint tendon and the upper medial aspect of the tibia.

Turning the probe axially demonstrates the medial retinaculum, which blends at its upper margin with the muscle fibres of vastus medialis obliquus.

Anterior structures

The patellar tendon or ligament is also an easily identifiable structure with the probe in the sagittal plane, and the structure can be traced from its origin on the inferior pole of the patella to its insertion in the tibial tubercle (Figs 2.7c and 2.7d). The tendon measures approximately 6 mm (anteroposterior) AP and 10 mm in lateral diameter. It is not uncommon to identify some expansion at its origin, and occasionally small areas of decreased reflectivity may be identified within it without indicating significant pathology. At its insertion the tendon, once again, expands to insert into the tibial tuberosity. Its superficial relationship is most often subcutaneous fat although, in its upper portion, a small quantity of fluid may be identified in the prepatellar bursa and inferiorly in the superficial component of the infrapatellar bursa. On the deep aspect of the ligament lies Hoffa's fat pad. The deep component of the infrapatellar bursa lies in a small triangle between the patellar tendon anteriorly, Hoffa's fat pad posteriorly and the tibia inferiorly.

Lateral structures

The iliotibial tract is identified as a well-defined structure with a typical appearance of a ligament or small tendon (Figs 2.7e and 2.7f). It can be easily traced to its insertion on Gerdy's tubercle on the anterolateral aspect of the tibia. Pathologically, the most important part of this structure is where it lies close to the lateral femoral condyle where it may become inflamed as a consequence of friction against the condyle. When the probe is rotated in the axial position and moved anteriorly, a further ligamentous condensation that can be traced to the lateral border of the patella can be identified. This is the lateral retinaculum.

More posteriorly, the lateral collateral ligament can be traced from lateral femoral condyle to its insertion into the fibular head. Rotating the inferior tip of the probe posteriorly brings the obliquely oriented ligament into plane. Its insertion lies close to the biceps tendon insertion and may be shared with it as a conjoined tendon. Occasionally, condensations representing the posterolateral corner ligaments can be seen. Most patients have a long and a short ligament. The long ligament is either a fabellofibular or arcuate ligament, the presence of a fabella discriminating the two. The short fibulo-popliteal ligament runs posteromedially to the long ligament.

The nerves of the anterior compartment comprise the geniculate arteries, veins and the genicular nerves. These have little clinical impact.

Posterior structures

Placing the patient prone is the best means of demonstrating the posterior anatomy. Broadly there are two muscle groups, medial and lateral, each overlying a femoral condyle and separated by the popliteal vessels and the posterior tibial nerve.

Keeping the probe in the coronal plane and moving posteriorly and with slight clockwise rotation the group of three muscles composing the pes anserinus is encountered. Rotating to the axial plane improves visualisation of the tendons in relation to one another (Fig. 2.8). The most anterior of these is the sartorius followed by, in sequence, the gracilis and the semitendinosus. All three insert as a conjoint tendon and the upper medial aspect of the tibia.

The superficial muscle laterally is the biceps femoris, which has also been previously described. With the probe in the axial plane, this muscle can be traced distally as it moves laterally and a little anterior to the insert in the head of the fibula (Fig. 2.8). The major deep muscle in this area is the lateral head of gastrocnemius, which arises in the lateral femoral condyle. As this extends distally over the femoral condyle it becomes separated from it, in some patients firstly by the origin of the plantaris muscle and in all patients, ultimately, by the popliteus muscle, which can be identified at the level of the tibial plateau.

The important nerve in this compartment is the common peroneal nerve. The lateral border of the lateral head of the gastrocnemius is the most useful landmark, and the common peroneal nerve can usually be located in close proximity to this (Fig. 2.9) and thence traced distally as it rounds the neck of the fibula and enters the peroneal compartment.

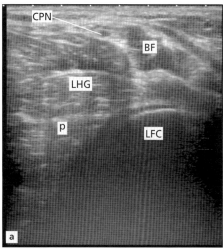

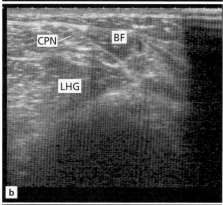

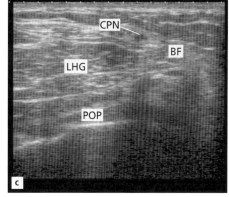

Fig. 2.9 Posterolateral aspect of the knee, following the common peroneal nerve (CPN). The principle two muscles are the lateral head of gastrocnemius (LHG) and biceps femoris (BF). (a) The plantaris muscle (P) may separate the lateral head of the gastrocnemius from the lateral femoral condyle (LFC). (b, c) As these muscles are followed more distally, the common peroneal nerve comes to a more superficial location but is still related to the lateral border of the gastrocnemius. The muscle deep to the gastrocnemius becomes the popliteus (POP).

Practical tip

The common peroneal nerve can be found at the back of the knee near the lateral head of the gastrocnemius muscle and then traced round the neck of the fibula and into the peroneal compartment.

THE CALF

The calf comprises four compartments, anterior, posterior and peroneal, with the posterior compartment being further divided into superficial and deep portions. The anterior compartment contains three muscles: the most medial is the tibialis anterior, in the middle is the extensor hallicus and laterally is the extensor digitorum. The principle vessels are the anterior tibial artery and deep peroneal nerve, which run between the extensor hallucis and digitorum (Fig. 2.10).

The peroneal compartment comprises the peroneal longus and brevis muscles with the

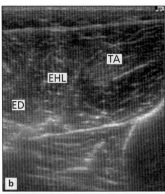

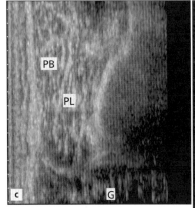

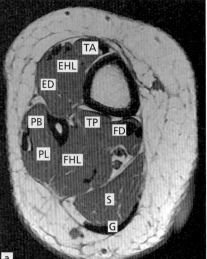

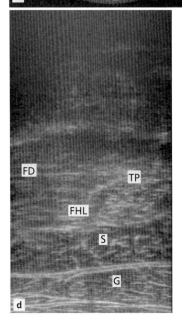

Fig. 2.10 The anterior compartment contains the tibialis anterior (TA), extensor hallicus longus (EHL) and extensor digitorum (ED). The peroneal compartment contains the peroneus brevis (PB) anterior to the peroneus longus (PL). The superficial posterior compartment contains the tendon of the gastrocnemius intimately related to the dorsal aspect of the soleus (S) and the deep compartment contains from medial to lateral the flexor digitorum (FD), tibialis posterior (TP), and flexor hallucis longus (FHL). The posterior tibial vessels and tibial nerve lie deep to the soleus.

brevis lying more anteriorly. The common peroneal nerve passes between them.

The posterior compartment is composed of superficial and deep groups. The superficial compartment contains the gastrocnemius and the soleus muscles. The gastrocnemius itself comprises two heads, the medial being the larger. The soleus forms the bulk of the superficial posterior compartment and, with the aponeurosis of the two heads of the gastrocnemius, form the Achilles tendon. The plantaris muscle and tendon arise form the posterolateral aspect of the lateral femoral condyle. The muscle belly is short, quickly giving rise to a long tendon, which runs along the medial aspect of the soleus, deep to the medial head of the gastrocnemius, to insert beside the Achilles tendon on the dorsum of the os calcis. Injuries to this structure are most commonly encountered at the musculotendinous junction. The deep posterior compartment contains, from medial to lateral, the tibialis posterior, flexor digitorum and flexor hallucis.

FOOT AND ANKLE

The hindfoot is one of the most common areas to be examined using ultrasound. As in many other joints, symptoms guide the ultrasound approach. Patients generally present with pain located posterior, inferior, medially or laterally, depending on the structures involved. Of these, the posterior and inferior are the most common. Symptoms in one of these compartments may reflect disease in the other; consequently they are best both examined together and are considered first. Patients who present with more global ankle symptoms rather than pain localised to a particular area probably require MRI for more complete assessment and in particular to assess the joint surfaces and bone.

Posterior hindfoot

The Achilles tendon is best examined with the patient supine and the legs extended over the edge of the couch (Fig. 2.11). The tendon is followed from its origin from the gastrocnemius and soleus to its insertion into the os calcis. The adjacent plantaris tendon is variable in its appearance. Usually it lies separate and anteriomedial to the Achilles tendon but in 20% of the population it blends into the medial

margin. Near the os calcis the pre-Achilles fat pad (Kager's triangle) separates the tendon from the muscles of the deep posterior compartment. The Achilles tendon has no true synovial sheath so physiological fluid is not seen. There is a paratenon surrounding the tendon, which can be seen as two echogenic lines outlining the tendon. Fluid within this space is unusual and is indicative of disease. Two bursae occur at the point of insertion: the retrocalcaneal bursa deep to the tendon separates it from the bursal process of the os calcis, and the superficial retro Achilles bursa, which is small and not always visible. Transversely the Achilles is elliptical in shape, flattening out near its insertion to cover the calcaneum like a cuff. The average AP diameter of the tendon is 5–6 mm, depending on the patient's physique. The anterior margin is usually flat or concave and any more than mild convexity should be regarded as abnormal.

> **Key point**
>
> The Achilles tendon has no true synovial sheath, so physiological fluid is not seen in an ultrasound image.

> **Key point**
>
> Depending on the patient's physique, the average (anteroposterior) AP diameter of the Achilles tendon is 5–6 mm.

Inferior hindfoot

Plantar fasciitis is a frequent cause of inferior heel pain especially in runners. The fascia is the tendinous aponeurosis of the intrinsic plantar foot muscles and has a fibrillar hyperechoic echotexture. It normally measures up to 4–4.5 mm in thickness. Transversely it may be difficult to identify but longitudinally its striated appearance can be recognised (Fig. 2.11). In nearly all cases of fasciitis, the thickening is most marked proximally and medially at the site of attachment to the os calcis, corresponding to clinical tenderness on the medial tubercle.

> **Key point**
>
> The plantar fascia normally measures up to 4–4.5 mm in thickness.

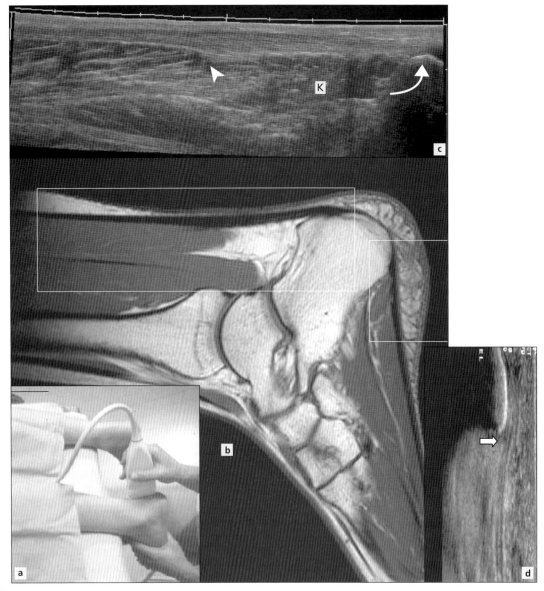

Fig. 2.11 Ultrasound imaging of the hindfoot. (a) The patient is shown in prone position with (b) a corresponding sagittal T1-weighted MRI. (c) A panoramic view of the Achilles tendon from muscle tendinous junction (arrowhead) to the insertion of os calcis (curved arrow). Kager's fat triangle (K) is seen anteriorly. No significant fluid is present in the pre-Achilles bursa. (d) The origin of plantar fascia from the os calcis (arrow).

Lateral hindfoot

The peroneal tendons that evert the foot are prone to subluxation, post traumatic entrapment and tendinopathy. They lie just posterior to the lateral malleous. The peroneus brevis tendon is located anterior to the peroneus longus and both slide within the retrofibular groove. The two tendons are best located initially in the axial plane (Fig. 2.12). Where careful examination is necessary to detect injury, which is often quite subtle. Particular attention should be paid to the peroneus brevis, which is the more commonly injured of the two. Both tendons should be followed as they round the lateral malleolus. At each level, the tilt of the probe should be adjusted to maximise the reflectivity from the tendons and remove anisotropic artefacts. Areas of decreased reflectivity that are persistent are likely to represent longitudinal split tears. Up to 3 mm of fluid within the common peroneal sheath just below the fibular is within normal limits; elsewhere only a trace should be seen. The peroneus longus inserts into the middle cuneiform and first metatarsal and the peroneus brevis inserts into the base of the fifth metatarsal. Fractures of the lateral malleolus or calcaneum can lead to damage of the peroneal retinaculum.

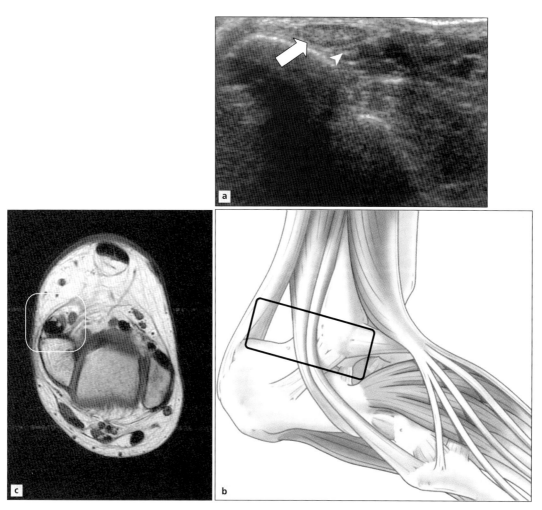

Fig. 2.12 (a) Axial-orientated view of the peroneal compartment showing the larger peroneus longus (arrow) posterior to the smaller and often eccentrically shaped peroneus brevis (arrowhead). (b) A schematic diagram indicating the probe position figuratively as a rectangle and (c) the corresponding axial T1-weighted MR Image are also shown.

A damaged retinaculum or shallow fibular groove can lead to subluxation or dislocation of the peroneal tendons where they come to lie lateral or anterior to the lateral malleolus. If not immediately apparent this can be demonstrated on dynamic scanning using inversion and eversion movements to precipitate subluxation. Longitudinal split tears of the peroneal tendons more commonly affect the peroneus brevis. Full thickness tears are rare.

> **Practical tip**
>
> The peroneii are best imaged in the axial plane. Careful assessment with probe tilting to remove anisotropy is necessary to exclude subtle longitudinal split tears. Full thickness tears are uncommon.

The peroneus quartus muscle is an accessory muscle located on the posterolateral aspect of the ankle, medial and posterior to the peroneal tendon group. It occurs in around 10% of the population. The commonest insertion site is into the os calcis but it can also insert into either the peroneus longus tendon, the peroneus brevis tendon or the cuboid. The peroneus quartus muscle is not to be confused with the peroneus tertius, which lies anterior to the lateral malleolus on the lateral aspect of the foot. It is closely related to the extensor digitorum longus muscle and inserts at the base of the fifth metatarsal. Its insertion point can be used to differentiate it from the extensor digitorum tendon of the fifth toe, which lies adjacent to it. Another variant that may be encountered is the peroneus digiti minimi, which extends from the peroneus brevis muscle to insert into the proximal phalanx of the fifth digit. It is relatively small in size and therefore rarely causes confusion or presents as a mass of unknown nature. Other muscle variants include a low-lying peroneus brevis musculotendinous junction that can even extend below the distal tip of the fibula.

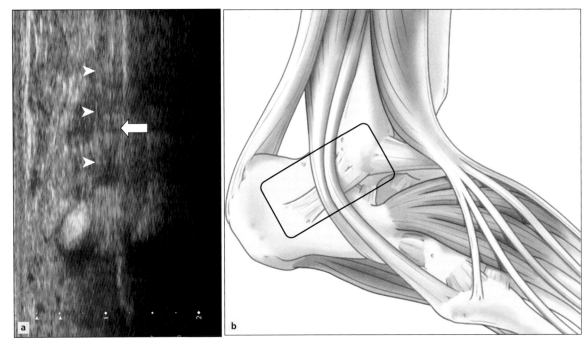

Fig. 2.13 Coronal-orientated image through the peroneal compartment. The calcaneofibular ligament (arrowheads) separates the peroneal tendons from the bony reflection of the underlying os calcis (arrow). Position of the probe is indicated schematically as a rectangle in (b).

Practical tip

The peroneus quartus muscle should not be confused with the peroneus tertius muscle, which can be found in front of the lateral malleolus.

As many as 85% of ankle sprains involve the lateral collateral ligaments. The anterior talofibular (ATaFL) and the calcaneofibular (CFL) ligaments are the two main components with the former most commonly injured. The posterior talofibular ligament is less frequently involved. The ATaFL runs almost horizontally from the anterior border of the fibular tip to the talus. It has an average length of 25 mm and width of 2 mm. Disruption of the ligament is seen as swelling, often appearing as a hypoechogenic soft tissue mass, inferior to the fibula. The ligament is scanned under stress with either internal rotation or anterior draw. In complete tears, the degree of abnormal movement is greater and the free ends of ruptured ligament can be seen dipping into the ankle joint on stress. Synovial hypertrophy may be seen within the anterolateral gutter in symptomatic patients. The CFL ligament lies deep to the peroneal tendons running from the apex of the lateral malleolus to a small tubercle on the lateral side of the os calcis (Figs 2.13 and 2.14).

Medial hindfoot

Key point

The posterior tibial tendon measures 4–6 mm in diameter and may be surrounded by up to 4 mm of fluid.

The posterior tibial tendon is the largest of the invertors of the foot measuring 4–6 mm in diameter and with up to 4 mm of physiological fluid around it. It runs immediately behind the medial malleolus. Tears occur most frequently just below the medial malleolus or at its insertion into the navicular. The flexor digitorum longus is half the diameter of the posterior tibial and the flexor hallucis longus is the smallest of the invertors. The flexor hallucis can also be identified by its lower musculotendinous junction and by its tendency to contain fluid within the synovial sheath. The flexor tendons are most easily located by axial scanning (Fig. 2.15).

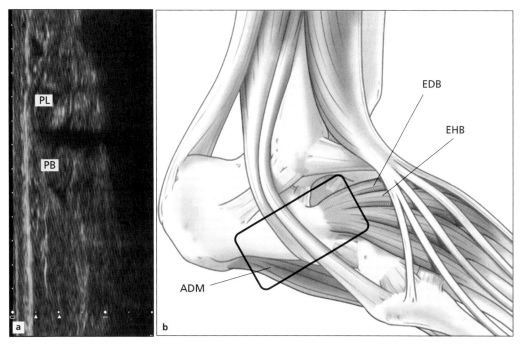

Fig. 2.14 Coronal-orientated section more distally than that of Fig. 2.13, and which picks up the extensor digitorum brevis (EDB), extensor hallicus brevis (EHB) and the dorsal lateral aspect of the foot.

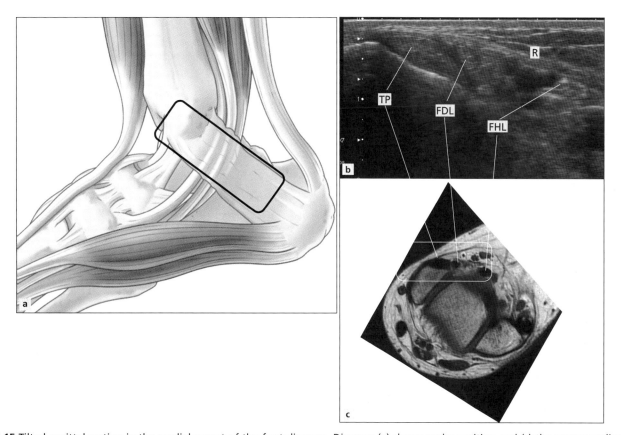

Fig. 2.15 Tilted sagittal section in the medial aspect of the foot diagram. Diagram (a) shows probe position and (c) the corresponding axial T1-weighted MR image. The posterior tibial vessels separate the flexor digitorum (FDL) from the flexor hallucis (FHL). Structures are all contained under the flexor retinaculum (R).

Longitudinal scanning is also important for a full assessment of the tendon but care must be taken with the technique to ensure that the correct tendon is identified. To locate the tibialis posterior tendon in the longitudinal plane, the probe is placed first at the lateral aspect of the medial malleolus so that only a bony contour is seen. It is then moved slowly posteriorly and angled slightly anterior so that it falls into the shallow groove occupied by the tibialis posterior tendon. Once identified, the tendon can be traced distally as it rounds the malleolus and moves towards its insertion on the medial aspect of the navicular. As the navicular is rounded, great care must be taken to stay on the tibialis posterior tendon. Even a small posterior movement will mean that the flexor digitorum tendon is encountered and may be followed erroneously into the foot. As the malleolus is rounded, a relatively sharp rotation of the probe is necessary to keep the tibialis posterior tendon in sight. Further confirmatory evidence is the more parallel course of the tibialis posterior tendon, its larger size and ultimately tracing it to its insertion into the navicular. With practice the pitfall of beginning on the tibialis posterior tendon and ending on the flexor digitorum tendon is easily avoided. As they round the malleolus, flexor digitorum and flexor hallucis are separated by the posterior tibial artery vein and nerve. All these structures lie deep to the flexor retinaculum, which prevents them subluxing anteriorly. More superficially and anteriorly, the long saphenous vein passes anterior to the medial malleolus. Rarely, congenital duplication of the tibialis posterior tendon and a common tendon sheath for the tibialis posterior and flexor digitorum can occur.

An accessory muscle, the accessory flexor digitorum longus, may be seen to pass through the tarsal tunnel adjacent to the flexor hallucis longus. Its distal attachment to the flexor digitorum usually helps to distinguish it from a significant mass.

Anterior hindfoot

The extensor tendons (anterior tibial tendon, extensor hallucis longus and extensor digitorum longus tendons) are easily examined anteriorly; however, pathology of these tendons is rare. Axial sections show the normal relationships of the tendons with the tibialis anterior most medial and the extensor digitorum lateral. The tibialis anterior and posterior lie "adjacent" to each other whilst the relationship of the extensor digitorum and hallucis are the reverse of their flexor counterparts.

A small amount of fluid is normally present in synovial joints and within the ankle this is usually distributed in the joint recesses. In asymptomatic people up to 3 mm of fluid in AP depth can be seen in the anterior recess (Fig. 2.16). More than this would indicate an effusion. Fluid is seen frequently in the posterior recess on MRI but assessment of the posterior recess is more difficult with ultrasound.

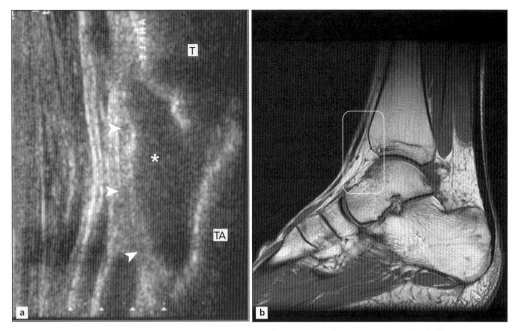

Fig. 2.16 Sagittal-orientated image of effused anterior ankle joint with corresponding T1 image of a different patient. The dorsal aspect of the talus (TA) is an easily recognised landmark and separate from the distal tibia (T). The anterior capsule is shown by the arrowheads with the reflective effusion beneath it (*).

THE MID-FOOT

As the long tendons described previously progress through the mid-foot they are joined by a number of short muscle groups. On the dorsum of the foot the short muscles tend to lie deep to the long tendons and comprise, from lateral to medial, the extensor digitorum brevis and extensor hallucis brevis. On the plantar aspect of the foot the short muscles tend to be superficial and are more numerous. From lateral to medial they comprise the abductor digiti minimi, flexor digitorum brevis, which lies superficial to flexor digitorum accessorius, and abductor hallucis. Overlying all of these is the continuation of the plantar fascia.

The bony anatomy in the mid-foot is complex and individual articulations can be much more difficult to identify than with MRI or CT. This is generally only of practical importance when injecting joints and, as this is usually carried out from the dorsal aspect of the foot, the bony anatomy will be described from this perspective.

The identification of individual joints is best carried out by placing the probe transversely across the dorsum of the foot and displaying a coronal image using true anatomical terminology. The neck of the talus is easily identified and is a good starting point. When the probe is moved distally, a two-bone section is achieved with the navicular the more medial and the cuboid lateral. Moving more distally again, four bones come into view, the more medial three representing the cuneiforms and the lateral still the cuboid (Fig. 2.17). Further progression distally identifies the five bones representing the five metatarsals. With this approach individual joints can be identified.

> **Practical tip**
>
> To identify the individual joints of the mid-foot, start with the easily identifiable neck of the talus, place the probe transversely across the top of the foot in order to obtain a coronal image of the region.

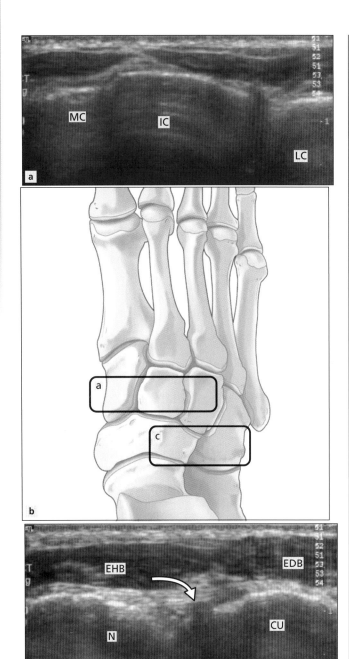

FOREFOOT

As one moves into the forefoot the dorsal anatomy changes relatively little when compared with the plantar anatomy where now four layers are identified. The first and more superficial layer comprises the adductor digiti minimi, flexor digitorum brevis and the abductor hallucis previously described. The second layer comprises the long flexors with their associated four lumbricals; the flexor accessorius also belongs to this layer. As in the hand the lumbricals pass to the hallux side of the toes. The third layer comprises the flexor digiti minimi and flexor hallucis brevis. The flexor hallucis brevis has two heads in which the sesamoids form.

The fourth layer sees the addition of the three plantar and four dorsal interossei in the anterior portion of the foot. As in the hand, the brevis tendons insert at the base of the middle phalanx with the exception of the first and fifth, which insert at the base of the proximal phalanx. Again, as in the hand, the brevis tendons split into two to create a tunnel to allow passage of the more distally inserting longus tendon.

As in the hand, the components of each synovial joint can be identified on good quality equipment. The pulleys are less well defined structures in the foot than they are in the hand but the collateral ligaments and plantar plate, injured in hyperextension as 'turf toe', can usually be identified.

Fig. 2.17 The different articulations of the foot can be quite difficult to recognise. The neck and head of the talus is quite characteristic in the sagittal plane and can be a useful landmark. Tracing distally from this and turning the probe axially allows the navicular (N)–cuneiform (CU) joint to be identified (curved arrow). The overlying muscles are extensor digitorum brevis (EDB) and extensor hallucis brevis (EHB). More anterior and medial to this, a typical three-bone section representing the three cuneiforms, medial (MC), intermediate (IC) and lateral (LC), can be achieved.

Ultrasound of the rotator cuff

3

Eugene G McNally

INTRODUCTION

The technique of ultrasound examination of the rotator cuff has been dealt with in chapter 1. This chapter deals specifically with the pathological findings that may be encountered within the supraspinatus, infraspinatus and subscapularis in patients with shoulder impingement and rotator cuff tear.

Shoulder pain is one of the commonest nontraumatic orthopaedic presentations to primary care, with only knee and back pain more common. A number of specific syndromes have been described which can usually be distinguished by a careful history and examination. One of these, the painful arc syndrome describes pain on lateral abduction, between 45° and 135°. This suggests impingement between the rotator cuff and the coracoacromial arch. Clinically, it needs to be distinguished from frozen shoulder, which is characterised by pain on multidirectional movement, and high arc impingement. These will be discussed in chapter 4.

> **Key point**
>
> Painful arc is most commonly due to impingement of the rotator cuff between humerus and coracoacromial arch on lateral abduction, and is usually easily distinguished from frozen shoulder clinically.

The pathological processes that account for painful arc begins with bursitis of the subacromial subdeltoid bursa, progressing to tendinopathy of primarily the supraspinatus tendon (SST). More advanced stages of the disease process include tears of the supraspinatus, which may propagate to tears of the infraspinatus and subscapularis. Bony changes also occur, including enthesopathy at the site of coracoacromial ligament insertion, whispy new bone formation at the site of SST insertion and irregular new bone formation in the upper portion of the bicipital groove. Chronic irritation of the biceps tendon as it moves through the groove can result in bicipital tendinopathy and rupture.

> **Key point**
>
> Dislocation of the biceps tendon can be due to rupture of the subscapularis muscle or following tears of the transverse ligament.

Although painful arc syndrome is common, the majority of cases are diagnosed clinically and most will respond to conservative treatment, usually a combination of physiotherapy and corticosteroid injection. Imaging is generally reserved for patients with atypical features in their clinical presentation or those who fail conservative treatment and surgery is being considered. The principal role of imaging is to determine what stage the disease has progressed to and consequently which form of surgery is to be undertaken. It is vital therefore that the imaging of rotator cuff disease be considered in conjunction with local surgical practices. In most cases, disease limited to bursitis and tendinopathy is treated by subacromial decompression. This procedure involves division of the coracoacromial ligament and burring of the undersurface of the acromium to increase the size of the space through which the rotator cuff moves during abduction. If a cuff tear is present, surgical repair of the tear will be considered in conjunction with subacromial decompression. The management of patients with partial rotator cuff tears is less clear. In most cases, these are treated as for bursitis and tendinopathy, however large partial tears or partial tears in throwing athletes may be treated by debridement or repair.

Ultrasound can also be used to define the nature and natural history of rotator cuff tears. Many patients with symptomatic rotator cuff tears are shown to have asymptomatic tears on the contralateral side. Only some of these will become symptomatic and fewer will have progression in the size of their tear. In a 5-year follow-up study, Yamaguchi and colleagues showed that half of 45 asymptomatic patients studied became symptomatic on follow up and less than half of the 23 patients re-examined by ultrasound showed tear progression (1).

> **Key point**
>
> It is vital that the imaging of rotator cuff disease be considered in conjunction with local surgical practices so that any ultrasound or MRI findings can directly impact the management of the patient.

Ultrasound has high accuracy in the diagnosis of cuff tears. Rotator cuff tears can be either full or partial thickness. A full thickness tear is a defect that allows communication between the subacromial subdeltoid bursa and the glenohumeral joint. Full thickness tears, although variable in appearance, demonstrate three common patterns. The free edge tear, the mid-substance tear and the massive tear, which is a combination of both. Partial thickness tears are so called because they only involve one or other of the surfaces of the supraspinatus tendon. Joint surface partial tears are more common than bursal surface partial tears.

> **Key point**
>
> A full thickness tear of the rotator cuff allows the subacromial subdeltoid bursa to come in contact with the glenohumeral joint.

> **Key point**
>
> Joint surface partial tears are more common than bursal surface partial tears.

Free edge tear

> **Key point**
>
> The anterior free edge is one of the most common tear patterns, particularly in younger individuals.

The anterior free edge is one of the most common tear patterns, particularly in younger individuals. The normal anterior free edge is examined with the probe in both transverse and coronal planes and is the area of the supraspinatus tendon that lies immediately adjacent to the anterior interval and biceps tendon. The characteristic findings in the anterior free edge tear are loss of the normal supraspinatus tendon substance, widening of the gap between the biceps tendon and supraspinatus tendon and exposure of a bare area of bone and cartilage where the tendon previously attached. These features are best appreciated on the axial section (Figs 3.1 and 3.2). It is important to follow the free edge down to and below its insertion the greater tuberosity in order to ensure that small tears are excluded.

The axial section is supported by additional signs best appreciated in the coronal plane. As outlined in Chapter 1, the normal subacromial subdeltoid bursa is convex upward in the coronal plane (Fig. 3.3) When a tear is present, the bursa sags into the space created by the tear (Figs 3.4–3.6) with the approximation of the

reflective line representing the subacromial subdeltoid bursa and the humeral head or humeral head articular cartilage. The ensuing concave upper border becomes an important sentinel for the underlying cuff tear.

> **Practical tip**
>
> In a coronally oriented image an important sign of a tear of the supraspinatus tendon is the sagging of the subacromial subdeltoid bursa into the space created by the tear.

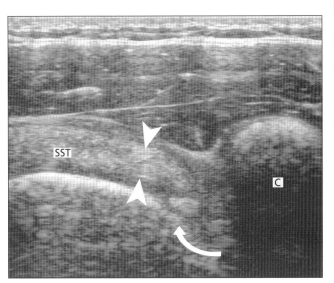

Fig. 3.1 Axial section through anterior shoulder showing reflective leading edge of coracoid (C) and humerus. Supraspinatus (SST) is shown with normal free edge between arrowheads adjacent to biceps (curved arrow)

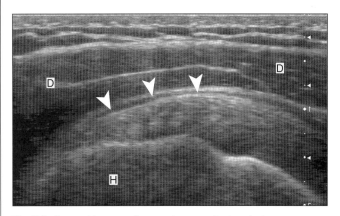

Fig. 3.3 Coronal image of normal supraspinatus, between deltoid (D) and humerus (H) with the SASD bursa overlying (arrowheads).

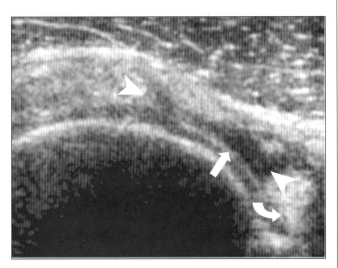

Fig. 3.2 Axially orientated image, anterior shoulder similar to Fig. 3.1 showing anterior free-edge tear. Note the increased distance between the biceps and SST when compared to Fig. 3.1, indicative of a tear. Biceps tendon (curved arrow). Note also the increased reflectivity from the surface of the humeral head cartilage (arrow) secondary to loss of acoustic attenuation in the presence of a cuff tear.

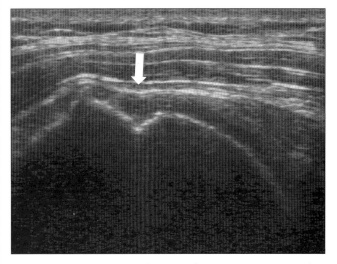

Fig. 3.4 Coronally orientated image of a supraspinatus tear. The orientation is similar to that of Fig. 3.3 but note the concave depression of the subacromial subdeltoid bursa (arrow), indicating a full thickness rotator cuff tear. The underlying humeral head also shows surface irregularity. The aetiology of this is poorly understood. Some authors advocate an impaction, particularly during overarm-throwing sports (posterosuperior impingement). Alternatively the bony irregularity may reflect traction on the surface attachment fibres.

In addition to these characteristic findings, a number of variations also occur. In some instances, the presence of excess fluid within the subacromial subdeltoid bursa can result in preservation of the humeral head subacromial deltoid distance. The tear is readily recognised by the presence of poorly reflective fluid (Fig. 3.7).

The presence of a transonic effusion increases sound throughput through the tear and results in a characteristic increased reflectivity from the surface of the humeral head articular cartilage

(Figs 3.2 and 3.8). This can also occur in the presence of a tear not distended with fluid. More difficult to recognise is the small defect that has been replaced by reflective debris or synovial thickening. In these instances a dynamic assessment is important to demonstrate

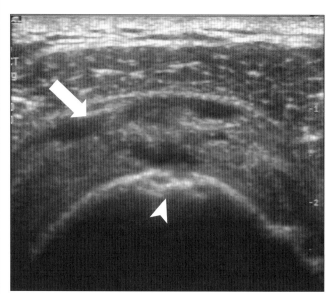

Fig. 3.7 Coronally orientated image of the supraspinatus tendon showing a fluid-filled cuff tear. Fluid can be seen at the joint surface (arrowhead) and at the bursal surface (block arrow). The communicating defect is not demonstrated convincingly on this static view. In these circumstances a dynamic assessment with alternating compression with the probe and a little shoulder movement can help to shown separation of the irregular and disrupted supraspinatus fibres and confirm the presence of a full thickness tear.

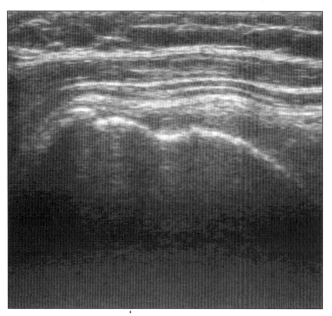

Fig. 3.5 Image of the supraspinatus tendon with orientation similar to that of Fig. 3.3. A further example of concave depression in the subacromial subdeltoid bursa indicative of a full thickness rotator cuff tear.

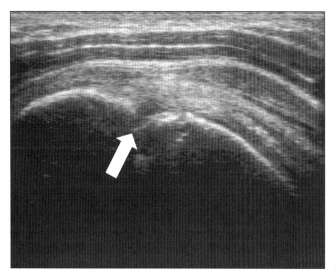

Fig. 3.6 Small full thickness tear on coronal image. Note irregular bony changes (arrow).

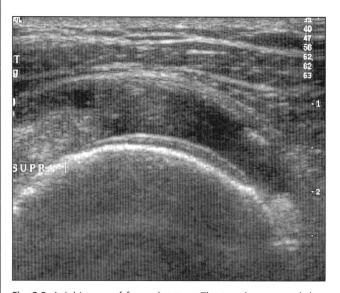

Fig. 3.8 Axial image of free-edge tear. The tear is acute and the SASD bursa is filled with fluid. The through-sound transmission in the area of the tear causes increased reflectivity from the cartilage surface. The cartilage under intact cuff does not demonstrate this sign.

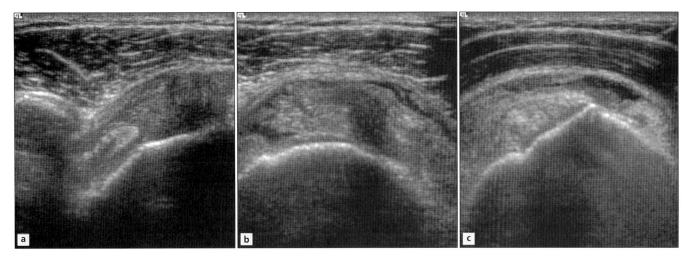

Fig. 3.9 Axial (a, b) and coronal (c) images of debris-filled full thickness tear. Heterogenous tissues, a relective articular surface and debris in the SASD bursa are clues to the tear, which can be confirmed on dynamic examination.

abnormal transmission of movement through the disorganised debris and improve visualisation of the tear (Fig. 3.9). If a suspicious tear is encountered, gentle movement of the probe and/or the patient's arm can help to elucidate the finding.

Occasionally, altered signal changes within the anterior free edge can be identified in the absence of volume loss or other signs of a tear. Interpretation of these signs can be difficult, particularly as in some scanning planes the presence of anisotropic artefact can create the spurious impression of a tear. The volume of tendon involved in these instances is usually small and in the author's view, the presence of normal supraspinatus volume is sufficient to exclude a significant rotator cuff tear.

> **Practical tip**
>
> If a suspicious lesion is encountered, gentle movement of the probe and/or the patient's arm can help to elucidate the finding.

Mid-substance tear

A second common type of supraspinatus tear is the mid-substance tear. The anterior and posterior portions of the tendon remain attached, but the intervening fibers are torn from their insertions. In the author's experience this is more commonly recognised in the older individual and may therefore be more the consequence of

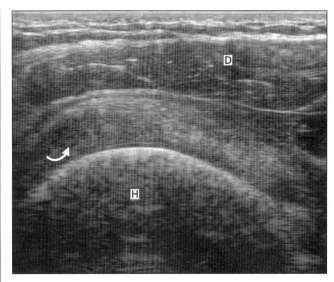

Fig. 3.10 Axially orientated image through mid-substance of supraspinatus. Four distinct layers can be identified including skin and subcutaneous fat, deltoid muscle (D), subacromial subdeltoid bursa separating deltoid from supraspinatus and the interface between supraspinatus and the leading edge of humerus (H). At the most posterior air portion of the supraspinatus, the more poorly reflective infraspinatus interface is just visible (curved arrow).

degeneration than trauma, though both tear types are multifactorial in their aetiology. This tear pattern is most easily visualised with the probe in the transverse plane but positioned more laterally than the plane used to identify the anterior free edge tear (Figs 3.10 and 3.11). Normal supraspinatus tissue can be identified anterior to this tear with normal supraspinatus and/or infraspinatus posterior. This normal tissue is referred to by some authors as the anterior and posterior pulleys.

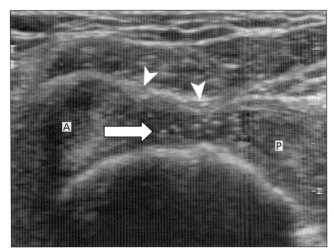

Fig. 3.11 Axially orientated image through supraspinatus mid-substance with orientation similar to that for Fig. 3.10 for comparison. Note the concave depression of the subacromial subdeltoid bursal interspace (arrowheads) into a full thickness tear that is partially filled by fluid (arrow). Note the intact anterior (A) portion and posterior (P) portion of supraspinatus.

Practical tip

A mid-substance tear of the supraspinatus tendon is most easily visualised with the probe in the transverse plane but positioned more laterally than when identifying an anterior free edge tear.

On older equipment or when low-frequency probes are used, a connective tissue bundle separating the anterior from posterior limbs of the deltoid muscle can cast alternating bands of reflectivity across the mid-portion of the supraspinatus and give the superious impression of a rotator cuff tear.

The massive tear

There is relatively little published on the natural history of small rotator cuffs tears, and the question of whether small tears propagate to massive tears and the rate at which they might do so have yet to be fully established. Once the supraspinatus becomes completely disrupted (Figs 3.12–3.14) the tear may extend into the infraspinatus. Isolated infraspinatus tears are uncommon, though may follow significant trauma, particularly motorcycle injuries. More common is isolated infraspinatus atrophy, which is seen in professional throwing athletes and is due to pressure on the suprascapular nerve either by repetitive compression or secondary to compression by a paralabral cyst. Anterior propagation of the massive tear leads to

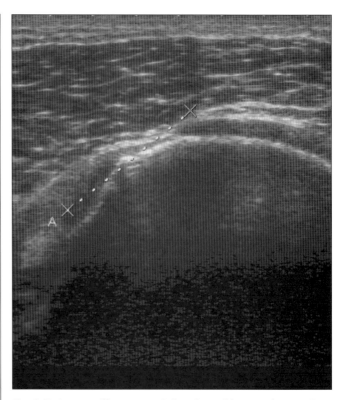

Fig. 3.12 Large cuff tear on axially oriented image. The tear is measured from the biceps tendon to where thinned cuff tissue is present.

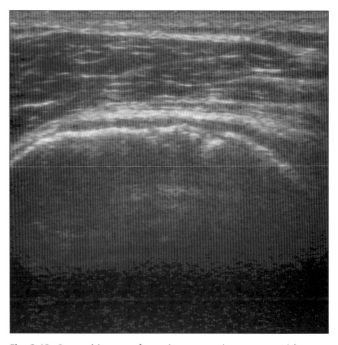

Fig. 3.13 Coronal image of massive supraspinatus tear with retraction.

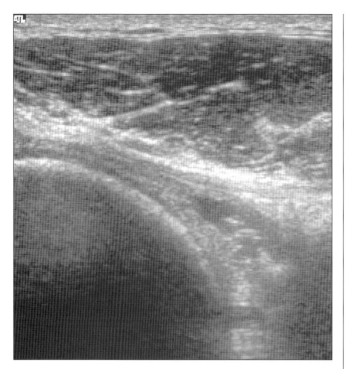

Fig. 3.14 Mid-substance tear taken with probe angles along the coracoacromial ligament. Note the humeral head articular cartilage in close proximity to the ligament, indicating a tear. A small amount of joint fluid is visible.

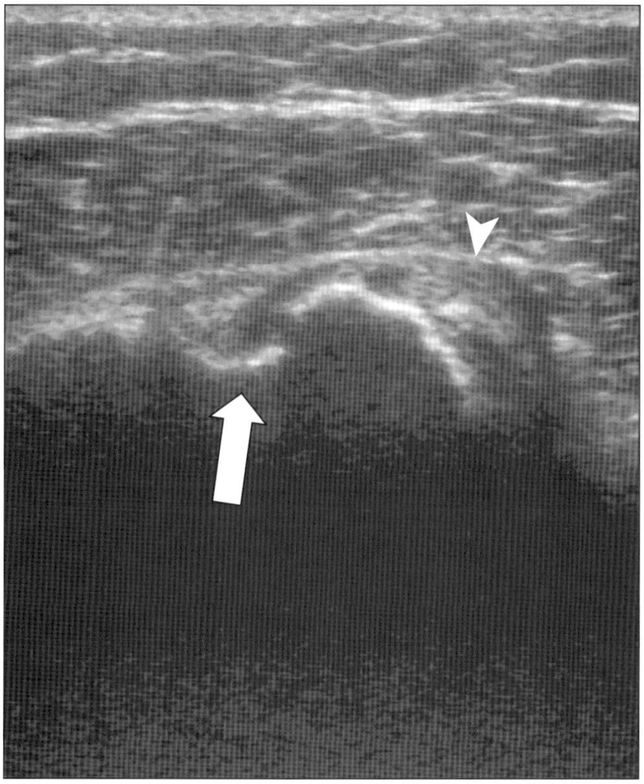

Fig. 3.15 End stage cuff arthropathy with associated subscapularis rupture and dislocation of the biceps tendon (arrowhead) from the now empty bicipital groove (arrow).

subscapularis rupture and medial displacement of the biceps tendon (Fig. 3.15). These features will be described in more detail in Chapter 4.

As SST tendinopathy progresses, changes are also taking place in the adjacent humeral head. Marked irregularity of the subchondral cortex and irregularity of the humeral head cortex at the supraspinatus attachment occurs (Fig. 3.16). This can result in large irregular humeral head defects. Similar changes may also be seen in the posterosuperior aspect of the humeral head in the overhead throwing athlete. These changes are seen in conjunction with posterosuperior labral injuries and partial tears of the joint surface of supraspinatus. Although a compressive aetiology has been previously supposed, there is evidence that the underlying lesion is tightening of the posterior limb of inferior glenohumeral ligament which leads to abnormal movement between the humeral head and glenoid and a rotational overuse injury to the supraspinatus and biceps tendon combined with traction injury to the humeral head and posterosuperior labrum. Bony changes also occur in the upper portion of the bicipital groove which becomes irregular and deep. A secondary bicipital tendinopathy may result from friction of the tendon against the irregular groove. The biceps tendon becomes frayed, may split logitudinally and ultimately rupture, leading to an 'empty groove'. The differential diagnosis on an empty groove is medial dislocation of the biceps tendon due to rupture of the transverse ligament and/or the subscapularis tendon. A careful search for the displaced tendon by moving the probe medially,

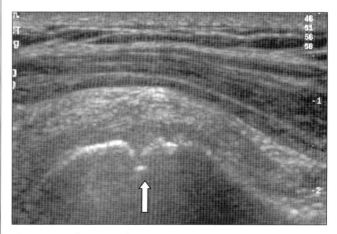

Fig. 3.16 Surface irregularity commonly seen during rotator cuff examination (arrow). The cause is uncertain with some authors suggesting an impaction aetiology and others an avulsive one. The irregularity is also seen in asymptomatic individuals.

in the axial plane, is necessary. In the final stages, the humeral head subluxes superiorly and will ultimately abut and erode the undersurface of the acromium. The more advanced stages glenohumeral arthropathy, which has sometimes been referred to as "cuff arthropathy", occurs. The full extent of glenohumeral cuff arthropathy cannot be appreciated on ultrasound, its radiological assessment is based predominantly on plain film findings.

In the presence of a massive rotator cuff tear, retraction of the free edge of the tendon occurs. This is usually to the level of the superior labrum, (Fig. 3.17) thus well below the acromium and difficult to appreciate using ultrasound. Ultrasound examination of the undersurface of the acromium is possible in some individuals, but reliable ultrasound findings have not been described. In view of this, assessment of the size of rotator cuff tears becomes more difficult and is frequently underestimated on ultrasound criteria (2). The ultrasound (US) estimation of the size of the cuff tear will differ from that estimated at surgery for other reasons, not least of which will be as a consequence of the different arm positions in which each of these assessments are taking place.

A massive rotator cuff tear with tendon retraction also results in atrophic changes within the supraspinatus muscle belly. These changes are readily appreciated on MR with loss of muscle bulk and increased signal on T1-weighted imaging reflecting atrophy (Fig. 3.18). A number

of studies have been directed at the assessment of supraspinatus muscle atrophy using ultrasound, but firm guidelines have yet to be established. Signs that have been used include overall increase reflectivity within the supraspinatus muscle. Quantitative measurements of this have not proved possible with ultrasound. A loss of reflectivity of the spine of the scapula has been described as a qualitative measurement of supraspinatus atrophy and fat replacement. The basis for this is increased sound resorption by the atrophic muscle results in decreased sound penetration and therefore decreased reflectivity from the bony surface. The thickness of the supraspinatus muscle can also be assessed although, as in other areas of ultrasound, it is difficult to define precisely the point of measurement to allow for reliable comparison and follow-up. The author has used the medial margin of the acromium as the baseline for measurement with assessment of muscle bulk made a fixed distance from this point. Comparative and longitudinal studies are necessary to establish the reliability of this measurement. In practice, the degree of muscle atrophy has less bearing on the difficulty of carrying out a repair than the overall size of

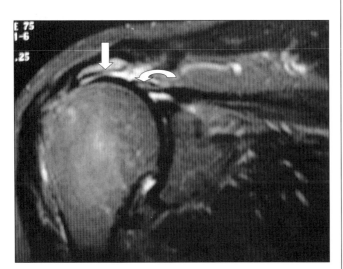

Fig. 3.17 Coronal fat-saturated image with large retracted supraspinatus tear. There is humero-acromial impingement with osseus oedema within the acromium (arrow). The retracted tendon end is detected at the superior glenoid margin (curved arrow).

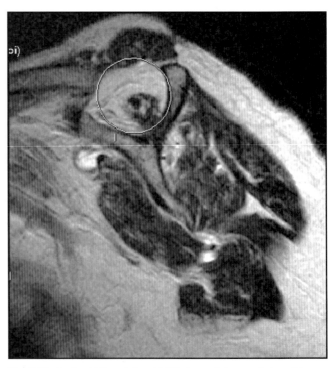

Fig. 3.18 Sagittal T1-weighted MRI through base of glenoid showing "Y" configuration. Between the spine of the acromium and the coracoid lies the supraspinatus muscle. In this case the muscle is grossly atrophic, being diffusely replaced by high signal fat (circle).

the cuff tear itself. Other criteria, including length of history, the presence or absence of symptoms, patient age and plain film findings of glenohumeral degeneration, are also more important in determining surgical outcome.

Partial tears and tendinopathy

A partial tear is defined as a tear that does not completely traverse the tendon it involves. In the case of the rotator cuff, they are therefore classified as either joint surface partial tears (Fig. 3.19) or the less common bursal surface partial tears. There are variable reports in the literature on the accuracy of ultrasound in the assessment of partial tears. Some of this variation may reflect the acute nature of some partial tears, which result from sporting injury, which are relatively easy to detect, versus more chronic lesions, which, in the absence of acute fluid, may be less obvious. There is also variation in the surgical definition and treatment of partial tears with many surgeons adopting a nonoperative stance (3). Population and patient differences probably apply to surgical decision making, with a more aggressive approach being taken with athletes who depend on their shoulder to compete.

For most patients, in the author's view, the division of cuff tears into partial and complete is somewhat spurious. A large area of tendon abnormality that happens to retain one or two thin fibres intact would officially be termed a partial tear, but in practice is much more likely to behave as a full thickness defect. Similarly a tiny pinhole defect, officially a full thickness tear, is unlikely to be considered for repair (Fig. 3.20). As imaging techniques improve and our ability to detect smaller and smaller lesions preoperatively increases, a re-evaluation of the currently accepted criteria and classifications may be appropriate. It is possible that a greater emphasis on the size of the abnormal area of cuff will be a better determinant of outcome than the full thickness/partial thickness classification. Throwing athletes are different from the general population and a more aggressive approach to the diagnosis and treatment of partial thickness rotator cuff tears is warranted. Partial tears in throwing athletes occur more posteriorly in the cuff than those in the general population and may be associated with tears of the superior or posterosuperior labrum. For these reasons assessment using MR arthrography is probably more appropriate if both lesions are to be detected. In some patients a bony notch can be found on plain films, many of which correspond to underlying partial rotator cuff tears (4). Although the aetiology is postulated as "internal instability", Nakagawa et al. argue that the absence of bursal-sided tears or correlation with objective measures of joint instability or posterosuperior labral injury argue against this. Instead they favour a shearing stress between the two tendons coupled with the known poorer healing of the joint surface of the tendon.

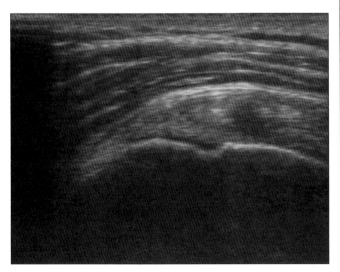

Fig. 3.19 Joint surface partial tear seen as an area of decreased reflectivity persistent on all projections and antianisotropic manoeuvres.

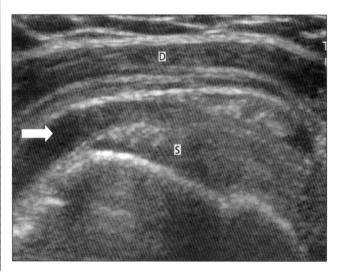

Fig. 3.20 Coronal-orientated image of supraspinatus. Poorly reflective fluid fills the subacromial subdeltoid bursa between the deltoid muscle (D) and supraspinatus (S). Subacromial subdeltoid fluid is seen as a poorly reflective crescenteric area (arrow).

The difference between partial tears and tendinopathy is also blurred and inter- and intraobserver variation in the diagnosis of these lesions is high. Chronic overuse superimposed on a background predisposition results in an area of mucoid degeneration within the tendon, leading to tendinopathy (Fig. 3.21). In many cases there is very little inflammatory response so that the term tendinitis is less appropriate. Imaging findings vary. In some cases, a grossly enlarged and heterogenous tendon on US allows for a more specific diagnosis of tendinopathy, but normal imaging appearances do not exclude the diagnosis. Calcific tendinopathy is a more specific and easily diagnosed form, with ultrasound demonstrating early calcification not apparent on plain radiographs (Fig. 3.22). This is discussed in more detail in Chapter 4.

Secondary signs of rotator cuff tears

> **Practical tip**
>
> Fluid in the subacromial subdeltoid bursa can help to outline the bursal surface of the supraspinatus tendon and help depict the margin of a tear.

Fluid in the subacromial subdeltoid bursa can help to outline the bursal surface of the supraspinatus tendon and help depict the margin of a tear. There have been variable reports of the incidence and usefulness of subacromial subdeltoid fluid in the presence of rotator cuff tear. In the author's view, although subacromial subdeltoid fluid is present in a high proportion of patients with a tear (Figs 3.23–3.26), in individual

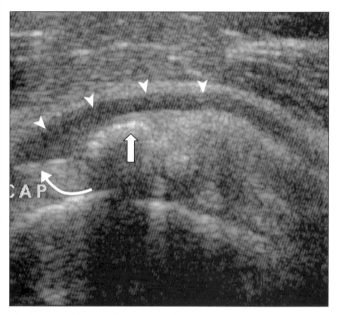

Fig. 3.22 Calcific tendinopathy prior to calcium aspiration. The needle (curved arrow) has penetrated the subacromial subdeltoid bursa and distended it with local anaesthetic (arrowheads). Note the reflective calcification within the cuff (arrow).

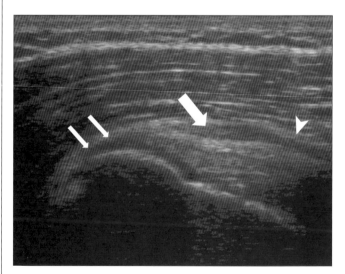

Fig. 3.23 Coronally orientated ultrasound of supraspinatus with arm in abduction. There is a thickening of the subacromial subdeltoid bursa (arrows), which is bunched up (large arrow) if the arm abducts, and the thickened bursa impinges on the coracoacromial ligament seen here in cross section as a reflective oval (arrowhead).

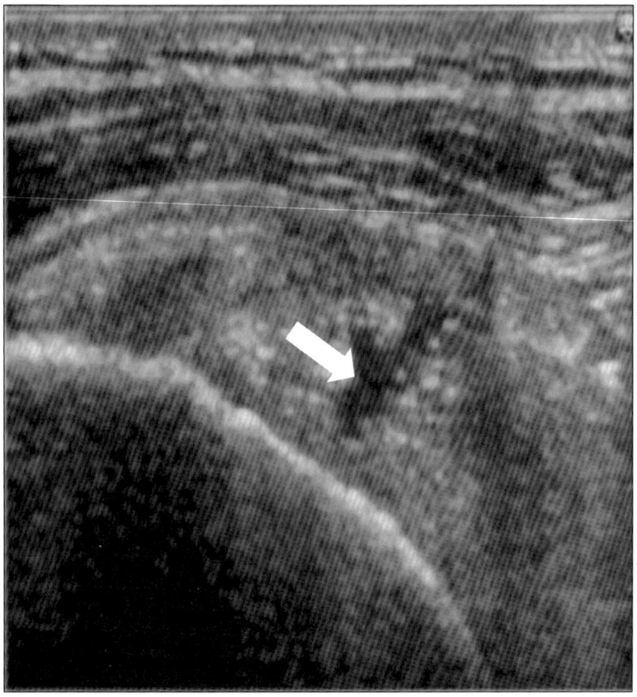

Fig. 3.21 Coronally orientated image of supraspinatus showing full thickness pin hole fluid-filled tear (arrow).

patients the diagnosis of a rotator cuff tear requires the presence of good primary signs. Despite this, there is a strong association and the presence of bursal fluid warrants a careful search if a tear is not initially obvious. Joint movement and variable probe pressure can be used to milk fluid into the tear. Similarly the presence of fluid

in the glenohumeral joint, as depicted by either a distension of the posterior joint space or fluid in the biceps tendon sheath (Figs 3.27 and 3.28), does not of itself confirm the presence of a rotator cuff tear. However, the presence of a large quantity of fluid in one compartment with no fluid in the other is a useful finding, indicating that a full thickness tear is unlikely since the presence of a defect would allow fluid to move readily from one compartment to the other.

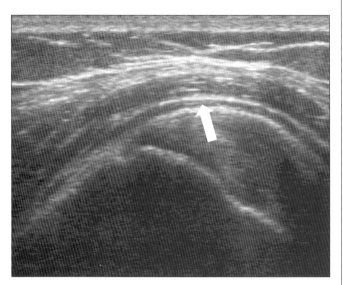

Fig. 3.24 A tiny quantity of subacromial subdeltoid bursal fluid just separates the supraspinatus tendon from the fatty and connective tissue marking the deltoid surface of the bursa. This is the target area for subacromial subdeltoid bursal injection where it is important to place the needle just deep to this reflective band rather than within it.

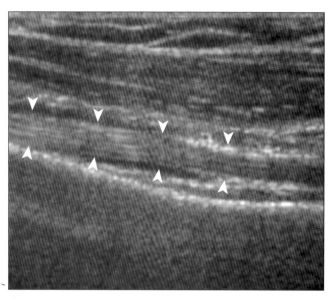

Fig. 3.26 Longitudinal view of biceps tendon (between arrowheads) within the groove in the proximal arm. Note the small quantity of fluid. This volume of fluid is normal. Fluid is most frequently identified at the distal end of the tendon close to musculotendinous junction.

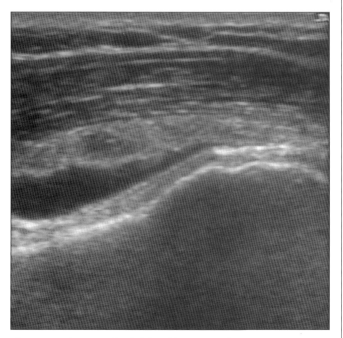

Fig. 3.25 Subacromial subdeltoid bursitis with synovitis.

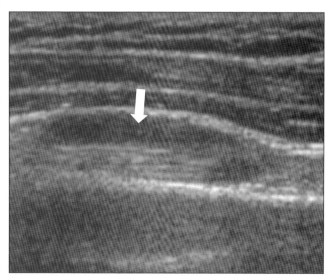

Fig. 3.27 Abnormal quantity of fluid within the biceps tendon sheath (arrow). Note that fluid within the biceps sheath may merely signify a glenohumeral effusion and does not necessarily indicate pathology within the biceps tendon.

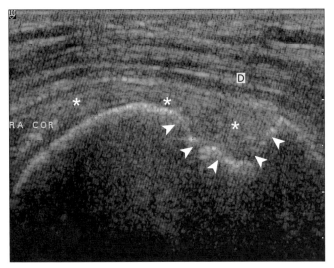

Fig. 3.28 Intact postoperative cuff repair. Note the large defect within the glenoid at the site of rotator cuff reinsertion (arrowheads). Intact tendon tissue (*) can be identified between the deltoid muscle (D) and in continuity with the bony defect.

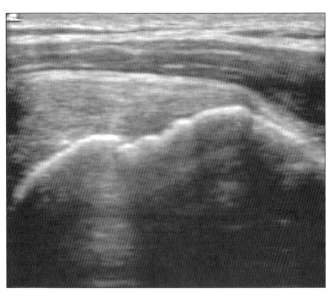

Fig. 3.29 Coronal image of post-cuff repair. Note the surgical bony defects and the substantial band of intact tissue that constitutes the repair.

If fluid is not present within the bursa it can be introduced and then used to detect more subtle tears. In a study of 113 patients, Lee *et al.* did not find that this technique, termed arthrosonography, improved diagnosis (5).

The presence of a tear of the biceps tendon is associated with rotator cuff tears in a high proportion of patients. With a prevalence of supraspinatous, infraspinatus and subscapularis tendon tears of 96.2, 34.6 and 47.1%, respectively in one study (6). Patients with biceps tendon tears were significantly more likely to also have subscapularis tendon tears. The long head of the biceps, the bicipital labral complex, the subscapularis tendon, the free edge of the supraspinatous tendon, the superior glenohumeral ligament, the coracohumeral and transverse ligaments all contribute to anterosuperior stability and a functioning anterior interval. Tears of any one of these structures may be associated with injuries to others, which should be carefully sought.

THE POSTOPERATIVE CUFF

One of the challenges of any form of postoperative imaging of the cuff is to differentiate between acceptable postoperative findings and those that may account for persistent symptoms. The imaging goals include the assessment of the coracoacromial ligament to determine whether it has been completely

divided and an examination of the cuff itself to detect new or recurrent tears. The dynamic capabilities of ultrasound offer distinct advantages over static imaging in that the amount of "functioning" cuff tissue can be assessed. Abnormal tissue on static examinations, particularly MRI, is frequently identified in asymptomatic individuals, suggesting that there is little correlation between postoperative tendinopathy or frank tendon defects and symptoms. By observing the repaired cuff during normal movements and particularly during cyclical ab- and adduction, the ultrasonologist can gain a much better idea of how the repaired fibres move together, whether there is disorganisation and opening of new complete or partial defects and whether the organised tissue comprises a reasonable mass of tissue (Figs 3.29 and 3.30) or represents little more than an intact tendinous band. Studies correlating this additional information with symptoms and postoperative arthroscopic findings are lacking.

DIAGNOSTIC IMPACT

The accuracy of ultrasound in the assessment of full thickness rotator cuff tears is well established in the literature. Studies carried out since 1986 show a consistent pattern with both high sensitivity and specificity particularly over the past five years, a trend reflecting improvements in ultrasand technology. Few of these studies

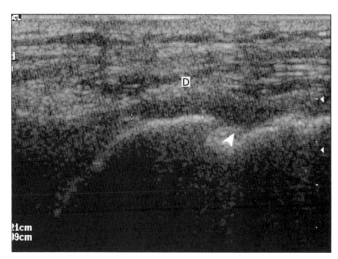

Fig. 3.30 Coronally orientated image following rotator cuff repair. A small bony defect is apparent (arrowhead). Compare with Fig. 3.28 and note the absence of reflective supraspinatus tissue between deltoid (D) and the humeral head, indicating a disruptive repair. The site of repair is replaced by poorly reflective fluid.

The accuracy of full thickness rotator cuff tears (RCT) on US using arthroscopic findings as the gold standard is summarised in Table 3.1. Two studies also compare US to MR and one to MR arthrography. Hodler *et al.* compared US to MR in 23 patients with suspected rotator cuff tears using arthrography as the gold standard. Sonography (SG) demonstrated 14 of 15 and MRI 10 of 15 rotator cuff tears, respectively. Sonography diagnosed 7 of 9 intact rotator cuffs correctly, MRI 8 of 9 (7). Swen and colleagues in a cohort of 21 patients found, for full-thickness rotator cuff tears (RCTs), the sensitivity was 0.81 for US and 0.81 for MRI. The specificity was 0.94 for US and 0.88 for MRI (8).

> **Key point**
>
> Accuracy in the detection of partial thickness tears is more variable than that of full thickness tears.

differentiate between tear size and overall accuracy despite the significant effect that size has on tear conspicuity. Massive full thickness tears are so obvious on ultrasound that less than 100% accuracy implies a poor technique or difficult patient. The inclusion of a high proportion of patients with this type of tear in any study is likely to improve accuracy figures without really reflecting either improved technology or technique. Conversely, some pinhole full thickness tears require some skill in their detection and 90% accuracy with this tear type is laudable.

Accuracy in the detection of partial thickness tears is more variable. Specificity is consistently high but with few exceptions sensitivity is consistently low, ranging from 13% in the study of Martin-Hervas *et al.* (9) to 94% from van Holsbeek *et al.* (10) (see Table 3.2). Possible explanations for this variation include variation in the definition of partial tear and tendinopathy, the patient population and the acute nature of the partial tears. Chronic degenerative partial tears with poorly defined irregular margins may be less conspicuous than sharply defined acute partial tears encountered in the athlete.

Table 3.1 **Full-thickness tears with arthroscopic correlation**

Author	Year	No. of patients	Sensitivity/specificity
Middleton *et al.* (12)	1986	106	91%
Crass *et al.* (13)	1988	500	>90%
Brandt *et al.* (14)	1989	38	75/43%
Burk *et al.* (15)	1989	10	63/50%
Paavolainen *et al.* (16)	1994	49	74/95%
Farin *et al.* (17)	1995	70	91%
van Moppes *et al.* (18)	1995	41	86/91%
Sonnabend *et al.* (19)	1997	117	PPV 95%
Read and Perko (20)	1998	42	100/97%
Swen *et al.* (8)	1999	21	81/94%
Martin-Hervas *et al.* (9)	2001	61	100%
Roberts *et al.* (21)	2001	24	80/100%
Chang *et al.* (22)	2002	422	92/100%

Table 3.2 **Partial-thickness tears with arthroscopic correlation**

Author	Year	No. of patients	Sensitivity/specificity
Paavolainen *et al.* (16)	1994	49	Unreliable
Farin *et al.* (17)	1995	98	78/100
van Holsbeek *et al.* (10)	1995	52	93/94
Sonnabend *et al.* (19)	1997	117	Insensitive
Read and Perko (20)	1998	42	46/97
Martin-Hervas *et al.* (9)	2001	61	13/68
Roberts *et al.* (23)	2001	24	71/100

In addition to the diagnosis of a tear an assessment of its approximate size is important for surgical planning. Implicit in some reports that note a difference between imaging and surgical assessment of tear size is the view that this represents an inherent inaccuracy in the imaging method in question. Small differences can, however, be accounted for by differences induced by arm position, which changes between MR, US and surgery. Muscle relaxation during anaesthesia may also account for some minor differences. Bryant *et al.* compared rotator cuff size using clinical assessment, US, MR and arthroscopy (2). US and MR provided similar estimates, underestimating actual cuff size by 30%. Arthroscopy estimations were under by 12%. Underestimation was less of an issue in a study by Farin *et al.*, where tears were underestimated in only 4% and overestimated in 7% of cases (11).

In many respects much of this literature fails to address an important issue in relation to cuff tear detection. Most tears are relatively easy to detect and some are difficult. In any one report, the accuracy is more dependent on the relative proportion of easy to difficult tears. If the study population is dominated by older patients with more chronic disease, massive cuff tears will predominate. In these cases, accuracy of less than 100% is unacceptable. In studies where the most common tear type is small, detection is dependent on careful scrutiny and the use of a variety of manoeuvres to enhance detection. Dynamic use of the probe with light compression, movement of the shoulder by varying degrees of internal rotation and the manipulation of any free fluid within the bursa to assist in tear detection can all help.

The diagnostic impact of shoulder ultrasonography remains in little doubt to those that use the technique. The increasing literature as outlined previously is also persuasive to those contemplating adding ultrasound to their diagnostic armamentarium. Perhaps most telling is the experience of those musculoskeletal radiologists who have the choice of using MRI or ultrasound in their practices. Most, including the author, appreciate that there is little difference between the techniques. Some patients are difficult to examine with either technique and the alternative is used to improve overall accuracy. The specific advantages of MRI are that it is more universally available, though this may change, can be done remotely by a radiographer/ technologist and be reported later by the radiologist either locally or by teleradiology. The hard copy images are better understood by referring clinicians and more usefully can be used to discuss and gain other opinions from colleagues. MR is obviously superior for visualising intra-articular structures where ultrasound has little or no role. Ultrasound equipment is much cheaper, more portable and preferable to a significant proportion of patients than MRI. It functions best when the referrer has a clear idea of the clinical problem and wishes only to determine the status of the rotator cuff. Its dynamic capability means that shoulder movement can be used to evaluate small tears effectively whilst the patient is being examined. When the MR examination is complete and the patient has left the department, further refinements in technique are not possible to better define a questionable abnormality. Ultrasound is also superior at correlating imaging findings with clinical symptoms. It is often argued that there is a long learning curve with ultrasound. It must also be recognised that equal skill is needed in the detection of small cuff tears on other imaging techniques and with arthroscopy.

THERAPEUTIC IMPACT AND IMPACT ON HEALTH

The role of ultrasound, and indeed MRI, in the surgical decision-making process for rotator cuff impingement has been outlined in the previous paragraphs. In our institution, the management of the patient with impingement that has failed to respond to conservative measures will be altered by the detection of a rotator cuff tear from arthroscopic subacromial decompression to arthroscopic, open or mini-open cuff repair. In some patients even the demonstration of a tear will not result in surgery if the tear is massive and the likelihood of functional restoration poor. Whilst this approach seems logical, it is based on the assumption that there is a link between the presence of a rotator cuff tear, the patient's symptoms and improvement following repair of that tear. The prevalence of asymptomatic cuff tears casts doubt on this logic, and the reasons why some tears are painful and some are not are poorly understood. Indeed most patients who undergo cuff repair also have a subacromial decompression and it is thus difficult to say in this group which of the procedures has had the better effect. The rehabilitation period following cuff repair, particularly with open procedures, is very much longer than that for subacromial decompression. The differences are less when the cuff repair is also carried out arthroscopically but the efficacy of arthroscopic cuff repair is still debated in the surgical community. That being the case, it seems reasonable to suggest that many patients with rotator cuff tears who have not responded to conservative therapy should undergo a trial of subacromial decompression and only undergo cuff repair should that prove unsuccessful in improving symptoms or if asymptomatic tear progression proves problematic. It is likely that there will be population differences with this as with any approach; for example, the approach to an elite athlete will be different from that to a sedentary individual. If this approach is to be adopted for the majority of patients, it is clear that the same surgical approach will be used for patients with impingement whether or not they have a tear, and consequently the need to diagnose a tear preoperatively, by any technique, is called into question.

REFERENCES

1. Yamaguchi K, Tetro AM, Blam O, Evanoff BA, Teefey SA, Middleton WD. Natural history of asymptomatic rotator cuff tears: a longitudinal analysis of asymptomatic tears detected sonographically. J Shoulder Elbow Surg 2001;10(3):199–203.
2. Bryant L, Shnier R, Bryant C, Murrell GA. A comparison of clinical estimation, ultrasonography, magnetic resonance imaging, and arthroscopy in determining the size of rotator cuff tears. J Shoulder Elbow Surg 2002;11(3):219–24.
3. Herman P, Wu M, Theodore J, Dubinsky, MD, Michael L, Richardson M. Association of shoulder sonographic findings with subsequent surgical treatment for rotator cuff injury. J Ultrasound Med 2003;22:155–161.
4. Nakagawa S, Yoneda M, Hayashida K, Wakitani S, Okamura K. Greater tuberosity notch: An important indicator of articular-side partial rotator cuff tears in the shoulders of throwing athletes. Am J Sports Med 2001;29(6):762–70.
5. Lee HS, Joo KB, Park CK, Kim YS, Jeong WK, Park DW, et al. Sonography of the shoulder after arthrography (arthrosonography): preliminary results. J Clin Ultrasound 2002;30(1):23–32.
6. Beall DP, Williamson EE, Ly JQ, Adkins MC, Emery RL, Jones TP, et al. Association of biceps tendon tears with rotator cuff abnormalities: Degree of correlation with tears of the anterior and superior portions of the rotator cuff. Am J Roentgen 2002;180:633–9.
7. Hodler J, Terrier B, von Schulthess GK, Fuchs WA. MRI and sonography of the shoulder. Clin Radiol 1991;43(5):323–7.
8. Swen WA, Jacobs JW, Algra PR, Manoliu RA, Rijkmans J, Willems WJ, et al. Sonography and magnetic resonance imaging equivalent for the assessment of full-thickness rotator cuff tears. Arthritis Rheum 1999;42(10):2231–8.
9. Martin-Hervas C, Romero J, Navas-Acien A, Reboiras JJ, Munuera L. Ultrasonographic and magnetic resonance images of rotator cuff lesions compared with arthroscopy or open surgery findings. J Shoulder Elbow Surg 2001;10(5):410–5.
10. van Holsbeeck MT, Kolowich PA, Eyler WR, Craig JG, Shirazi KK, Habra GK, et al. US depiction of partial-thickness tear of the rotator cuff. Radiology 1995;197(2):443–6.
11. Farin PU, Kaukanen E, Jaroma H, Vaatainen U, Miettinen H, Soimakallio S. Site and size of rotator-cuff tear. Findings at ultrasound, double-contrast arthrography, and computed tomography arthrography with surgical correlation. Invest Radiol 1996;31(7):387–94.
12. Middleton WD, Reinus WR, Totty WG, Melson CL, Murphy WA. Ultrasonographic evaluation of the rotator cuff and biceps tendon. J Bone Joint Surg Am 1986;68(3):440–50.
13. Crass JR, Craig EV, Feinberg SB. Ultrasonography of rotator cuff tears: A review of 500 diagnostic studies. J Clin Ultrasound 1988;16(5):313–27.
14. Brandt TD, Cardone BW, Grant TH, Post M, Weiss CA. Rotator cuff sonography: A reassessment. Radiology 1989;173(2):323–7.
15. Burk DL, Karasick D, Kurtz AB, Mitchell DG, Rifkin MD, Miller CL, et al. Rotator cuff tears: Prospective comparison of MR imaging with arthrography, sonography, and surgery. Am J Roentgen 1989;153(1):87–92.
16. Paavolainen P, Ahovuo J. Ultrasonography and arthrography in the diagnosis of tears of the rotator cuff. J Bone Joint Surg Ser A 1994;76(3):335–40.
17. Farin PU, Jaroma H. Acute traumatic tears of the rotator cuff: Value of sonography. Radiology 1995;197(1):269–73.
18. van Moppes FI, Veldkamp O, Roorda J. Role of shoulder ultrasonography in the evaluation of the painful shoulder. Eur J Radiol 1995;19(2):142–6.
19. Sonnabend DH, Hughes JS, Giuffre BM, Farrell R. The clinical role of shoulder ultrasound. Aust N Z J Surg 1997;67(9): 630–3.

20. Read JW, Perko M. Shoulder ultrasound: Diagnostic accuracy for impingement syndrome, rotator cuff tear, and biceps tendon pathology. J Shoulder Elbow Surg 1998;7(3):264–71.
21. Roberts CS, Walker JA, Seligson D. Diagnostic capabilities of shoulder ultrasonography in the detection of complete and partial rotator cuff tears. Am J Orthoped 2001;30:159–62.
22. Chang CY, Wang SF, Chiou HJ, Ma HL, Sun YC, Wu HD. Comparison of shoulder ultrasound and MR imaging in diagnosing full-thickness rotator cuff tears. Clin Imaging 2002;26(1):50–4.
23. Roberts CS, Walker JA, Seligson D. Diagnostic capabilities of shoulder ultrasonography in the detection of complete and partial rotator cuff tears. Am J Orthoped 2001;30(2):159–62.

Ultrasound of the shoulder

4

Wayne Gibbon

INTRODUCTION

The present chapter is based on nearly 15 years experience of shoulder sonography. A wide range of sonographic shoulder abnormalities may be demonstrated in addition to the more familiar ones seen in the rotator cuff. This chapter will concentrate on these associated conditions and differential diagnosis of shoulder conditions, excluding the rotator cuff. It will also provide information as to the necessary dynamic sonographic techniques and normal sonographic anatomy and some examples of more common conditions alluded to in this text.

The important requirement for shoulder ultrasound as an examination tool reflects the fact that clinical assessment has been shown to have a low accuracy in the diagnosis of periarticular shoulder lesions (1).

> **Key point**
>
> The necessity for shoulder ultrasound as an examination tool is a reflection of the poor accuracy of clinical assessment in diagnosing periarticular shoulder lesions.

STERNOCLAVICULAR JOINT

The most common presentation of sternoclavicular joint pathology is as a painless, hard lump. The majority of these are "silent" subluxations and typically occur in middle-aged/elderly females. These subluxations are usually unilateral and the proximal end of the clavicle can be seen to lie more anteriorly than the (manubrium) sternum on the contralateral normal side. The transducer should be placed oblique transversely across the sternoclavicular joint and along the line of the clavicle from an anterior approach.

In this position a prominent step will be seen between the anteriorly placed medial end of the clavicle and the normally sited sternum when compared to the normal joint where the clavicle is only minimally "proud" of the sternal surface. In such patients the clavicle usually subluxes superiorly as well as anteriorly. Due to the orientation of the thoracic inlet at this point it is usually possible to scan the sternoclavicular joints in the coronal as well as anterior transverse planes. In patients with sternoclavicular joint subluxation a prominent step is again seen on the pathological side in this coronal plane, confirming the cephalad migration of the medial end of the clavicle relative to the superior surface of the manubrium.

In patients with acute traumatic dislocations of the sternoclavicular joint this dislocation may be either anterior or posterior. If anterior the appearances are similar to those of silent or idiopathic subluxation except for a variable associated soft-tissue haematoma. In posterior dislocation the "step" is reversed. Acute traumatic posterior dislocations of the sternoclavicular joints are prone to have associated injury to the great vessels lying immediately behind. In these circumstances colour Doppler imaging may be useful in assessing possible vascular compromise/injury.

The sternoclavicular joints are synovial and as such may be involved in more generalised synovium-based conditions, particularly rheumatoid arthritis (Fig. 4.1). In these circumstances there again is usually anterior–superior subluxation but with a slightly low echogenicity of a soft-tissue mass surrounding the medial end of the clavicle and lying between the clavicle and sternum. Centrally within this synovial mass there is usually anechoic synovial fluid, which may be aspirated if necessary should symptoms be very acute, and differentiation from septic arthritis required. Ultrasound can also be used to guide percutaneous synovial biopsy should this be necessary. A "cutting" biopsy needle may be passed obliquely across the anterior part of the synovial mass under direct ultrasound guidance so as to avoid "overpenetration" of the joint with potential damage to the adjacent great vessels in the root of the neck.

ACROMIOCLAVICULAR JOINT

Normal anatomical appearances

The acromioclavicular joint is usually best scanned from above in the longitudinal coronal

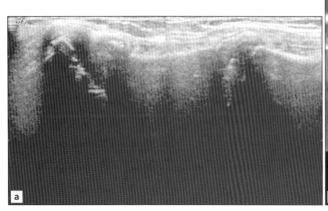
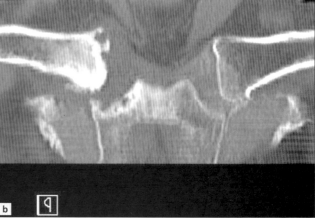

Fig. 4.1 Sternoclavicular joint arthropathy. (a) Transverse section ultrasound images of both sternoclavicular joints showing widening of the right joint space compared to the left with associated irregularity of articular surface contours and increased soft tissue interposed between bone ends consistent with subluxation secondary to an erosive arthropathy. (b) Corresponding CT coronal reconstruction of sternoclavicular joints.

plane along the long axis of the distal clavicle. In this plane both distal clavicle and acromial surfaces are flat with the acromial side being slightly deeper (i.e. further away from the transducer surface than the clavicle). If this gap is accentuated, particularly in patients with acromioclavicular joint dislocation (and to a lesser extent subluxation), but also occasionally in normal individuals, then it may be difficult to maintain good even transducer contact. This problem, however, is usually overcome by using a slightly thickened layer of "contact" gel. Lying between the articular bone ends is a soft-tissue "gap" of variable distance. This is usually filled with synovium. Deep to this gap there is a further interface reflecting the deep or inferior acromioclavicular ligament and the supraspinatus musculoskeletal junction (best appreciated during shoulder abduction).

The superficial/superior acromioclavicular ligament is usually well seen as a thin echogenic band of coronally orientated collagen bundles extending from the distal centimeter or so of the superior superficial surface of the distal clavicle and bridging the joint to insert into the acromion process of the scapula, covering much of its superior superficial surface. It has a flat or mildly convex superficial surface.

Occasionally a notch or fissure may be seen extending across the surface of the acromion. In these circumstances an axial conventional radiograph to assess the possible presence of an os acromiale, which is a failure of normal secondary ossification fusion that can predispose to subacromial impingement, is suggested.

The normal mean ultrasonographic distance of the joint capsule from the bone rim is 2.2 ± 0.5 mm in 21–32-year-olds and 2.9 ± 0.7 mm in 37–81-year-olds (2). The normal mean width of the joint space is 4.1 ± 0.9 mm and 3.5 ± 0.9 mm for these same age groups.

> **Practical tip**
>
> The normal mean ultrasonographic distance of the acromioclavicular joint capsule from the bone rim is 2.2 ± 0.5 mm in 21–32-year-olds and 2.9 ± 0.7 mm in 37–81-year-olds. The normal mean width of the joint space is 4.1 ± 0.9 mm and 3.5 ± 0.9 mm for these same age groups.

Joint degeneration (osteoarthrosis)

The acromioclavicular joint is a synovial joint that is prone to injury both acutely and chronically during repetitive abduction beyond 90° and as such is prone to hyaline cartilage degeneration or osteoarthrosis. Sonographically, as with other joints there is reduction in joint space width and osteophyte formation, the latter feature being seen as superficial marginal bony prominences on either the distal clavicular or acromial, or both sides of the joint. Occasionally small extra interfaces apparently deep to the surface of the bone at articular margins may be seen representing through transmission of sound through the thinned roof of a subarticular cyst/geode. There may be an associated synovitis with the hypoechoic soft tissue, normally lying in the acromioclavicular joint space at rest, starting to bulge the superior joint capsule/superficial acromioclavicular ligament, producing a variable degree of convexity of this surface when scanned from in the coronal plane.

Impingement

Acromioclavicular joint impingement is a common cause of "high-arc" shoulder impingement, i.e. impingement at greater than 90° of abduction. Pain occurs on both active and passive movement and the patient is able to point directly and very specifically to the painful point, which in this instance is immediately below the ultrasound transducer when the acromioclavicular joint is being visualised.

> **Practical tip**
>
> When assessing sonographically for acromioclavicular joint impingement, the best scanning results have been achieved in the author's experience by simply asking the patient to put their hand on their opposite shoulder.

When clinically assessing the acromioclavicular joint impingement pain is best elicited with the arms in the "swallow-tail" position, i.e. with the patient's elbows extended and shoulders fully adducted to 60° or more of extension behind their back. When assessing sonographically, however, it is the author's experience that it is easier to simply ask the patient to put their hand on their opposite shoulder. This full shoulder adduction in minor flexion/internal rotation is both a more comfortable position for the patient and an easier position for maintaining transducer contact during movement. The joint is then scanned "dynamically" during movement from the neutral rest position with the patient's arm at their side into the position of full anterior adduction.

Practical tip

The acromioclavicular joint can be scanned "dynamically" during movement of the patient's arm from the neutral rest position at their side into that of full anterior adduction.

Key point

During adduction in normal shoulders the acromioclavicular joint space is slightly reduced and the acromion is elevated from its rest position, while in patients with acromioclavicular joint impingement the joint space is markedly or completely reduced with the normal interposing soft tissue being extruded superiorly.

In normal shoulders during adduction there is only slight reduction of the acromioclavicular joint space and "elevation" of the acromion from its rest position. In patients with acromioclavicular joint impingement during adduction the joint space is markedly or completely reduced with the normal interposing soft tissue being extruded superiorly (and presumably inferiorly) so as to cause a prominent convexity of the superior joint capsule and acromioclavicular ligament (Fig. 4.2). At the same time the acromion is elevated greater than normal during adduction and may even "override" the distal end of the clavicle in severe cases. Increased transducer pressure at the time usually reproduces the patient's characteristic pain.

In patients with severe degenerative changes there may be no effective joint space at rest and a bulging of extruded soft tissue may be visualized sonographically even in the neutral position. In these circumstances dynamic joint movement is only minimal; however, it is still possible to reproduce typical symptoms and the patient is able to specifically localise the pain to the site of the applied ultrasound transducer.

It should be remembered that similar osteophytes occurring inferiorly (inferior Neer osteophytes), not visible on ultrasound due to lack of appropriate acoustic window, and bulging of inferior capsule may predispose to subacromial impingement. Therefore it is not surprising that there should be an association between acromioclavicular joint disease/ impingement and rotator cuff disease/ impingement.

Geyser phenomenon

Geyser phenomenon relates to a conventional arthrographic finding in patients with full thickness rotator cuff tears. Arthrographic contrast may be seen in some individuals to pass from the glenohumeral joint via a full thickness supraspinatus tendon tear into the subdeltoid and the normally interconnecting subacromial bursa. Contrast can then pass from this bursa or along the adjacent potential space into the acromioclavicular joint, causing it to progressively bulge its superior joint capsule (Fig. 4.3). If pronounced, it can result in a diverticulum extending into the supraclavicular fossa and it is this upward extension as a "blow hole" phenomenon that resulted in the term "geyser phenomenon". It is not uncommon for these abnormalities to present as a supraclavicular mass rather than shoulder problem per se and the skeletal sonologist should be aware of this condition as a potential differential diagnosis for such masses. The presence of an associated, usually massive, full thickness rotator cuff tear should heighten awareness of this diagnostic possibility. Failure to recognise this may result in an unnecessary or inappropriate operative procedure. In such shoulders scanning in the sagittal plane through the acromioclavicular joint may allow demonstration of a communication between the bulging superior joint capsule and a deep defect in the rotator cuff.

Subluxation/dislocation

Acromioclavicular subluxation is due to rupture, avulsion or stripping of the weak superficial/ superior and deep/inferior acromioclavicular ligaments but with an intact coracoclavicular ligament. In an acromioclavicular dislocation

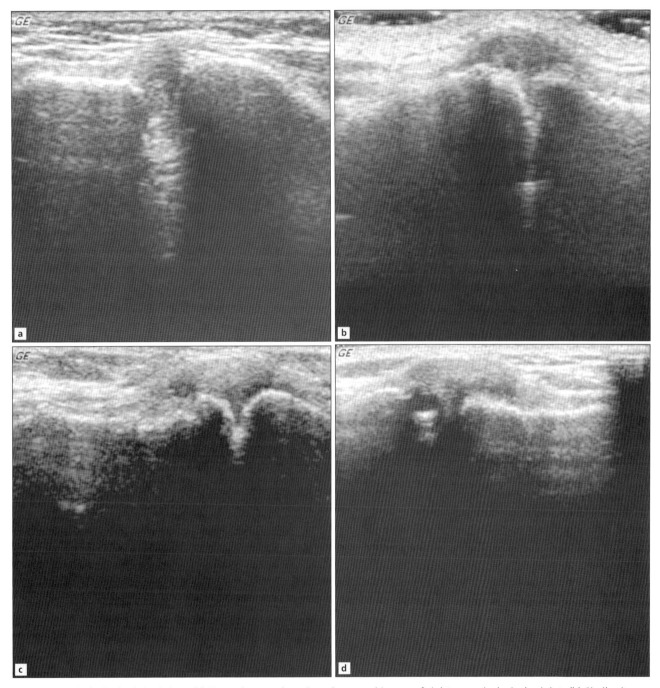

Fig. 4.2 Acromioclavicular joint injury. (a) Normal coronal section ultrasound image of right acromioclavicular joint. (b) Similar image in a patient with acromioclavicular joint impingement performed with the arm in full adduction showing marked reduction in joint space with upward extrusion of thickened synovium and superior joint capsule. (c) Another patient with absence of joint space in the neutral arm position and early marginal osteophyte formation. (d) Subchondral cyst formation at articular margin secondary to chronic impingement.

there is additional rupture of the much stronger coracoclavicular ligament. This latter ligament affectively holds the weight of the upper limb and its failure results in marked acromioclavicular joint separation. The coracoclavicular ligament is best demonstrated in the anterior sagittal plane by first locating the bony prominence of the coracoid process

1–2 cm or so medial to the humeral head in the transverse plane. On finding the coracoid process the transducer can be rotated into the sagittal plane so as to show both the rounded bony surfaces of the coracoid (below) and distal third of the clavicle (above). In this scan plane the coracoclavicular ligament can be seen as an echogenic vertical or oblique vertical band, which

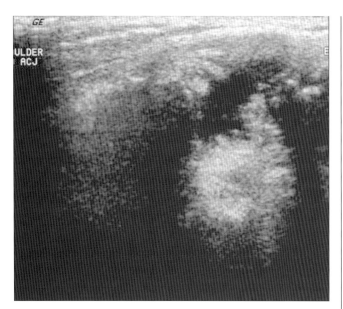

Fig. 4.3 Sonographic geyser phenomenon. There is fluid distension and superior concavity of the superior joint capsule of the right acromioclavicular joint due to extrusion of fluid from the subacromial space through a full thickness rotator cuff tear (not shown).

is broader than it is thick and which contains vertically orientated, densely packed echoes reflecting the contained collagen bundles.

Practical tip

The coracoclavicular ligament is best demonstrated in the anterior sagittal plane by first locating the bony prominence of the coracoid process 1–2 cm or so medial to the humeral head in the transverse plane. On finding the coracoid process the transducer can be rotated into the sagittal plane so as to show both the rounded bony surfaces of the coracoid (below) and distal third of the clavicle (above).

Key point

The mean AC (acromioclavicular) index (AC joint width of uninjured side/AC joint width of injured side) for Tossy-I instability determined by ultrasound was 1.0; mean indices of 0.49 and 0.5 were determined for Tossy-II injury by ultrasound and X-ray, respectively, and those of 0.21 and 0.2, respectively, for Tossy-III instability.

In acromioclavicular subluxations there is a widening of the distance between the distal end of the clavicle and acromion with increased transducer distance to acromion (depth) (Fig. 4.4). The reliability of ultrasound examination of AC joint instability is equal to that of radiographic measurement especially if an acromioclavicular index is calculated (AC index = AC joint width of uninjured side/AC joint width of injured side) (3). The mean AC index for Tossy-I instability determined by ultrasound was 1.0; mean indices of 0.49 and 0.5 were determined for Tossy-II injury by ultrasound and X-ray, respectively, and of 0.21 and 0.2, respectively, for Tossy-III instability. Statistical analysis showed significant differences between the mean AC indices of all three groups ($P < 0.0001$). Any deformity may be significantly reduced by supporting the arm in acute injuries or active shoulder abduction in more chronic injuries (limited due to pain acuteness). The defect in the superficial acromioclavicular ligament may be demonstrated sonographically in acute cases. Alternatively there may be a very oedematous ligament at either end containing a small echogenic focus with acoustic shadowing reflecting a small bone fragment from osseoligamantous avulsion injury.

In dislocations the distance between the coracoid and clavicular surfaces increases and this too may be accurately assessed sonographically (4). Usually in these injuries the coracoclavicular ligament is thickened heterogenously and may exhibit a defect usually in its central third but not uncommonly at one or other end/bony attachment. A variable haematoma may be seen in the surrounding soft tissues, depending on the timescale following the injury. Tears of the deltoid and trapezius muscles and their common fascia are easily detectable in high-grade injuries of the acromioclavicular joint using sonography (5).

Post-traumatic acro-osteolysis is an unusual sequellae of acromioclavicular joint injury whose pathogenesis is not fully understood. Sonographically it can be seen as marked irregularity of the distal clavicular bone surface with associated joint synovitis. The appearances are, however, not pathonemonic and it must be differentiated radiographically from conditions such as primary inflammatory arthropathy or osteomyelitis.

Erosive arthropathy

The acromioclavicular joint is not an uncommon site of involvement in rheumatoid arthritis, psoriatic arthropathy and other inflammatory

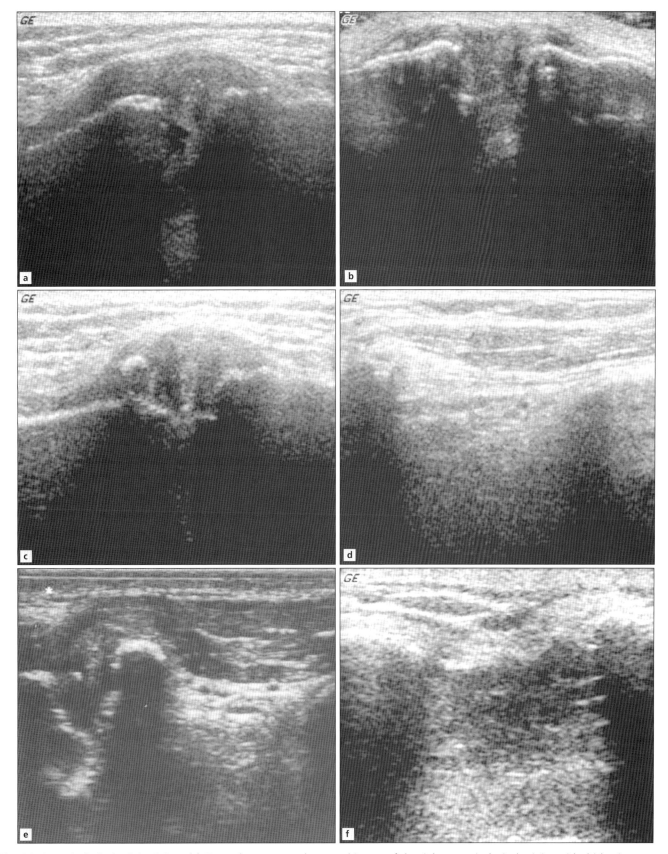

Fig. 4.4 Acromioclavicular joint injury. (a) Coronal transverse ultrasound image of the right acromioclavicular joint with thickening and oedema of the superficial acromioclavicular ligament but with minimal joint widening consistent with a minor joint subluxation injury. (b) More marked acromioclavicular joint space widening without acromial depression in an injury more significant than that in Fig. 4.1a. (c) Another patient with acromioclavicular joint subluxation, in this case also exhibiting bony avulsion of the distal insertion of the superficial acromioclavicular ligament. (d) Normal sagittal ultrasound image of corococlavicular ligamant. (e) Avulsion of the bony attachment of the corococlavicular ligament from its clavicular end with interposed haematoma in a patient with acute acromioclavicular joint dislocation. (f) Corresponding widening of acromioclavicular distance and tear/redundancy of the superficial acromioclavicular ligament in the same patient as that in (e).

arthropathies as well as septic arthritis. In all of these condition there is usually a florid synovitis and hyperaemia on colour Doppler imaging, which is readily demonstrable sonographically at an early stage in the disease process. At a later stage there may be focal, irregularly margined, defects in adjacent bone surfaces, reflecting bone erosion (Fig. 4.5). If clinical doubt as to possible infection exists, needle aspiration under ultrasound-guidance may improve diagnostic yield.

To detect soft-tissue changes in arthritic acromioclavicular joints MRI is better than ultrasound and for revealing bony surface changes, CT is the best method with radiography being least sensitive but most specific (2). Ultrasound can detect acromioclavicular joint changes reliably and is able to exclude joint inflammation. It is able to exclude joint inflammation when the ultrasonographic distance of the joint capsule from the bone rim is <3 mm. Effusion in the AC joint may reflect inflammation, but may also be a sign of degeneration.

Infection in the acromioclavicular joint is uncommon, but is seen in increased frequency in immune-compromised patients and intravenous drug users. A normal glenohumeral joint on ultrasound in a patient suspected of having a septic shoulder should prompt careful review of the acromioclavicular joint (6). Aspiration of the acromioclavicular joint is easily performed under ultrasound guidance.

Interventional procedures

In addition to needle aspiration for microbiological assessment ultrasound may be used to guide needle placement for other diagnostic/therapeutic procedures. Although the joint is largely superficial it can be difficult to guarantee correct site of needle placement using clinical landmarks alone. Ultrasound guidance ensures that the precise site of the needle tip is known so that if no pus can be aspirated or no therapeutic benefit is gained from injection of local anesthetic or corticosteroids the operator has greater confidence in any negative results. The author has found injection of Marcaine® 0.5% in 1 ml with triamcinolone 40 mg particularly useful in patients with high-arc shoulder impingement secondary to symptomatic acromioclavicular arthropathy both in confirming the diagnosis prior to possible surgical acromioplasty or lateral clavicle excision and in providing short- to medium-term symptomatic relief.

SUBACROMIAL SUBDELTOID (SASD) BURSAL DISEASE

Subacromial impingement

The anatomy of the subacromial subdeltoid bursa is complex but ultrasound examination is able, at least in part, to help understand this complexity (7). The subacromial bursa communicates with

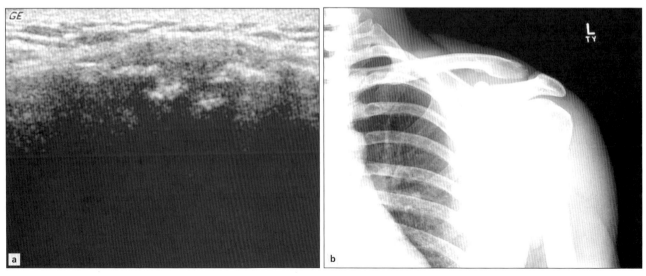

Fig. 4.5 Erosive arthropathy of the acromioclavicular joint. (a) Coronal transverse ultrasound image, and (b) corresponding radiograph showing marginal bone erosion of both sides of joint.

the subdeltoid bursa in the vast majority of individuals and therefore may be effectively considered as the same physical entity i.e. the SASD bursa. The two most common ultrasound manifestations of bursitis are fluid within the bursa (Figs 4.6 and 4.7) and thickening of the synovial lining without much free fluid, though it must be recognised that the bursa frequently appears completely normal on ultrasound but injected and inflamed at arthroscopy. Patients with bursitis complain of pain on abduction as the inflamed bursa is compressed. There are probably three points where this bursa can be compressed—beneath the acromioclavicular joint, at the lateral margin of the acromion and at the coracoacromial ligament. The absence of

a good acoustic window limits demonstration of impingement at the inferior surface of the acromioclavicular joint and inferior Neer marginal osteophytes are better demonstrated using tailored conventional radiographs, MRI or multiplanal reconstructions of volumetric data sets generated by multislice CT. Such impingement can, however, be extrapolated from the changes most readily seen sonographically over the superior surface of the acromioclavicular joint (see the previous section). Impingement on the lateral acromion and coracoacromial ligament, however, is very well demonstrated sonographically.

In many respects the static features of subacromial impingement are those of rotator

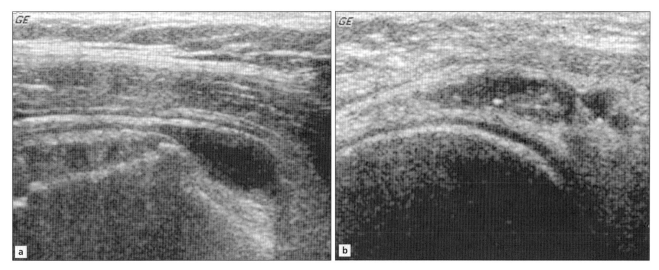

Fig. 4.6 Subacromial subdeltoid bursitis secondary to subacromial impingement. (a) Coronal ultrasound image of left shoulder with dependent fluid distension of the subdeltoid component of the bursa. (b) Coronal image in same patient showing focal thinning of the rotator cuff and irregular synovial thickening of the subdeltoid bursal wall showing the bursitis to be secondary to subacromial impingement and partial thickness tear of the superficial surface of the supraspinatus tendon.

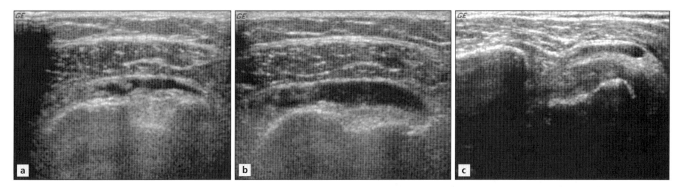

Fig. 4.7 Subdeltoid bursal distension secondary to subacromial impingement. (a) Transverse section ultrasound image at level of the bicipital groove showing mild fluid distension with the arm in the neutral position and (b) same image with the arm in active abduction with increased bursal distension due to subacromial impingement. (c) Coronal ultrasound image of left shoulder showing extruded fluid into the subdeltoid bursa with glenohumeral abduction.

cuff tendinopathy and are described elsewhere (Chapter 3).

In brief they are:

- Irregular tendinosis and fraying of the superficial surface of particularly the anterior rotator cuff tendons in the region of the rotator cuff interval ± intra-articular portion of the long head of the biceps tendon;
- Synovial thickening or fibrosis of the walls of the SASD bursa with variable fluid distension depending on disease activity and arm position;
- Spurring of the lateral margin of the acromion and irregularity of the bone surface of the greater humeral tuberosity ± "whispy" supraspinatus tendon entheseal calcification; and
- Thickening of the coracoacromial ligament.

The dynamic sonographic features of subacromial impingement are the three B's:

- "Ballottement" of synovial fluid from the subacromial bursa beneath the acromial arch into the subdeltoid portion of the bursa;
- "Bunching" of the SASD bursa or rotator cuff tendons on the lateral acromial margin or coracohumeral ligament; and
- "Blocking" of active glenohumeral abduction.

> **Key point**
>
> Dynamic scan criteria ("ballottement" of synovial fluid from the subacromial bursa beneath the acromial arch into the subdeltoid portion of the bursa; "bunching" of the SASD bursa or rotator cuff tendons on the lateral acromial margin or coracohumeral ligament; and "blocking" of active glenohumeral abduction) can correctly diagnose subacromial impingement with a sensitivity of 0.79 and a positive predictive value of 0.96.

> **Practical tip**
>
> Performing the dynamic study of subacromial impingement from the front allows one to easily see the patient's face and gain information about the discomfort produced by shoulder movements.

Dynamic scan criteria can correctly diagnose impingement with a sensitivity of 0.79 and a positive predictive value of 0.96 (8). The authors perform the dynamic study by looking for subacromial impingement from the front so that it is easier to see the patient's face and gain information as to the discomfort produced by the shoulder movements. Initially the patient sits on the edge of the bed or chair with their arm in full internal rotation and adduction behind their back (or as close to full as pain allows). The patient then abducts, externally rotates and slightly flexes the shoulder actively out to their side. As they do so the rotator cuff is scanned in the oblique coronal plane to the body/true coronal plane to the supraspinatus tendon. It is usually best to have a consistent reference point such as the lateral border of the clavicle or the coracoacromial ligament to ensure reproducibility. The supraspinatus should smoothly glide beneath the acromion and ligament without catching or producing a palpable "click". If active movement becomes limited by pain before the supraspinatus fully disappears from view the examiner should take the full weight of the patient's arm and then continue the abduction passively, allowing the arm to externally rotate and flex slightly as they do so. Such a passive movement should be used to take the shoulder to approximately 90° of abduction, after which time the deltoid muscle rather than rotator cuff is the prime mover and no further pain should be felt from active abduction (unless there is additional "high-arc" impingement at the acromioclavicular joint).

> **Practical tip**
>
> When the patient abducts, externally rotates and slightly flexes the shoulder actively out to their side, scan the rotator cuff in the oblique coronal plane to the body/true coronal plane to the supraspinatus tendon.

> **Key point**
>
> In normal circumstances, when a person abducts, externally rotates and slightly flexes their shoulder actively out to their side, the supraspinatus tendon should smoothly glide beneath the acromion and ligament without catching or producing a palpable "click".

> **Practical tip**
>
> The ballotement of fluid from the subacromial to the subdeltoid part of the SASD bursa during active abduction may be confirmed by scanning with the transducer in the transverse axis at the level of the mid-bicipital groove.

Fluid ballottement from the subacromial to subdeltoid part of the SASD bursa may be seen initially during active abduction when scanning along the long axis of the supraspinatus tendon. This fluid extrusion may then be confirmed by scanning with the transducer in the transverse axis at the level of the mid-bicipital groove. This groove acts as a consistent reference point for assessment of, what may at times be very subtle, bursal distension. Repeating the motion whilst scanning, or asking the patient to do so prior to scanning, tends to increase the volume of bursal fluid probably, at least in part due to the irritation of the synovial walls of the SASD bursa. A similar increase in the SASD bursal (and glenohumeral and bicipital sheath) synovial fluid has been shown in asymptomatic handball players up to 16–20 h after training with full reversibility by 22–24 h after the stress (9).

A particular variation on the process of subacromial impingement is impingement due to large areas of rotator cuff calcification. Soft-tissue calcification is relatively inert biologically and does not usually produce inflammatory reaction (unless in evolution or dissolution). Large areas of calcification within the rotator cuff, particularly the supraspinatus tendon more than the subscapularis tendon, may, however, become symptomatic due to their "mass effect". The fact that they increase the tendon thickness, and probably reduce tendon compressibility, means that such calcification produces or exacerbates subacromial impingement. This results in inflammation of the SASD bursa, and colour Doppler imaging often shows associated hyperaemia around the area of calcification. The correlation between colour Doppler ultrasonographic findings and clinical symptoms in such cases has been reported as being good ($P < 0.01$) (10). The above further compromises the subacromial space, producing a vicious cycle of symptoms. This cycle may be broken by reducing the bulk of calcification (e.g. aspiration) (11), reducing the bursal distension/synovitis (e.g. steroid injection) (12) or increasing the subacromial space surgically (e.g. acromioplasty). Ultrasound-guided fine-needle multiple punctures and/or aspiration showed marked improvement of patients' clinical condition with more than 50% size reduction of calcific plaque at a follow-up ultrasound study, suggesting it to be an effective treatment for symptomatic rotator cuff calcification (13).

It is interesting that following surgical acromioplasty the calcification decreases in size or disappears completely, inferring that the impingement has a significant part to play in the initial generation of this dystrophic tendon calcification. The above, coupled with the risks of symptomatic deterioration from bursal crystal spillage (see the next section), is the reason why the author prefers in such circumstances, at least in the first instance, to attempt ultrasound-guided bursal steroid injection rather than calcium aspiration or barbotage.

Arthropathy-associated bursitis

The SASD bursa has the same predisposition to synovium-based conditions seen elsewhere in the body, especially rheumatoid arthritis and crystal arthropathy, infection and more rare conditions such as pigmented villo-nodular synovitis (PVNS) and synovial osteochondromatosis (Fig. 4.8).

In general if an extremely florid SASD bursitis is evident sonographically then causes other than chronic subacromial impingement such as rheumatoid arthritis or subacute/low-grade sepsis should be sought. Crystal-related bursitis can be extremely painful and can rapidly go on to a "frozen shoulder" due to the pain severity. If there is "bursal chondrocalcinosis" due to calcium pyrophosphate or mixed crystal deposition the bursal fluid contents may be extremely echogenic due to the extra-interfaces and as such may need to be differentiated from similarly echogenic bursal haemorrage (as may occur in trauma, haemophilia or synovial angiomatous malformation). In such circumstances the study may be difficult due to severity of pain of even minimal transducer pressure. If ultrasound-guided aspiration, foraging or barbotage of symptomatic rotator cuff calcification is being performed care should be taken to minimise crystal spillage into the SASD bursa as this can produce quite severe postintervention pain.

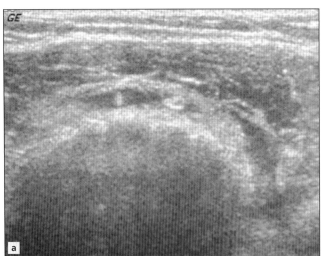
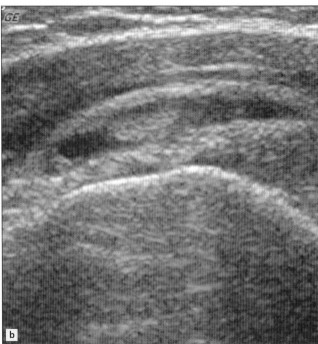

Fig. 4.8 Synovial osteochondromatosis of the subdeltoid bursal. (a, b) Ultrasound images showing multiple echogenic foci of varying shapes and sizes are present within the fluid distended bursa.

> **Practical tip**
>
> When performing ultrasound-guided aspiration, foraging or barbotage of symptomatic rotator cuff calcification, care should be taken to minimise crystal spillage into the SASD bursa as this can produce quite severe postintervention pain.

If a condition is thought, for clinical or other reasons, to be involving the glenohumeral joint and there is palpable swelling clinically in region of the shoulder joint then two inferences can be made. Firstly, the swelling is likely to be related to florid SASD bursitis as fluid distension or synovial thickening of the glenohumeral joint is not usually palpable due to the tight constraints of the surrounding joint capsule and rotator cuff. Secondly, there is likely to be either concurrent disease in both the SASD bursa and glenohumeral joint, there is continuity/extension of disease process via a full thickness defect in the rotator cuff, or both of these processes exist. Therefore, a septic arthritis originating in the glenohumeral joint will rapidly extend into the SASD bursa and from there potentially the acromioclavicular joint via a full thickness rotator cuff tear (or visa versa) (14). Similarly any injection into the SASD bursa will rapidly pass via the cuff tear into the glenohumeral joint. The fact that this passage of fluid occurs with shoulder movement can be confirmed on dynamic ultrasound examination where the effect of glenohumeral abduction is to widen the rotator cuff tear and distend the SASD bursa. This can be seen for naturally occurring joint and bursal fluid but is also the basis of "arthrosonography" where injecting contrast medium (or saline) into the glenohumeral joint and subacromial bursa significantly improves the diagnostic yield of rotator cuff ultrasonography (15) with a resulting 97% sensitivity and 95% specificity (16).

SASD bursal injection

Injection of this bursa can be very readily performed under direct ultrasound-guidance. The author prefers to have the patient lying in the decubitus position with their symptomatic shoulder uppermost and their arm lying at their side. After preparing and cleaning the area appropriately so as to maintain good aseptic conditions a 3 cm 23 G needle (or in larger patients 5 cm 22 G paediatric "spinal" needle) is passed in a horizontal sagittal plain so that its tip comes to lie on the surface of the supraspinatus tendon. The 7–10 Mhz linear-array ultrasound transducer (preferably a lightweight combination of scan-head and connection lead) is prepared for sterility. It is then placed in the required long axis so that the needle can be correctly guided parallel to its surface. This maximises the echogenicity and perspicuity of the fine needle. The procedure is performed under local anaesthetic infiltration. Once the suprapinatus tendon surface has been reached a further bolus of 1–2 ml of local anaesthertic is injected under direct ultrasound vision to ensure that there is no intratendinous injection, good bursal distension and rapid migration of fluid in the bursa from SD to SA components. It also acts as a diagnostic test for subacromial impingement, i.e. whether it subsequently takes away shoulder symptoms in the immediate short term. Triamcinolone (40 mg) or a similarly injectable long-activity steroid is then injected again under direct sonographic vision. The crystalline nature of this injectate and its contained microbubbles produced by prior agitation means that the fluid is echogenic and therefore its correct distribution easily confirmed.

ADHESIVE CAPSULITIS (FROZEN SHOULDER)

"Frozen shoulder", or more correctly adhesive capsulitis, is not an uncommon but probably significantly overdiagnosed, painful shoulder condition. It is usually a self-limiting condition but may take 1–2 years to disappear. In an adhesive capsulitis these is marked reduction in certain shoulder movements. External rotation is the first movement to be limited and last to recover. It produces both an active and passive painful block to abduction. Beyond this point of "block" any further shoulder abduction produced is not gleonohumeral but scapulothoracic movement and this limitation of movement largely persists even under general anaesthsia. An adhesive capsulitis is characterised arthrographically by a reduction in the overall joint capacity and failure to fill normally connecting bursae such as the subscapularis bursa.

Using arthrography as a gold standard sonography has a reported sensitivity of 91%, a specificity of 100% and an accuracy of 92% for detecting adhesive capsulitis, showing dynamic sonography to be a reliable technique for the diagnosis of this condition (17). At the time of ultrasound study the first sign of a true frozen shoulder is the difficulty found in obtaining good images of the subscapularis tendon. This is because to obtain such images the humerus should be externally rotated so as to bring the subscapularis parallel to the linear-array transducer surface. The reduced range of external rotation in an adhesive capsultis means that the subscapularis tendon is angled obliquely to the transducer and therefore image quality is limited and overall echogenicity artefactuality reduced due to the resulting anisotropy (beam obliquity artefact). On dynamic scanning during shoulder abduction there is failure of normal retraction of the rotator cuff below the acromial arch, which is painful and cannot be overcome passively by the investigator. When looking at the patient clinically the shoulder may appear to abduct a degree more with assisted passive motion; however, the ultrasound image is unchanged. That is, the glenohumeral joint has not moved and the additional abduction movement has occurred between the scapular and chest wall. Thirdly there may be increased fluid in the dependent portion of the bicipital tendon sheath presumably due to expression of synovial fluid out of the glenohumeral joint proper. Finally, sonographic examination may demonstrate the particular underlying condition that has predisposed to the secondary adhesive capsulitis, e.g. subacromial impingement, rotator cuff tear or crystal arthropathy.

Subacromial impingement is a potential trigger for a secondary frozen shoulder. Therefore where this impingement predominates, a shoulder may exhibit active limitation of active shoulder abduction, which may be partly overcome by passive abduction (typical subacromial impingement) only to reach a total block to further active and passive movement (typical frozen shoulder). Indeed if the subacromial impingement is predisposed to by acromioclavicular joint impingement, dynamic features of all three conditions and their corresponding dynamic sonographic signs described previously may, not uncommonly, be present in the same painful shoulder.

Hydrostatic overdistension is a therapeutic technique that has been used quite widely as treatment for adhesive capsulitis. Although the author prefers to do this under fluoroscopic/arthrographic control for better "global" visualisation of contrast (distension fluid) spread this can be successfully performed under ultrasound guidance, minimising the necessity for ionising radiation and water-soluble contrast agent administration.

LONG HEAD OF BICEPS

Sonographic abnormalities of the biceps tendon or the soft tissue surrounding the biceps tendon have been found in 5.3% of patients examined for shoulder pain (18).

Normal sonographic anatomy

The long head of the biceps tendon normally lies in the bony channel between the greater humeral tuberosity (laterally) and lesser tuberosity (medially). It is kept in the groove by a combination of these bony walls and the transverse bicipital ligament that bridges them superficially. This ligament is in continuity with the subscapularis tendon as it inserts into the lesser tuberosity and to a lesser extent the supraspinatus tendon as it inserts into the greater tuberosity. If the walls of this groove are shallow there appears to be an increased incidence of medial displacement of the biceps tendon (19). If the groove is narrow with steep/sharp walls then there is an apparent increased risk of tendon degeneration and tear. The normal tendon within the groove is slightly elliptical in cross section with internal echoes from fibres orientated longitudinally along the biceps tendon. The transversely orientated bicipital ligament appears as a thin echogenic band with a transversely orientated internal fibrillar pattern. The synovial sheath of the long head of the biceps tendon is effectively an out-pouching from the synovial lining of the glenohumeral joint and covers the tendon as it passes below the bicipital ligament and for a variable distance below this ligament. The tendon takes its blood supply from this sheath via a vincula, which although not normally seen may be readily visible when the bicipital tendon sheath is distended with fluid. At its distal end the long head of the biceps tendon can be followed right down to its musculotendinous junction where it flares out and becomes indistinguishable from the muscle belly. The proximal end is more difficult to visualise. Sequentially altering the orientation of the transducer, as the tendon changes from its vertical to horizonal alignment, as it courses over the superior humeral surface, does allow visualisation of its intra-articular path. However, in adults it is not usually possible to see its insertion into the superior glenoid labrum and as such ultrasound has a limited role in assessing possible superior labral anterior–posterior tears (SLAP lesions) except perhaps for a Grade-4 tear where there is associated tendon rupture propagating distally.

Tendinopathy

The long head of the biceps is particularly prone to injury and disease both in combination with the rotator cuff and due to its part intra-articular course, many other conditions involving the shoulder joint itself.

Repeated minor trauma results in tendinosis of the bicipital tendon. The tendon becomes thickened and more rounded in cross section and its echogenicity becomes heterogenous and decreased. Intrasubstance tears may develop with a longitudinally orientated hypoechoic or aneachoic central area starting to split the tendon sagittally (Fig. 4.9). These longitudinal intrasubstance tears are usually at the level of the bicipital groove (unless part of a SLAP lesion) as opposed to most transverse tears, which tend to occur in the tendons intra-articular section. It is possible that the longitudinal tears reflect impingement onto the medial wall of the bicipital groove and the more proximal transverse tears

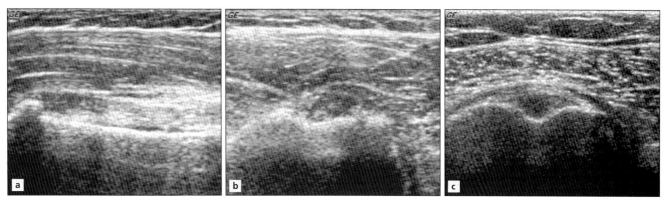

Fig. 4.9 Long head of biceps tear. (a) Longitudinal ultrasound imaging through the long axis of the biceps tendon showing a hypoechoic band within the proximal tendon consistent with a partial thickness tear. (b) Transverse ultrasound image through the bicipital groove with a "2-part" biceps tendon appearance due to a longitudinal partial thickness tear. (c) Third patient with absence of the biceps tendon in the bicipital groove but intact transverse bicipital ligament.

subacromial impingement of glenohumeral joint disease (e.g. rheumatoid arthritis). In the presence of a complete tear the remaining tendon usually retracts distally under the pull of the biceps brachialis muscle, exhibiting a variable degree of redundancy and "waviness" as it does so. It is not uncommon, however, for the tendon to become adherent to the walls of the bicipital grove, which limits the degree of distal tendon retraction. Therefore, the intra-articular course of the biceps tendon should be followed for as long as possible to avoid missing proximal "minimally retracted" tears. In general the degree of biceps muscle atrophy is less for long head of biceps tendon tears in the shoulder than the atrophy seen in lower tendon tears at the elbow. This reflects the fact that the short head of the biceps tendon is very rarely involved in disease or injury and therefore this reduces the degree of muscle dysfunction.

Occasionally, rather than becoming thickened the long head of the biceps tendon becomes thinned and atrophic following injury, although more commonly this atrophy tends to be seen in full thickness tears with resulting loss of tendon loading. It is possible that even without full thickness tears having occurred, this atrophy in "tendinosis" reflects a previous tear with partial healing. In full thickness tears with tendon retraction the tendon sheath may contract on itself and the bicipital groove fill with other echogenic debris. Care should be taken not to misdiagnose this as bicipital tendon atrophy. This can usually be avoided by comparison with the contralateral shoulder (assuming this to be normal, which is often not the case in tendon overuse injuries).

Tenosynovitis

> **Practical tip**
>
> To distinguish between sheath synovitis and complex synovial fluid containing internal echoes, synovium is noncompressible while the latter can be balloted away by increased transducer pressure.

In both cases of significant bicipital tendinosis and tears there is usually associated synovitis within the bicipital tendon sheath. It may be difficult to differentiate sheath synovitis from complex synovial fluid containing internal echoes (Fig. 4.10). In general, however, synovium is noncompressible while synovial fluid can be balloted away by increased transducer pressure. Colour Doppler characteristics can also assist with the differential diagnosis (Fig. 4.11). Also synovial fluid tends to accumulate naturally under gravity at the lowermost end of the tendon sheath, ballooning out below the less distensible transverse bicipital ligament. Synovitis may also accumulate in this region; indeed in chronic severe rheumatoid arthritis this sheath may propagate distally almost as far as the elbow joint. However, unlike with synovial hypertrophy, scanning fluid with the limb elevated allows drainage of fluid towards the shoulder joint, confirming its fluid nature.

> **Practical tip**
>
> Another way to confirm a synovial mass as fluid is to elevate the limb while scanning, which allows the fluid, unlike synovial hypertrophy, to drain towards the shoulder joint.

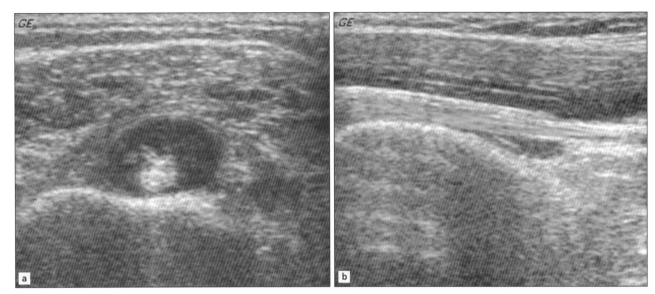

Fig. 4.10 Fluid distension of the long head of biceps tendon sheath. Two separate patients with marked (a) and more subtle (b) fluid distension showing the dependent nature of the fluid and its tendency to be less marked at the level of the transverse bicipital ligament due to the ligament's relative nondistendability.

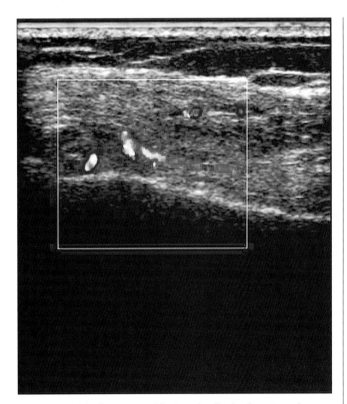

Fig. 4.11 Bicipital tenosynovitis. Longitudinal colour Doppler image along the length of the biceps tendon in the bicipital groove shows marked hyperaemia and synovial thickening consistent with synovitis. The long head of biceps tendon itself is generally hypoechoic, consistent with associates tendionopathy.

Due to the continuity of the sheath with the glenohumeral joint itself, bicipital tenosynovitis or bicipital sheath fluid accumulation may reflect intra-articular disease rather than bicipital pathology per se (in a similar way that Baker's cyst synovitis or fluid distention usually reflects knee joint pathology rather than local bursal dysfunction).

It is for this same reason and the dependent nature of the sheath that it is not uncommon for "intra-articular" loose bodies to be lodged in the bicipital tendon sheath and should not be confused with tendon calcification, which is most unusual at this tendon site (Fig. 4.12). Also mineralization of the transverse ligament can occasionally be observed (18) and this too should not be confused with loose body formation or calcific tendonitis.

Medial tendon subluxation/dislocation

The long head of the biceps tendon may migrate medially during external rotation. Dynamic scanning of a shoulder during maximal external rotation will detect 86% of cases of subluxation. Static scanning alone, however, can detect approximately the same percentage of dislocations due to their more fixed nature (20).

If the tendon lies on the anterior/medial wall of the bicipital during humeral external rotation but relocates centrally with internal rotation this is termed a medial subluxation (21) (Fig. 4.13). If the tendon comes fully out of the groove this is then termed a medial dislocation (Fig. 4.14). A dislocated tendon can relocate with internal rotation but it is the author's experience that this

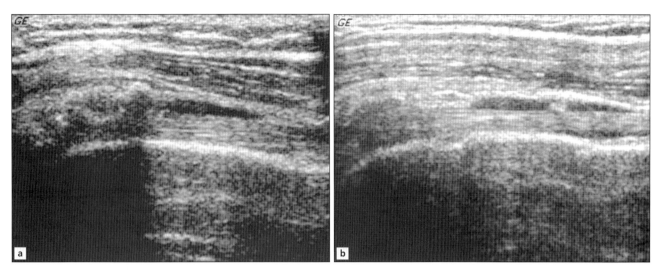

Fig. 4.12 Loose bodies in biceps tendon sheath. (a, b) Longitudinal ultrasound images along the long axis of the same biceps tendon at the level of and just distal to the transverse bicipital ligament. Multiple echogenic areas, some exhibiting acoustic shadowing, are seen along the length of the biceps tendon sheath. The altered appearances between scan images (a, b) emphasises the true "loose" nature of these partially calcified bodies.

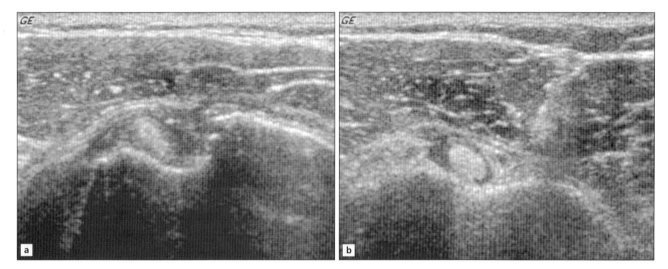

Fig. 4.13 Medial subluxation of the long head of the biceps tendon. Transverse ultrasound images through the right bicipital groove in two different patients. In (a) the transverse ligament has been stripped away from the lesser tuberosity of the humerus, allowing the biceps tendon to potentially migrate between the ligament and bone (and therefore, as the condition progresses, below the subscapularis tendon). In (b) the transverse ligament has been torn at its anterior end, allowing the biceps tendon to potentially migrate through the defect in the ligament (and therefore, as the condition progresses, superficial to the subscapularis tendon).

is a most unusual occurrence. When the tendon dislocates, it usually does so in continuity with its tendon sheath. There are essentially three patterns of medial biceps tendon dislocation:

- Medial migration superficial/anterior to the subscapularis tendon—This occurs when the transverse bicipital ligament is ruptured, allowing the tendon to pass over the top of the subscapularis tendon. This is probably the most common pattern of medial dislocation.
- Medial migration deep/posterior to the subscapularis tendon—This occurs when the subscapularis tendon and the transverse

bicipital ligament are sheared off the lesser tuberosity in continuity, allowing the biceps tendon to pass between them and the underlying humerus.
- Medial migration into the substance of the subscapularis tendon due to the severe tendinosis the subscapularis tendon has developed. This is extremely unusual.

There is a high association between rotator cuff tear and biceps tendon subluxation or dislocation (19). In most cases of dislocation there has been shown to be an associated complete rupture of the subscapularis tendon (21).

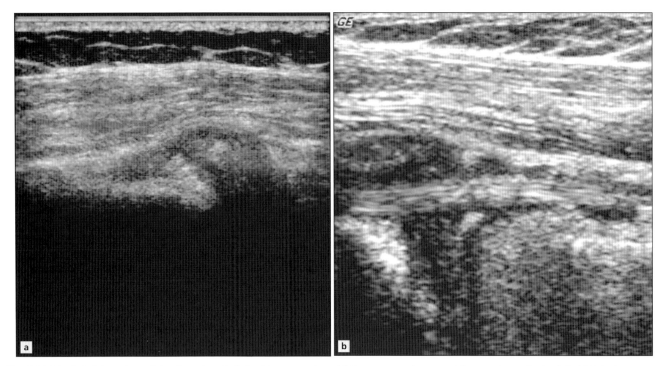

Fig. 4.14 Medial dislocation of the long head of the biceps tendon. (a) Transverse ultrasound image through the left bicipital groove shows an empty groove and the biceps tendon lying superficial to the lesser tuberosity of the humerus. (b) Corresponding sagittal section along the biceps tendon performed in full external rotation shows that the tendon no longer has any part of the humeral shaft lying beneath it due to the degree of the tendon's medial displacement.

Also when medially dislocated, the empty bicipital grove may be seen by the unwary sonologist and diagnosed as a full thickness bicipital tendon tear with retraction. Therefore, great care must be taken in these circumstances to ensure that a medially placed tendon has not been missed.

GLENOHUMERAL SUBLUXATION/DISLOCATION

When comparing sonography and arthroscopy in differentiating abnormal labrum (tear or degeneration) from normal labrum sonography has a sensitivity of 63–88%, specificity of 67–98% and accuracy of 88% (22, 23). Therefore, ultrasonography may be valuable in the detection of anterior labral (Bankart) lesions even in patients with recent shoulder dislocation although, at the presnt time, the true clinical value is unclear.

Sonography would seem to have a role diagnosing complications of shoulder dislocation. In patients with persistent pain after proximal humeral head fractures or cases where a question exists as to the degree of fragment displacement diagnostic ultrasound investigation may yield useful additional information (24). These avulsion fractures of the supraspinatus insertion (greater tuberosity) or occasionally subscapularis insertion (lesser tuberosity) usually show between 1- and 8 mm displacement and this may be clinically significant. This is due to the fact that the displacement may precipitate or accentuate subacromial impingement. In such cases, during dynamic examination, impingement of the supraspinatus tendon between the acromion and the greater tuberosity fracture fragment may be observed.

> **Key point**
>
> Sonography performed on patients with shoulder dislocations has been reported to demonstrate rotator cuff lesions in approximately 29–32% of traumatic shoulder dislocations.

Sonography performed on patients with shoulder dislocations has been reported to demonstrate rotator cuff lesions in approximately 29–32% of traumatic shoulder dislocations (25, 26). The incidence of tears in patients with first dislocation is higher than that for recurrent dislocations. Also following shoulder dislocations women appear to rupture the rotator cuff more often than men.

If a patient is unable to elevate the affected arm more than 90° in the scapular plane 2 weeks after dislocation, there should be a particularly high suspicion of rotator cuff tear (77%) (26).

Sonographically, humeral impaction injuries (Hill–Sachs lesions) (Figs 4.15 and 4.18) occur in approximately 80% of traumatic dislocations and bony avulsions of the greater tuberosity in about 10% (25) (Figs 4.16 and 4.17). When compared to either CT-arthrography or arthroscopy as the "gold standard", ultrasonography has been shown to have a sensitivity of 95–96%, specificity of 92–93% and diagnostic accuracy of 94–95% for Hill–Sachs lesions (27, 28). In comparison to normal subjects there is a significant increase in downward subluxation demonstrable sonographically in patients with multidirectional instabilities (29).

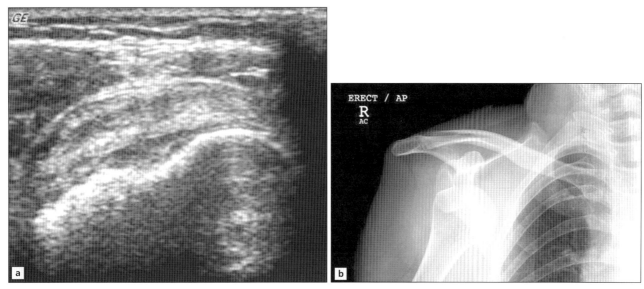

Fig. 4.15 Acute glenohumeral dislocation. (a) Oblique coronal ultrasound image along the long axis of the posterior part of the supraspinatus tendon. The tendon is hypoechoic, heterogenous and thickened, and fluid extends below the tendon between it and a roughened area of the humeral head. The appearances reflect tendon contusion over an area of minor Hill–Sach-type injury. (b) Conventional radiograph from 1 week previously showing the acute shoulder dislocation, which had been relocated by the time of the ultrasound study.

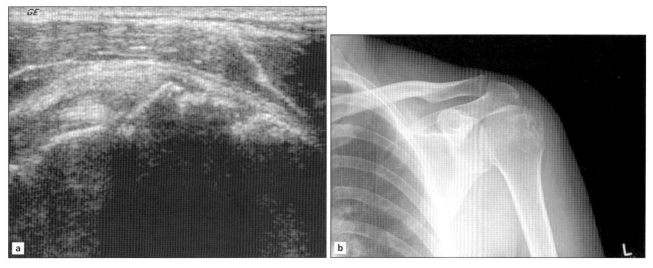

Fig. 4.16 Avulsion fracture of the greater tuberosity of the humerus. (a) Oblique coronal ultrasound image along the long axis of the anterior part of the supraspinatus tendon, showing marked irregularity of bone surface laterally at site of rotator cuff insertion. (b) Corresponding conventional radiograph performed immediately after the ultrasound examination confirms the sonographic bony abnormality to be a partial avulsion of the rotator cuff osseotendinous junction.

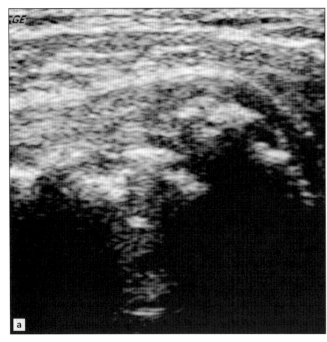
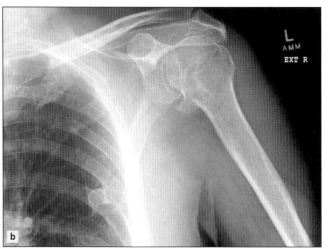

Fig. 4.17 Avulsion fracture of the lesser tuberosity of the humerus. (a) Transverse ultrasound image along axis of the subscapularis tendon on the anterior aspect of the proximal humerus shows marked irregularity of the bone surface of the lesser tuberosity of the humerus. (b) Corresponding conventional radiograph performed immediately after the ultrasound examination confirms the sonographic bony abnormality to be a partial avulsion of the subscapularis osseotendinous junction/lesser tuberosity of the humerus.

Traumatic pseudoaneurysm of the axillary artery after shoulder dislocation has also been demonstrated using colour Doppler imaging (30).

INFLAMMATORY ARTHROPATHIES

Sonography is able to reveal inflammatory conditions at early stages of rheumatoid arthritis when no radiographic changes are seen. The most common ultrasound finding is SASD bursitis in 69% of shoulders. In these patients synovitis may be demonstrated in the glenohumeral joint in 58% of shoulders, biceps tendinitis in 57% and similar changes in the supraspinatus tendon in 33% (31).

Practical tip

The mean distance between the humerus and the joint capsule when measured sonographically at the axilla with the humerus in 90° abduction is 2.4 ± 0.5 mm. Intrasynovial effusion can be suspected if the distance is 3.5 mm or more, or the difference between both sides is 1 mm or more.

The mean distance between the humerus and the joint capsule when measured sonographically at the axilla with the humerus in 90° abduction is 2.4 ± 0.5 mm. Intrasynovial effusion can be suspected if the distance is 3.5 mm or more, or the difference between both sides is 1 mm or more (32). It has been shown that in patients with rheumatoid arthritis ultrasound had a sensitivity of 100% and specificity of 100% for the detection of effusion/hypertrophy in the glenohumeral joint when validated by surgical findings, a sensitivity of 93% and a specificity of 83% for effusion/hypertrophy in the subacromial subdeltoid bursa, a sensitivity of 100% and a specificity of 83% for effusion/hypertrophy in the biceps tendon sheath, a sensitivity of 83% and a specificity of 57% for rotator cuff tear and a sensitivity of 70% and a specificity of 100% for biceps tendon rupture (33).

In a comparative imaging study of the shoulders of patients with rheumatoid arthritis ultrasound depicted humeral erosions in 92% of shoulders examined compared to 96% using MRI, 77% using CT and 73% for conventional radiography (33) (Fig. 4.19). This same study showed that both MRI and ultrasound were superior to CT in detecting small erosions while conventional radiography frequently missed small erosions. Also ultrasound was the most

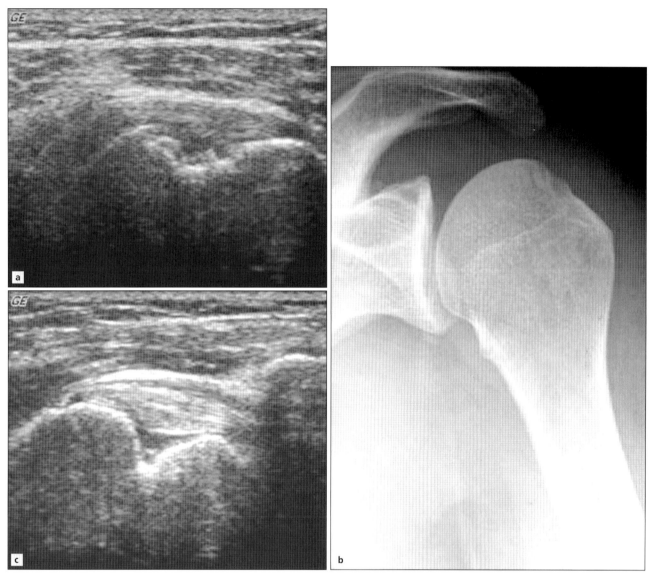

Fig. 4.18 Hill–Sach lesion and adhesive capsulitis. (a) Oblique coronal ultrasound image performed during shoulder abduction along the long axis of the posterior part of the supraspinatus tendon showing marked irregularity of bone surface medially, consistent with an impaction fracture (Hill–Sach lesion). (b) The rotator cuff has failed to migrate fully below the acromion during attempted active and passive abduction manoeuvres, consistent with a true "frozen shoulder". (c) Corresponding conventional radiograph confirms the bony defect on the humeral head, i.e. Hill–Sach lesion, and avulsion fracture inferior to the glenoid margin, i.e. bony Bankart lesion, secondary to previous glenohumeral dislocation.

sensitive method for showing greater tuberosity surface erosions whereas for large erosions there was little difference between sonography and either MRI or CT.

Gompels and Darlington, in as early as 1981, published a case report of a patient with advanced rheumatoid arthritis who presented with bilateral shoulder dislocation due to septic arthritis where ultrasonography was particularly helpful in guiding a 20 G needle to fluid collections within the debris-filled joint capsules and in facilitating successful aspiration (34). They also showed how ultrasound could provide a painless, noninvasive and safe method of serial assessment of the joints

after therapy. Massive synovial proliferation is occasionally seen in the bursae of patients with inflammatory arthritis; however, such rheumatoid involvement of the subacromial subdeltoid bursa in adults is uncommon, and it is still rarer in children. When it does occur, then sonography clearly shows the location and nature of the soft-tissue swelling (35).

It is not uncommon for the shoulder to be involved in the seronegative spondyloarthopathies, particularly ankylosing spondylitis and psoriatic arthritis. Any erosions produced tend to be shallow and immediately at the attachment of soft tissue such as the

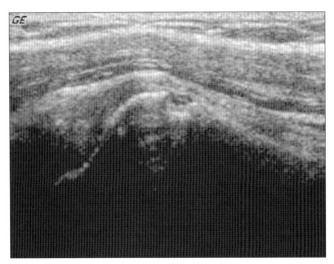

Fig. 4.19 Erosive arthropathy of the glenohumeral joint. A small irregular bone defect is present in the lesser tuberosity of the humerus, seen in a sagittal ultrasound image in a patient with suspected sero-negative arthritis.

supraspinatus tendon insertion, i.e. subentheseal erosions. This is in contradistinction to the deeper erosions of rheumatoid arthritis, which tend to occur at "bare areas" such as the junction between the humeral head and joint capsule.

The shoulder is involved in approximately a third of adults with haemophilia. Rotator cuff tears/tendinosis and to a lesser extent bicipital tendonitis are a common component of this shoulder haemophilic arthropathy according to the evidence from ultrasound studies (36).

Synovial osteochondromatosis of the glenohumeral joint and SASD bursa are rare conditions; however, the ultrasound appearance of them have been described in isolated case reports (37) (Fig. 4.8).

GLENOID LABRAL CYSTS

The glenoid labrum can develop a degenerative cystic abnormality analogous to the meniscal cyst that not uncommonly occurs in the knee. Ultrasonographic examination has shown these glenoid labral cysts to be an anechoic cystic lesion ranging from 3 to 30 mm in diameter and at a range of different shoulder sites including:

- between the deltoid muscle and the subscapularis tendon;
- between the deltoid muscle and the biceps tendon;
- below the coracoacromial ligament; and
- over the suprascapular notch area.

Patients with symptomatic glenoid labral cysts usually complain of pain located over the suprascapular notch due to the fact that they are at an anatomical site that is predisposed to suprascapular nerve entrapment (38). Muscle weakness may also be present due to atrophy of the supraspinatus and infraspinatus muscles. The main symptom, that of pain, may be significantly improved by sonographically guided aspiration with a success rate of 86% (39).

> **Practical tip**
>
> The pain caused by a glenoid labral cyst can be significantly reduced by sonographically guided aspiration with a success rate of 86%.

MUSCLE TEARS

More than likely all of the muscles in the region have been reported as having isolated tears (40); however, probably the most common to tear, especially due to physical/sporting activity, is the pectoralis major muscle. This originates from three "heads", i.e. clavicular, sternal and costal, which combine to form a broad fan-shaped muscle origin. The muscle significantly tapers to form an insertion into the margin of the biciptal groove, having more medially formed the anterior wall of the axilla. This muscle's large bulk combined with the rapid reduction in thickness over a fulcrum (shoulder joint) means that it is particularly prone to tear in the region of the medial border of the axilla. Tears of the pectoralis major muscle are often sports-related, e.g. weightlifters during "bench-pressing" or rugby players making a tackle in such a way that there is a forcible block to shoulder flexion with it in abduction. The sonographic appearances of these tears are the same as those seen elsewhere in the skeleton. The important points in functional terms are the precise site of tears and its effective percentage of cross-sectional area, both of which are eminently resolved sonographically. The percentage tear rather than tear size is important with such a fan-shaped muscle; for example, a 4 cm tear may be insignificant in prognostic terms if it is close to its sternal attachment, whereas that same 4 cm tear may constitute a significant injury when occurring close to its humeral insertion.

SHOULDER MASSES

The sonographic appearances of benign and malignant, primary and secondary, bony and soft-tissue masses in the pain are no different than elsewhere in the skeleton. This should not, however, be forgotten when sonographically examining a patient's shoulder, especially if their symptoms are slightly atypical, and the investigator should always be alert to the possibility of their existence either in isolation or concurrent with more common shoulder conditions such as rotator cuff tears. A rotator cuff tear may be seen in approximately 80% of 80-year-olds' shoulders, the majority of which are more or less symptomatic; therefore, their presence should not distract the sonologist from an alternative diagnosis.

COMPLICATIONS OF ORTHOPAEDIC METALWARE

Although metalware produces a variable posterior reverberation echo and complete acoustic shadowing the surface of implanted metalware is often clearly visualised sonographically and also superficial and adjacent to the soft tissues (Fig. 4.20).

Intramedullary nails are commonly used for fixation of humeral shaft fractures and are usually inserted proximally via the superior surface of the greater tuberosity. Accordingly if left "proud" of the bone surface or otherwise irritating the adjacent rotator cuff these tendons may become markedly degenerate. Also due to the anatomical site of insertion postoperative infection will often result in both intra-articular and SASD bursal infection.

The correlation of sonographic and clinical results following shoulder arthroplasty demonstrated that patients with an excellent clinical result showed no or only a few pathological findings on sonography compared with those with a moderate or poor result (41).

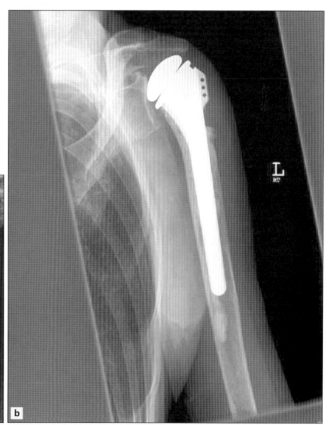

Fig. 4.20 Rotator cuff defect in patient following shoulder arthroplasty. (a) Oblique coronal ultrasound image shows the surface contours and typical metal reverberation artefact of the surgical prosthesis. There is no identifiable normal supraspinatus tendon superficial to the prosthesis. (b) Corresponding conventional radiograph shows upward migration of the shoulder prosthesis consistent with a large full thickness rotator cuff defect.

AMYLOID

Real-time, high-resolution ultrasound is a relatively sensitive (72%) and highly specific (97%) noninvasive adjunct to the clinical diagnosis of beta 2m amyloidosis in patients receiving long-term haemodialysis (42).

Sonographically in patients on chronic haemodialysis and clinical findings suggestive of amyloidosis:

- The mean rotator cuff thickness in the patients with amyloidosis is significantly greater than that in the normal group ($P < 0.0001$).
- The synovial sheath of the long head of the biceps tendon is usually thickened.
- The subacromial subdeltoid bursa is thickened.
- Intra- or periarticular nodules are common (43).

Increased thickness of the joint capsule and echogenic proliferation of the synovia are also commonly observed (44).

Of particular interest is the involvement of the subscapularis tendon in dialysis-related amyloidosis, which is unusual in mechanical cuff tendinopathy. Repeat ultrasonography can become an important way to follow-up progression of shoulder dialysis-related amyloidosis in haemodialysed patients (45).

REFERENCES

1. Naredo E, Aguado P, De Miguel E, Uson J, Mayordomo L, Gijon-Banos J, Martin-Mola E. Painful shoulder: Comparison of physical examination and ultrasonographic findings. Ann Rheum Dis 2002;61(2):132–6.
2. Alasaarela E, Tervonen O, Takalo R, Lahde S, Suramo I. Ultrasound evaluation of the acromioclavicular joint. J Rheum 1997;24(10):1959–63.
3. Kock HJ, Jurgens C, Hirche H, Hanke J, Schmit-Neuerburg KP. Standardized ultrasound examination for evaluation of instability of the acromioclavicular joint. Arch Orthopaed Trauma Surg 1996;115(3–4):136–40.
4. Sluming VA. Technical note: Measuring the coracoclavicular distance with ultrasound—A new technique. Br J Radiol 1995;68(806):189–93.
5. Heers G, Hedtmann A. [Ultrasound diagnosis of the acromioclavicular joint]. Orthopäde 2002;31(3):255–61.
6. Widman DS, Craig JG, van Holsbeeck MT. Sonographic detection, evaluation and aspiration of infected acromioclavicular joints. Skeletal Radiol 2001;30(7):388–92.
7. van Holsbeeck M, Strouse PJ. Sonography of the shoulder: Evaluation of the subacromial–subdeltoid bursa. Am J Roentgen 1993;160(3):561–4.
8. Read JW, Perko M. Shoulder ultrasound: Diagnostic accuracy for impingement syndrome, rotator cuff tear, and biceps tendon pathology. J Shoulder Elbow Surg 1998;7(3):264–71.
9. Kruger-Franke M, Fischer S, Kugler A, Rosemeyer B. [Stress-related clinical and ultrasound changes in shoulder joints of handball players]. Sportverletzung Sportschaden 1994;8(4):166–9.
10. Chiou HJ, Chou YH, Wu JJ, Hsu CC, Huang DY, Chang CY. Evaluation of calcific tendonitis of the rotator cuff: role of color Doppler ultrasonography. J Ultrasound Med 2002;21(3):289–95.
11. Bradley M, Bhamra MS, Robson MJ. Ultrasound guided aspiration of symptomatic supraspinatus calcific deposits. Br J Radiol 1995;68(811):716–9.
12. Wolk T, Wittenberg RH. [Calcifying subacromial syndrome—Clinical and ultrasound outcome of non-surgical therapy]. Z Orthop Ihre Grenzgeb 1997;135(5):451–7.
13. Chiou HJ, Chou YH, Wu JJ, Huang TF, Ma HL, Hsu CC, Chang CY. The role of high-resolution ultrasonography in management of calcific tendonitis of the rotator cuff. Ultrasound Med Biol 2001;27(6):735–43.
14. Lombardi T, Sherman L, van Holsbeeck M. Sonographic detection of septic subdeltoid bursitis: a case report. J Ultrasound Med 1992;11(4):159–60.
15. Fermand M, Hassen CS, Ariche L, Samuel P, Postel JM, Blanchard JP, Goldberg D. Ultrasound investigation of the rotator cuff after computed arthrotomography coupled to bursography. Joint Bone Spine Rev Rhumat 2000;67(4):310–4.
16. Lee HS, Joo KB, Park CK, Kim YS, Jeong WK, Kim YS, Park DW, Kim SI, Park TS. Sonography of the shoulder after arthrography (arthrosonography): Preliminary results. J Clin Ultrasound 2002;30(1):23–32.
17. Ryu KN, Lee SW, Rhee YG, Lim JH. Adhesive capsulitis of the shoulder joint: Usefulness of dynamic sonography. J Ultrasound Med 1993;12(8):445–9.
18. Wurnig C. [Sonography of the biceps tendon]. Z Orthop Ihre Grenzgeb 1996;134(2):161–5.
19. Levinsohn EM, Santelli ED. Bicipital groove dysplasia and medial dislocation of the biceps brachii tendon. Skeletal Radiol 1991;20(6):419–23.
20. Farin PU, Jaroma H, Harju A, Soimakallio S. Medial displacement of the biceps brachii tendon: Evaluation with dynamic sonography during maximal external shoulder rotation. Radiology 1995;195(3):845–8.
21. Walch G, Nove-Josserand L, Boileau P, Levigne C. Subluxations and dislocations of the tendon of the long head of the biceps. J Shoulder Elbow Surg 1998;7(2):100–8.
22. Taljanovic MS, Carlson KL, Kuhn JE, Jacobson JA, Delaney-Sathy LO, Adler RS. Sonography of the glenoid labrum: A cadaveric study with arthroscopic correlation. Am J Roentgen 2000;174(6):1717–22.
23. Schydlowsky P, Strandberg C, Galbo H, Krogsgaard M, Jorgensen U. The value of ultrasonography in the diagnosis of labral lesions in patients with anterior shoulder dislocation. Europ J Ultrasound 1998;8(2):107–13.
24. Jerosch J, Muller G. [Sonographic findings in radiologically non-displaced proximal humerus fractures]. Ultraschall Medizin 1991;12(1):36–40.
25. Weishaupt D, Berbig R, Prim J, Bruhlmann W. [Ultrasound findings after shoulder dislocation]. Ultraschall Medizin 1997;18(3):129–33.
26. Berbig R, Weishaupt D, Prim J, Shahin O. Primary anterior shoulder dislocation and rotator cuff tears. J Shoulder Elbow Surg 1999;8(3):220–5.
27. Pancione L, Gatti G, Mecozzi B. Diagnosis of Hill-Sachs lesion of the shoulder. Comparison between ultrasonography and arthro-CT. Acta Radiologica 1997;38(4 Pt 1):523–6.

28. Jerosch J, Marquardt M. [The value of sonographic diagnosis for the demonstration of Hill-Sachs lesions]. Z Orthopad Ihre Grenzgeb 1990;128(5):507–11.
29. Jerosch J, Marquardt M, Winkelmann W. [Ultrasound documentation of translational movement of the shoulder joint. Normal values and pathologic findings]. Ultraschall Medizin 1991;12(1):31–5.
30. Zieren J, Kasper A, Landwehr P, Erasmi H. [Traumatic pseudoaneurysm of the axillary artery after shoulder dislocation]. Chirurg 1994;65(11):1058–60.
31. Alasaarela EM, Alasaarela EL. Ultrasound evaluation of painful rheumatoid shoulders. J Rheum 1994;21(9):1642–8.
32. Koski JM. Axillar ultrasound of the glenohumeral joint. J Rheum 1989;16(5):664–7.
33. Alasaarela E, Leppilahti J, Hakala M. Ultrasound and operative evaluation of arthritic shoulder joints. Ann Rheum Dis 1998;57(6):357–60.
34. Gompels BM, Darlington LG. Septic arthritis in rheumatoid disease causing bilateral shoulder dislocation: Diagnosis and treatment assisted by grey scale ultrasonography. Ann Rheum Dis 1981;40(6):609–11.
35. Ruhoy MK, Tucker L, McCauley RG. Hypertrophic bursopathy of the subacromial-subdeltoid bursa in juvenile rheumatoid arthritis: Sonographic appearance. Ped Radiol 1996;26(5):353–5.
36. MacDonald PB, Locht RC, Lindsay D, Levi C. Haemophilic arthropathy of the shoulder. J Bone Joint Surg Br Vol 1990;72(3):470–1.
37. Campeau NG, Lewis BD. Ultrasound appearance of synovial osteochondromatosis of the shoulder. Mayo Clinic Proc 1998;73(11):1079–81.
38. Antoniadis G, Richter HP, Rath S, Braun V, Moese G. Suprascapular nerve entrapment: experience with 28 cases. J Neurosurg 1996;85(6):1020–5.
39. Chiou HJ, Chou YH, Wu JJ, Hsu CC, Tiu CM, Chang CY, Yu C. Alternative and effective treatment of shoulder ganglion cyst: ultrasonographically guided aspiration. J Ultrasound Med 1999;18(8):531–5.
40. Dragoni S, Giombini A, Candela V, Rossi F. Isolated partial tear of subscapularis muscle in a competitive water skier. A case report. J Sports Med Phys Fitness 1994;34(4):407–10.
41. Westhoff B, Wild A, Werner A, Schneider T, Kahl V, Krauspe R. The value of ultrasound after shoulder arthroplasty. Skeletal Radiol 2002;31(12):695–701.
42. Kay J, Benson CB, Lester S, Corson JM, Pinkus GS, Lazarus JM, Owen WF Jr. Utility of high-resolution ultrasound for the diagnosis of dialysis-related amyloidosis. Arthritis Rheum 1992;35(8):926–32.
43. Cardinal E, Buckwalter KA, Braunstein EM, Raymond-Tremblay D, Benson MD. Amyloidosis of the shoulder in patients on chronic hemodialysis: Sonographic findings. Am J Roentgenol 1996;166(1):153–6.
44. Rapp-Bernhardt U, Milbradt H, Bernhardt TM, Dohring W. [Ultrasound diagnosis of soft tissue changes in dialysis-associated amyloidosis]. Ultraschall Medizin 1997;18(2):91–4.
45. Sommer R, Valen GJ, Ori Y, Weinstein T, Katz M, Hendel D, Korzets A. Sonographic features of dialysis-related amyloidosis of the shoulder. J Ultrasound Med 2000;19(11):765–70.

Ultrasound of the elbow

5

Ian Beggs

JOINT EFFUSIONS, CYSTS AND BURSAE

> **Key point**
>
> Although radiographs can detect 5–10 ml of fluid within the elbow joint, sonography is more sensitive and can detect 1–3 ml.

Joint effusions are recognised on lateral radiographs of the elbow by elevation of the anterior and posterior fat pads when the joint contains 5–10 ml of fluid. Sonography is more sensitive than radiographs and can detect 1–3 ml of fluid (1). Effusions are best detected by examining the olecranon fossa (Fig. 5.1a) with the elbow flexed (1). The fluid (Fig. 5.1b) elevates the echogenic fat pad (2). Fluid can be distinguished from pannus (Fig. 5.2), which is relatively echogenic and incompressible (3). Septic arthritis can be excluded by showing absence of joint fluid or confirmed by using ultrasound-guided aspiration if fluid is present (4, 5).

Synovial cysts and ganglia may develop from the elbow joint, commonly from the anterior capsule, and extend distally (6). Cysts may be multiloculated and have a stalk.

The cubital or bicipito–radial bursa lies between the distal biceps tendon and the radial tuberosity (7). Enlargement of the bursa most often results from repetitive minor trauma and can compress the median, radial or posterior interosseous nerves or impair movement (7). Ultrasound shows a cystic mass (Fig. 5.3) in close proximity to the distal biceps tendon. Transverse scans with the forearm supinated may be best (3). The bursa is well defined and fluid-filled but may be septate or thick-walled or have echogenic contents (3, 7, 8). The bursa may envelop the biceps tendon, simulating tenosynovitis, but the tendon does not have a sheath. The characteristic site, wedged between the biceps tendon and the radial tuberosity, distinguishes the bursa from a ganglion (7).

Olecranon bursitis is also due to repetitive trauma. It produces a subcutaneous fluid-filled mass superficial to the olecranon process (Fig. 5.4). Colour Doppler ultrasound may show

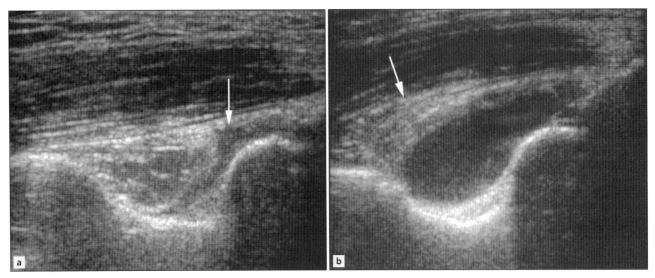

Fig. 5.1 (a) Longitudinal scan of olecranon fossa shows small effusion (arrow) between fat pad and bone. (b) A large joint effusion elevates the posterior fat pad (arrow).

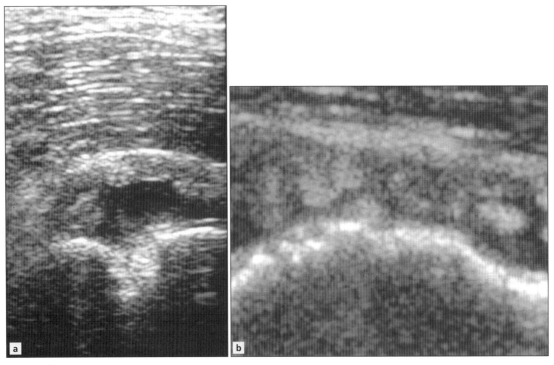

Fig. 5.2 (a) Echogenic synovial thickening is easily distinguished from anechoic fluid. (b) Echogenic pannus occupies the joint space: there is almost no synovial fluid.

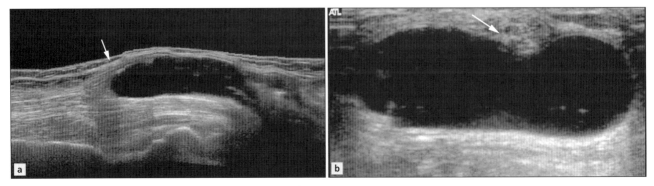

Fig. 5.3 (a) Longitudinal scan shows distal biceps tendon (arrow) elevated by bicipito-radial (cubital) bursa. (b) Transverse scan showing large cubital bursa deep to biceps tendon (arrow). (Both images courtesy of Dr Simon Ostlere.)

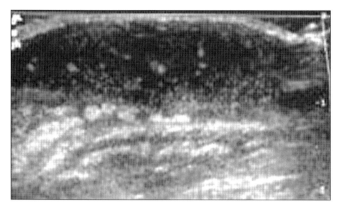

Fig. 5.4 Longitudinal scan of infected olecranon bursitis: the fluid contents are echogenic.

peripheral hyperaemia (9). The bursal wall may be thickened and irregular, especially in septic bursitis (3).

LOOSE BODIES

The elbow is the second most common site of loose bodies (10). They present with pain, locking or restricted movement. Removal restores function and prevents osteoarthritis. Most loose bodies are small. They are frequently undetectable on radiographs, even if calcified.

Practical tip

When the elbow is flexed to 90° there is a "soft spot" on the lateral aspect of the elbow that lies between the radial head, capitellum and proximal ulna and distant from the ulnar nerve. Injection of 12–15 ml of saline at this site is safe and produces an ultrasound arthrogram that shows otherwise occult loose bodies, increases conspicuity in equivocal cases and confirms if radiographic opacities are intra- or extra-articular.

In the presence of joint fluid, ultrasound shows an echogenic, intra-articular focus surrounded by fluid (11, 12) (Fig. 5.5) but in many cases the joint is dry (13). Injection of 12–15 ml of saline into the joint demonstrates loose bodies that are undetectable in dry joints, increases conspicuity in equivocal cases and confirms whether radiographic opacities are intra- or extra-articular (13). The injection (Fig. 5.6) is made with the elbow flexed to 90° and the hand pronated. In this position there is a "soft spot" on the lateral aspect of the elbow that lies between the radial head, capitellum and proximal ulna and distant

from other structures such as the ulnar nerve. After injecting local anaesthetic into the overlying skin and subcutaneous tissues it is easy to manipulate the needle into the soft spot perpendicular to the skin. The intra-articular position of the needle is confirmed when the local anaesthetic runs freely into the joint without discomfort. As joint distension is uncomfortable, no more than 15 ml should be injected in total and this should include some local anaesthetic (13). This approach can also be used to aspirate joint fluid for diagnostic purposes and to inject steroids.

The ultrasound examination should include the coronoid and olecranon fossae, deep to the collateral ligaments and around the radial head and annular ligament, all potential sites of loose bodies.

MRI and CT are alternative techniques for detecting loose bodies. Their accuracies are also increased when a joint effusion or intra-articular contrast is present (14, 15).

BICEPS RUPTURE

The distal tendon of the biceps brachii muscle is about 7 cm long and inserts on the medial aspect of the radial tuberosity. The lacertus fibrosus is an aponeurosis that extends from the musculotendinous junction to the medial deep fascia of the forearm and lies superficial to the brachial artery and median nerve (3). The biceps tendon can be difficult to see on sonographic examination because of the effect of anisotropy as it curves laterally and dives deeply to insert on the radial tuberosity (3, 9).

Rupture of the distal biceps tendon is uncommon and is usually due to attempting to lift a heavy weight. Complete rupture of the tendon usually produces an immediate popping sensation, pain and a clinically palpable defect and is not a diagnostic problem. However, if the aponeurosis remains intact and the muscle is not retracted or clinical examination is hampered by soft-tissue swelling, imaging may be required to confirm the diagnosis. Early surgery improves clinical outcome.

For ultrasound examination, the elbow should be slightly flexed and the forearm maximally supinated. Longitudinal scans require a slight inferolateral angulation while transverse scans should be perpendicular to the long axis of the

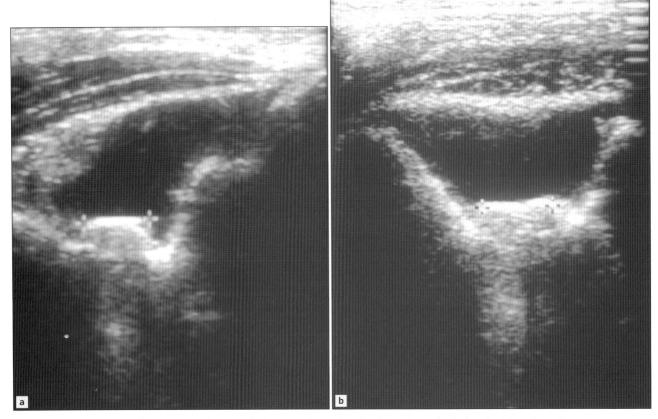

Fig. 5.5 Longitudinal (a) and transverse (b) scans of olecranon fossa showing large loose body (marked by calipers).

Technique

- Aseptic, LA, 19G needle
- Radio-capitellar joint
- 12–15 ml saline
- 7.5 and 13.5MHz

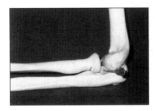

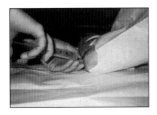

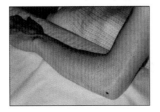

Fig. 5.6 Elbow injections are made at the palpable "soft spot" on the lateral aspect of the flexed elbow. The injection of saline should be stopped when the patient complains of discomfort. (Reprinted with permission from Miller JH, Beggs I. Detection of intraarticular bodies of the elbow with saline arthrosonography. Clin Radiol 2000;56:231–4.)

forearm but "heel-toed" into the interosseous space (16). Complete rupture of the tendon with muscle retraction produces a defect (Fig. 5.7) at the expected site of the tendon. The gap is filled with fluid or haematoma (Fig. 5.8) and the retracted tendon edge (Fig. 5.9) may be visible (3,

16). Retraction is greater when the aponeurosis is disrupted (3, 16). Longitudinal scans are probably most useful in demonstrating complete ruptures (16). A partial tear shows a thick, wavy, echogenic tendon that can be followed all the way to the radial tuberosity (16). The alterations in texture and thickness are seen on transverse and longitudinal scans but the wavy contour is appreciated only on longitudinal scans. It may not be possible to distinguish between a partial tear and tendinosis, which also produces tendon thickening, although a wavy contour suggests a partial tear (16).

Practical tip

Longitudinal scans of the biceps tendon require a slight inferolateral angulation while transverse scans should be perpendicular to the long axis of the forearm but "heel-toed" into the interosseous space.

The diagnosis of distal biceps tendon rupture may be obvious on ultrasound. However, the tendon is frequently difficult to see on ultrasound because of anisotropy. Despite claims about the accuracy of sonographic diagnosis of biceps

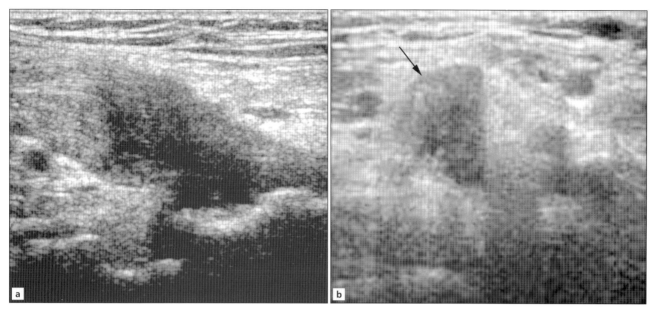

Fig. 5.7 Longitudinal (a) and transverse (b) scans of cubital fossa show fluid (arrow) at the site of the torn biceps tendon.

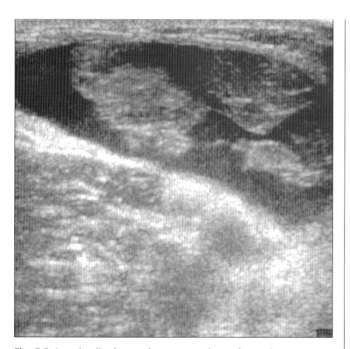

Fig. 5.8 Longitudinal scan shows extensive, echogenic haematoma at site of disrupted biceps tendon.

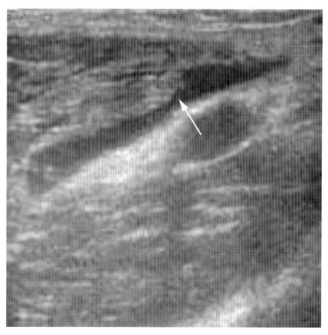

Fig. 5.9 Longitudinal scan shows retracted tendon edge (arrow).

tendon rupture (16, 17), if there is any doubt about the diagnosis, MRI should be used (3, 18, 19) and is probably the first choice investigation.

TRICEPS RUPTURE

The triceps tendon originates in the triceps muscle and inserts on the olecranon process.

Rupture usually results from a fall on an outstretched hand. A bone fragment may remain attached to the tendon. Ultrasound shows a wavy, retracted tendon surrounded by fluid (20). Due to the proximity of the tendon and the cubital tunnel, triceps rupture may cause acute ulnar nerve compression (21). Partial rupture produces a small fluid-filled defect or an hypoechoic segment (Fig. 5.10) in the tendon (9).

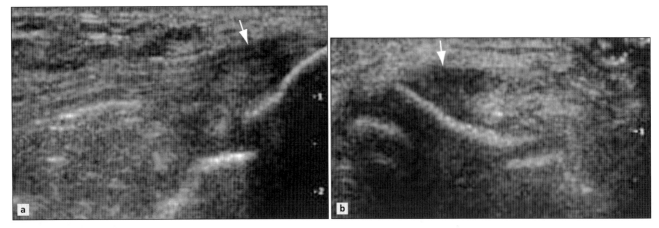

Fig. 5.10 Longitudinal (a) and transverse (b) scans of partial rupture of triceps tendon following hyperextension injury three days previously. The ruptured segment of tendon appears hypoechoic and swollen (arrows).

EPICONDYLITIS

The common extensor tendon originates from the anterolateral surface of the lateral humeral epicondyle and is beak-shaped. The individual components cannot be identified but the extensor carpi radialis brevis comprises most of the deep fibres and the extensor digitorum most of the superficial fibres. The extensor digiti minimi and carpi ulnaris contribute only small amounts to the common tendon (22).

Tennis elbow or lateral epicondylitis is thought to be due to repetitive microtrauma during supination of the forearm and dorsiflexion of the wrist (22) that results in breakdown of collagen fibres with the tissue necrosis and fibrosis (23). Cyclical damage and repair ensue (24). Inflammation is absent (25).

Predisposing causes include tennis, throwing activities and occupational trauma. Patients present with lateral elbow pain exacerbated by the underlying activity. The diagnosis is usually straightforward and most cases resolve with conservative management, including rest, physiotherapy, anti-inflammatories and steroid injections. Imaging is only needed in nonresponders.

Key point

Diagnosis of epicondylitis is usually straightforward and most cases resolve with conservative management, including rest, physiotherapy, anti-inflammatories and steroid injections. Imaging is only needed in nonresponders.

Ultrasound has shown that the deep fibres are predominantly involved and that few cases involve the superficial or posterior fibres. Focal hypoechoic areas superimposed on normal tendon may represent areas of focal degeneration (22). Diffuse reduction in echogenicity (Fig. 5.11a) with loss of the normal fibrillar architecture probably represents diffuse tendinopathy (22). Anechoic clefts represent partial or complete tears (5, 22). Tendon swelling, thickening of peritendinous tissues, foci of calcification (Fig. 5.11b) in the tendon, a bursa adjacent to the tendon and hyperostosis on the epicondyle may also be present (22, 26). Although colour and power Doppler ultrasound have been reported to show no abnormality (22), neovascularity may be present (Fig. 5.12). The radial collateral ligament lies immediately deep to the common extensor tendon and appears as a thin, echoic band. It is commonly thickened or partially or completely ruptured in severe cases of lateral epicondylitis (22, 27).

The common flexor tendon lies on the medial aspect of the elbow joint and arises from the medial epicondyle. It is shorter and thicker than the common extensor tendon. Medial epicondylitis or "golfer's elbow" is also the result of repeated microtrauma. The sonographic findings are virtually identical to those of lateral epicondylitis (28). There are no studies that assess US vs MRI in the diagnosis of epicondylitis. However, studies that compare operative findings with US or MRI suggest that they are of similar diagnostic accuracy (22, 27).

The ulnar collateral ligament is stronger than the radial collateral ligament and, like it, appears as a thin echogenic band. It may be injured

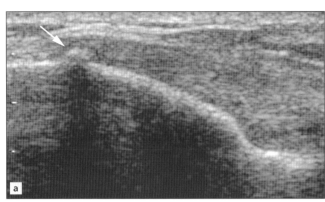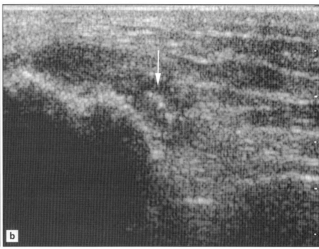

Fig. 5.11 Longitudinal scans of epicondylitis showing swollen, hypoechoic common tendon origin with arrowed hyperostosis (a) and intrasubstance calcification (b). (Both images courtesy of Dr Simon Ostlere.)

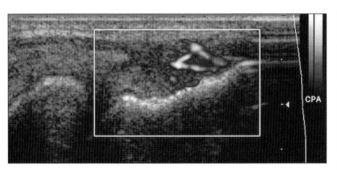

Fig. 5.12 Colour Doppler shows neovascularity at swollen common tendon origin. (Image courtesy of Dr Simon Ostlere.)

by repeated valgus stress or dislocation. Degeneration or tears of the ulnar collateral ligament can occur without injury to the overlying common flexor tendon (3). Ultrasound can demonstrate thickening and calcification in the injured ligament. Stress radiography has been used for the diagnosis of ulnar collateral ligament disruption, with a greater than 0.5 mm medial jointopening being suggestive of injury (29). The dynamic capability of ultrasound can reproduce this sign (30) and offers one advantage over MRI, which is an effective means of demonstrating UCL injuries.

ULNAR NERVE AND CUBITAL TUNNEL

The ulnar nerve runs in the cubital tunnel on the posterior aspect of the elbow. The boundaries of the cubital tunnel are the olecranon and the medial epicondyle and its roof is a fibrous band or retinaculum, Osborne's fascia (31). Small

footprint transducers provide the best delineation of the cubital tunnel; larger transducers need a stand-off (3). Entrapment of the ulnar nerve results in medial elbow pain and sensory or motor disturbance in the fourth and fifth fingers.

The normal ulnar nerve appears oval and speckled on transverse scans; it appears less echogenic than at other sites because of the effect of anisotropy as it curves round the elbow (3).

Key point

Transverse scans of the elbow during flexion demonstrate medial dislocation of the ulnar nerve in 20% of normal elbows, confirming previous clinical studies.

Transverse scans during flexion demonstrate medial dislocation of the ulnar nerve in 20% of normal elbows (32), confirming previous clinical studies (33). Repeated friction on dislocation may cause neuritis and functional deficit. Dislocation of the medial triceps muscle belly and ulnar nerve over the medial epicondyle on flexion can also be observed using ultrasound (34). Symptomatic ulnar dislocation results in swelling (Fig. 5.13) of the nerve (34, 35).

Ultrasound can also show compression of the ulnar nerve in the cubital tunnel by, for example, a thickened retinaculum, ganglion, anomalous anconeus muscle or bony spur. The nerve is narrowed at the level of compression and swollen proximally with loss of the normal fascicular pattern (36, 37).

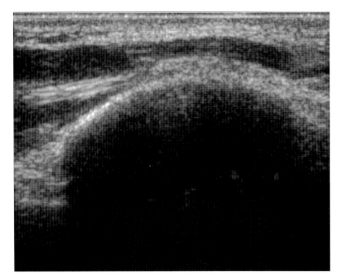

Fig. 5.13 Longitudinal scan of swollen and hypoechoic ulnar nerve.

CHILDREN

Ultrasound can be used in children to detect and assess fractures (38). A cortical break, haemarthrosis or displacement of bone or physis may be seen (38–41). Extension of fractures of the lateral condyle of the humerus through the articular cartilage indicates instability (42). In pulled elbow, when the radial head slips below the annular ligament, ultrasound shows a slight increase in the distance between the radial head and the capitellum (43).

> **Practical tip**
>
> In pulled elbow, when the radial head slips below the annular ligament, ultrasound shows a slight increase in the distance between the radial head and the capitellum.

Early osteochondritis dissecans results in flattening of the cortical bone. The margins of the bone fragment can be defined. The overlying articular cartilage remains intact (44). Unossified medial epicondyle avulsion can be difficult to diagnose in very young children. Ultrasound has been used to detect injury (45). The severity of the injury and any associated displacement may be assessed. In older children, occult injuries to the radial neck may create a diagnostic dilemma. These fractures are less common than supracondylar fractures but are difficult to assess in the immature skeleton on radiography

but relatively easy on ultrasound where a discontinuity at the proximal radial physis may be seen.

REFERENCES

1. De Maeseneer M, Jacobson JA, Jaovisidha S, Lenchik L, Ryu KN, Trudell DR, Resnick D. Elbow effusions: distribution of joint fluid with flexion and extension and imaging implications. Invest Radiol 1998;33:117–25.
2. Miles KA, Lamont AC. Ultrasonic demonstration of the elbow fat pads. Clin Radiol 1989;40:602–4.
3. Martinoli C, Bianchi S, Giovagnorio F, Pugliese F. Ultrasound of the elbow. Skeletal Radiol 2001;30:605–14.
4. Lim-Dunham JE, Ben-Ami TE, Yousefzadeh DK. Septic arthritis of the elbow in children: the role of sonography. Pediatr Radiol 1995;25:556–9.
5. Jacobson JA, van Holsbeeck MT. Musculoskeletal ultrasonography. Orthop Clin North Am 1998;29:135–67.
6. Steiner E, Steinbach LS, Scharkowski P, Tirman PFJ, Genant HK. Ganglia and cysts around joints. Radiol Clin North Am 1996;34:395–425.
7. Liessi G, Cesari S, Spaliviero B, Dell'Antonio C, Avventi P. The US, CT and MRI findings of cubital bursitis: a report of five cases. Skeletal Radiol 1996;25:471–5.
8. Spence LD, Adams J, Gibbons D, Mason MD, Eustace S. Rice body formation in bicipito-radial bursitis: ultrasound, CT and MRI findings. Skeletal Radiol 1998;27:30–2.
9. Lin J, Jacobson JA, Fessell DP, Weadock WJ, Hayes CW. An illustrated tutorial of musculoskeletal sonography: Part 2, upper extremity. Am J Roentgen 2000;175:1071–9.
10. Morrey BF. Loose bodies. In: Morrey BF, editor. The elbow and its disorders, 2nd ed. Philadelphia: WB Saunders; 1993:860–71.
11. Frankel DA, Bargiela A, Bouffard JA, Craig JG, Shirazi KK, van Holsbeeck MT. Synovial joints: evaluation of intraarticular bodies with US. Radiology 1998;206:41–4.
12. Bianchi S, Martinoli C. Detection of loose bodies in joints. Rad Clin N Am 1999; 37:679–90.
13. Miller JH, Beggs I. Detection of intraarticular bodies of the elbow with saline arthrosonography. Clin Radiol 2000;56:231–4.
14. Quinn SF, Haberman JJ, Fitzgerald SW, Traughber PD, Belkin RI, Murray WT. Evaluation of loose bodies in the elbow with MR imaging. J Magn Reson Imag 1994;4:169–72.
15. Brossmann J, Preidler K-W, Daenen B, Pedowitz RA, Andresen R, Clopton P, Trudell D, Pathria M, Resnick D. Imaging of osseous and cartilaginous bodies in the knee: Comparison of MR imaging and MR arthrography with CT and CT arthrography in cadavers. Radiology 1996;200:509–17.
16. Miller TT, Adler RS. Sonography of tears of the distal biceps tendon. Am J Roentgen 2000;175:1081–6.
17. Weiss C, Mittelmeier M, Gruber G. Do we need MR images for diagnosing tendon ruptures of the distal biceps brachii? The value of ultrasonographic imaging. Ultraschall Med 2000;21:284–6.
18. Falchook FS, Zlatkin MB, Erbacher GE, Moulton JS, Bisset GS, Murphy BJ. Rupture of the distal biceps tendon: evaluation with MR imaging. Radiology 1994;190:659–63.
19. Fitzgerald SW, Curry DR, Erickson SJ, Quinn SF, Friedman H. Distal biceps tendon injury: MR imaging diagnosis. Radiology 1994;191:203–6.
20. Kaempffe FA, Lerner RM. Ultrasound diagnosis of triceps tendon rupture: a report of 2 cases. Clin Orthop 1996;332:138–42.
21. Duchow J, Kelm J, Kohn D. Acute ulnar nerve compression syndrome in a powerlifter with triceps tendon rupture: a case report. Int J Sports Med 2000;21:308–10.

22. Connell D, Burke F, Coombes P, McNealy S, Freeman D, Pryde D, Hoy G. Sonographic examination of lateral epicondylitis. Am J Roentgen 2001;176:777–82.

23. Chard MD, Cawston TE, Riley GP, Gresham GA, Hazleman BL. Rotator cuff degeneration and lateral epicondylitis: a comparative histological study. Ann Rheum Dis 1994;53:30–4.

24. Nirschl RP, Perrone FA. Tennis elbow. The surgical treatment of lateral epicondylitis. J Bone Joint Surg Am 1979;61:832–9.

25. Regan W, Wold LE, Coonrad R, Morrey BF. Microscopic histopathology of chronic refractory lateral epicondylitis. Am J Sports Med 1992;20:746–9.

26. Maffulli N, Regine R, Carrillo F, Capasso G, Minelli S. Tennis elbow: an ultrasonographic study in tennis players. Br J Sports Med 1990;24:151–5.

27. Bredella MA, Tirman PFJ, Fritz RC, Feller JF, Wischer TK, Genant HK. MR imaging findings of lateral ulnar collateral ligament abnormalities in patients with lateral epicondylitis. Am J Roentgen 1999;173:1379–82.

28. Ferrara MA, Marcelis S. Ultrasound of the elbow. J Belge Radiol 1997;80:122–3.

29. Rijke AM, Goitz HT, McCue FC, Andrews JR, Berr SS. Stress radiography of the medial elbow ligaments. Radiology 1994;191:213–6.

30. De Smet AA, Winter TC, Best TM, Bernhardt DT. Dynamic sonography with valgus stress to assess elbow ulnar collateral ligament injury in baseball pitchers. Skeletal Radiol 2002;31:671–6.

31. O'Driscoll SW, Horii E, Carmichael SW, Morrey BF. The cubital tunnel and ulnar neuropathy. J Bone Joint Surg Br 1991;73:613–7.

32. Okamoto M, Abe M, Shirai H, Ueda N. Morphology and dynamics of the ulnar nerve in the cubital tunnel. Observations by ultrasonography. J Hand Surg (Br) 2000;25:85–9.

33. Childress HM. Recurrent ulnar-nerve dislocation at the elbow. Clin Orthop 1975;108:168–73.

34. Jacobson JA, Jebson PJL, Jeffers AW, Fessell DP, Hayes CW. Ulnar nerve dislocation and snapping triceps syndrome: diagnosis with dynamic sonography-report of three cases. Radiology 2001;220:601–5.

35. Chiou HJ, Chou YH, Cheng SP, Hsu CC, Chan RC, Tiu CM, Teng MM, Chang CY. Cubital tunnel syndrome: diagnosis by high-resolution ultrasonography. J Ultrasound Med 1998;17:643–8.

36. Okamoto M, Abe M, Shirai H, Ueda N. Diagnostic ultrasonography of the ulnar nerve in cubital tunnel syndrome. J Hand Surg (Br) 2000;25:499–502.

37. Martinoli C, Bianchi S, Gandolfo N, Valle M, Simonetti S, Derchi LE. US of nerve entrapments in osteofibrous tunnels of the upper and lower limbs. RadioGraphics 2000;20:S199–S217.

38. Markowitz RI, Davidson RS, Harty MP, Bellah RD, Hubbard AM, Rosenberg HK. Sonography of the elbow in infants and children. Am J Roentgen 1992;159:829–33.

39. Dias JJ, Lamont AC, Jones JM. Ultrasonic diagnosis of neonatal separation of the distal humeral epiphysis. J Bone Joint Surg Br 1988;70:825–8.

40. Davidson RS, Markowitz RI, Dormans J, Drummond DS. Ultrasonographic evaluation of the elbow in infants and young children after suspected trauma. J Bone Joint Surg Am 1994;76:1804–13.

41. Lazar RD, Waters PM, Jaramillo D. The use of ultrasonography in the diagnosis of occult fracture of the radial neck. A case report. J Bone Joint Surg Am 1998;80:1361–4.

42. Vocke-Hell AK, Schmid A. Sonographic differentiation of stable and unstable lateral condyle fractures of the humerus in children. J Pediatr Orthop B 2001;10:138–41.

43. Kosuwon W, Mahaisavariya B, Saengnipanthkul S, Laupattarakasem W, Jirawipoolwon P. Ultrasonography of pulled elbow. J Bone Joint Surg Br 1993;75:421–2.

44. Takahara M, Shundo M, Kondo M, Suzuki K, Nambu T, Ogino T. Early detection of osteochondritis dissecans of the capitellum in young baseball players. Report of three cases. J Bone Joint Surg Am 1998;80:892–7.

45. May DA, Disler DG, Jones EA, Pearce DA. Using sonography to diagnose an unossified medial epicondyle avulsion in a child. Am J Roentgen 2000;174:1115–7.

Ultrasound of the hand and wrist

6

Stefano Bianchi, Carlo Martinoli, Michel Cohen and Nathalie Boutry

The recent technical developments of ultrasound (US) equipment, particularly the increase in the transducers frequency and the decrease in the size of the probes, allow an accurate dynamic assessment of the small structures of the hand and wrist. The goals of this chapter are to describe the US pathological findings of the most common disorders of the hand and wrist. We will review the US appearance of rheumatoid arthritis and other inflammatory conditions, traumatic lesions, entrapment neuropathies and finally expansible lesions.

RHEUMATOID ARTHRITIS AND OTHER INFLAMMATORY DISORDERS

Rheumatoid arthritis (RA) is characterised by chronic synovitis, resulting in bone and cartilage damage. The diagnosis of RA is based on clinical, laboratory and radiological findings. So far, plain radiography was the mainstay for both diagnosis and monitoring of RA. Nevertheless, the first radiological changes, i.e. bone erosions, occur late in the disease process, from 6 to 24 months after symptom onset. Furthermore, conventional radiographs provide only indirect information about synovial inflammation. Recently, powerful and expensive new drugs, the so-called disease-modifying antirheumatic drugs (DMARDs), have been developed to prevent progression of joint destruction and long-term disability. Therefore, early detection of RA and identification of patients with aggressive disease as well as evaluation of therapeutic response are clearly required.

Magnetic resonance imaging (MRI) of the hand and wrist joints has been reported as the technique of choice for the detection of synovitis and bone erosions in patients with early RA (1, 2). MRI, however, is an expensive imaging modality for the evaluation of a common rheumatic disorder such as RA. In contrast, US allows low-cost imaging and is widely available. Furthermore, recent technological advances in musculoskeletal ultrasound, especially high frequency linear-array transducers in the 10- to 15-MHz range, have greatly improved the visualisation of superficial structures such as the small distal joints and

Rheumatoid arthritis and other inflammatory disorders

Synovitis
Bone erosions
Cartilage damage
Tenosynovitis and tendon rupture
Rheumatoid nodules
Differential diagnosis

Traumatic conditions

Bone trauma
Capsulo ligamentous lesions
Tendons disorders
Tears of the retinacula
Other lesions

Entrapment neuropathies

Carpal tunnel syndrome
Guyon tunnel syndrome.

Tumours and tumour-like lesions

General considerations, technique of examination and guidelines for US report
Ganglia
Giant tumour of tendon sheath
Lipomas
Pseudoaneurysms
Nerve tumours
Glomus tumours

Miscellaneous conditions

nowadays, US can exquisitely demonstrate early inflammatory changes such as synovitis, bone erosions and cartilage loss. Other abnormalities associated with RA (i.e. tenosynovitis, tendon rupture and rheumatoid nodules) can be detected with US.

Synovitis

Synovitis is the earliest change occurring in RA. It is characterised by proliferation of the synovial membrane (pannus) associated with synovial hyperaemia in active synovitis.

Pannus

Sonographic findings include joint cavity widening and synovial membrane thickening, with or without associated joint effusion. US helps to differentiate joint effusion from synovial proliferation. Joint effusion is anechoic, expelled from the region by compression with the transducer. Conversely, hypertrophic synovium is hypoechoic relative to the surrounding soft tissues and pressure from the transducer can deform it but not express it (Fig. 6.1). In metacarpo-phalangeal joints (MCP), the dorsal or the volar metacarpal synovial recesses appear enlarged and their proximal extremities are seen to bulge. Less frequently, synovitis can be associated with distension of the dorsal or volar phalangeal recesses (Fig. 6.2). Backhaus *et al.* (3) found US to be even more sensitive (53%) than MRI (41%) in the detection of synovitis in patients with early RA. It should be noted,

however, that these authors used a 7.5-MHz transducer.

Synovial hyperaemia

Colour or power Doppler US is valuable in distinguishing between hypervascular and fibrous pannus. In active synovitis, increased vascular flow is demonstrated throughout the pannus on colour or power Doppler images (Fig. 6.3). For optimal detection of synovial hyperaemia, standardisation and correct adjustment of Doppler settings such as the pulse repetition frequency (PRF), the colour gain and the flow optimisation parameters are major prerequisites. Usually, the colour gain is set just below the disappearance of noise artefacts from cortical bone, and machine settings are optimised

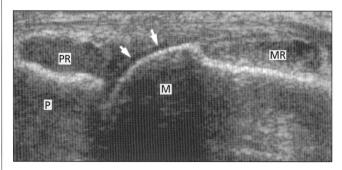

Fig. 6.2 Dorsal longitudinal sonogram of a MCP joint in a patient with early RA shows distension of metacarpal and phalangeal synovial recesses by synovial proliferations. Arrows indicate the cartilage of the metacarpal head as a thin, hypoechoic layer. P = phalangeal base, M = metacarpal head, PR = phalangeal synovial recess, MR = metacarpal synovial recess.

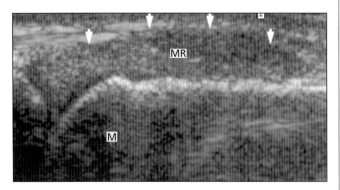

Fig. 6.1 Dorsal longitudinal sonogram of a MCP joint in a patient with early RA. Note the intra-articular synovial pannus appearing as a homogeneous hypoechoic structure widening the joint cavity (arrows). The cartilage of the metacarpal head and the bone surface appears normal without evidence of either cartilage thinning or bone erosions. M = metacarpal head, MR = metacarpal synovial recess.

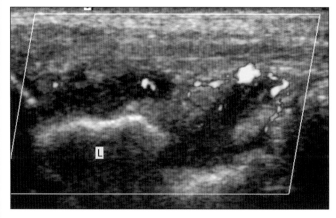

Fig. 6.3 Power Doppler longitudinal sonogram of the dorsal surface of the wrist in a patient with early RA shows synovitis. Note the anechoic fluid distension at the radiocarpal and midcarpal joint as well as the peripheral hypoechoic synovial pannus, which shows internal flow signals related to hypervascularity. L = lunate.

for detection of low-velocity blood flow. Synovial hyperaemia can be observed using either colour or power Doppler imaging, the latter being more sensitive to slow flow but also to motion artefacts. When spectral Doppler is used, the arterial perfusion of the pannus shows a persistent diastolic flow. However, in most studies, the visual assessment of hyperaemia is qualitative, which may result in interobserver variability. In the near future, the use of software programs dedicated to quantitative assessment of the synovial perfusion will probably reduce the subjective nature of US studies.

Schmidt *et al.* (4) and Walther *et al.* (5) have compared colour and power Doppler findings with histopathologic data of the synovial membrane from patients with osteoarthritis and RA of the knee, respectively. Doppler US was able to differentiate between nondestructive, noninflammatory synovial proliferation (in osteoarthritis) and destructive, inflammatory synovial proliferation or pannus (in RA). Furthermore, there was a significant correlation between the intensity of perfusion seen on Doppler images and the degree of vascularity seen histologically.

By using contrast-enhanced MRI as a reference method, Steuer *et al.* (6) and Szkudlarek *et al.* (7) showed that power Doppler US is reliable for assessing inflammatory activity in the MCP joints of RA patients. In Szkudlarek *et al.*'s study (7), power Doppler US had a sensitivity of 88.8% and a specificity of 97.9%.

Several authors (7–10) have investigated the relation between (colour/power) Doppler US findings and clinical data (number of tender and swollen joints). Most of them (8–10) found significant differences between finger joints with active RA and those with inactive RA with regard to the extent of the pannus and its vascularization. The erythrocyte sedimentation rate (ESR) also correlated with the vascularization of the synovial membrane. Conversely, in Szkudlarek *et al.*'s study (7), power Doppler US findings and clinical assessment of joint swelling and tenderness were weakly correlated.

Microbubble-based US contrast agents may be of value in the assessment of disease activity (10). Klauser *et al.* (10) found that contrast-enhanced colour Doppler US significantly improves the detection of intra-articular vascularization in the finger joints of patients with RA. The precise role

of US contrast agents in RA, however, is yet to be fully defined.

Doppler US has shown promise in the assessment of therapeutic response in patients with RA (11). A significant decrease in pannus vascularization is observed after treatment (steroid therapy or TNF-α), reflecting the improvement in terms of symptoms and disease activity variables (ESR, C-reactive protein).

Bone erosions

US can detect bone erosions of the finger joints in patients with early RA (12). Bone erosions appear as a cortical defect with irregular margins on longitudinal and transverse US scans (Fig. 6.4). In the wrist joints, the most common sites for erosions are lunate, triquetrum and capitate. Another common site for bony changes is the styloid process of the ulna. In MCP joints, the metacarpal heads are more frequently involved than the phalangeal bases. The radial aspect of

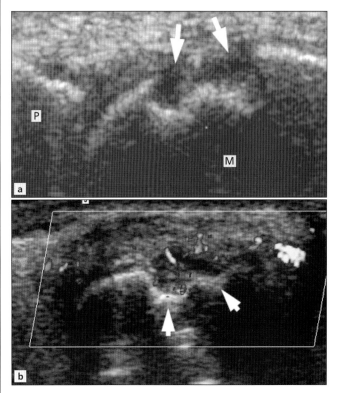

Fig. 6.4 (a) Longitudinal sonogram of the ulnar aspect of the fifth MCP joint in a patient with RA clearly depicts a large bilobated bone erosion filled by pannus (arrows). P = phalangeal base, M = metacarpal head. (b) Power Doppler longitudinal sonogram of the radial aspect of the second metacarpal head in a patient with RA shows synovial proliferations inside the articular space. Please note the hypervascular pannus filling two small bone erosions of the metacarpal head (arrows).

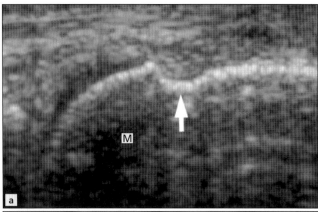

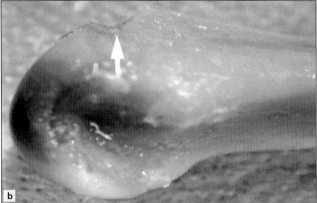

Fig. 6.5 (a) Dorsal longitudinal sonogram of the second MCP joint in a volunteer shows a pseudo-erosion (arrow). M = metacarpal head. (b) Corresponding anatomic inspection shows the metacarpal notch where the metacarpal synovial recess inserts (arrow).

the second metacarpal head is a key target of the erosive process.

Potential diagnostic pitfalls are due to "erosion-like" defects located on the dorsal side of the nonthumb metacarpal heads and on the ulnar side of the fifth metacarpal head (Fig. 6.5). Anatomic correlation demonstrates that they correspond to the bone notches where the metacarpal synovial recesses insert. Sonographically, these pseudo-erosions typically appear as well-defined bone defects on both longitudinal and transverse US scans with regular cortical margins. They are not found at the radial aspect of the metacarpal heads or at the phalangeal bases. Both location and their morphological features are helpful in distinguishing between anatomic variants and bone erosions.

From Wakefield *et al.*'s study (13), it emerges that US is superior to plain radiography in detecting bone erosions of finger joints affected by RA. In patients with early RA, US detected

6.5-fold more erosions than conventional radiographs did, in 7.5-fold the number of patients. In patients with late disease, these differences were 3.4- and 2.7-fold, respectively. Furthermore, intra- and interobserver reliability was good. In contrast, Backhaus *et al.* (3) did not find US to be better than radiography in detecting bone erosions; US had a sensitivity of 11% by comparison with radiography (16%) and MRI (43%) in patients with different inflammatory joint diseases, including RA. A transducer with a small surface area, such as a "hockey stick" transducer, can be advantageous when the finger joints are evaluated, because it allows better visualisation of different aspects of the joints. However, it should be noted that US is limited in evaluation of wrist joints.

Cartilage damage

US can provide reliable, albeit incomplete information about articular cartilage integrity. To date, however, little information is available on US imaging findings in patients with early RA. In the wrist joints, US evaluation of the cartilage is limited. In contrast, the hyaline cartilage of the metacarpal heads is well seen on US images. It can be explored on either the dorsal side or the volar side. A mild palmar flexion (15°) helps to demonstrate the dorsal aspect of the cartilage. The phalangeal cartilage cannot be identified with US imaging. In our experience, the mean thickness of the metacarpal head cartilage is 0.8 mm (range, 0.4–1.4 mm).

In the MCP joints, US pathological changes include irregularity of the normally smooth cartilage surface and cartilage thinning. Loss of definition of the cartilaginous layer and loss of the normal, hyperechoic linear reflection between the joint cavity and the cartilage are the earliest changes to occur in cartilage damage (Fig. 6.6).

Tenosynovitis and tendon rupture

Tenosynovitis, inflammation of the synovial lining of the tendon sheaths, is a common finding in an RA hand. Hand and wrist might be involved in up to 64 to 95% of patients with this condition. The extensor carpi radialis, the extensor digitorum, the extensor carpi ulnaris and the flexor digitorum tendons are frequently involved (Fig. 6.7).

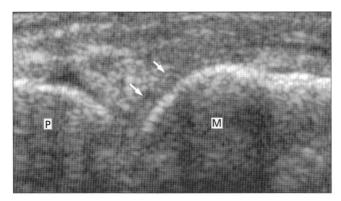

Fig. 6.6 Dorsal longitudinal sonogram of the second MCP joint in a patient with early RA shows loss of cartilage–joint cavity interface and indistinctness of the cartilage margins (arrows). P = phalangeal base, M = metacarpal head.

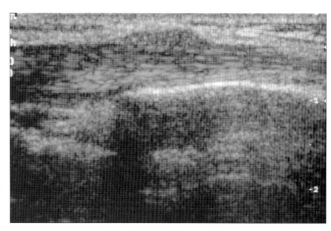

Fig. 6.8 Sagittal sonogram of de Quervain's sclerosing tenosynovitis. (Note focal reflective thickening of tendon sheath).

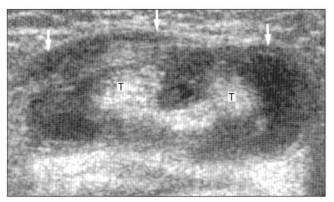

Fig. 6.7 Transverse sonogram of the second extensor compartment of the wrist in a patient with early RA shows tenosynovitis. Note the distension (arrows) of the tendon sheath with synovial proliferation and to a lesser degree by effusion. T = extensor carpi radialis tendons.

At sonography, distension of the tendon sheath with fluid (exudative tenosynovitis), hypoechoic synovial proliferation (proliferative tenosynovitis) or both may be evident. Hyperaemic changes also can be seen with Doppler sonography in the tendon sheath. The tendon itself is usually normal in echotexture. Indeed, partial and eventually complete tendon tears occur in advanced RA. However, high-frequency US is a sensitive method for detecting subtle intrinsic tendon abnormalities such as loss of the normal fibrillar echotexture or blurring of the tendon margins. Sclerosing (de Quervain's) tenosynovitis differs from the more common variants in that there is often less fluid and more tenosynovial thickening. Classicially this entety affects the first extensor compartment (Fig. 6.8).

Rheumatoid nodules

Rheumatoid nodules usually occur in RA patients with positive rheumatoid factor tests. They are found in 17% of patients in the finger tendons, only in flexor tendons (14). Sonographically, rheumatoid nodules typically appear as small (<1 cm), oval shaped, well-defined, hypoechoic nodules (14). They may be located centrally within the substance of the tendon itself, eccentrically attached to the tendon margin or may develop in subcutaneous tissues.

Differential diagnosis

Unfortunately, the US findings do not define specific types of arthritis. However, dactylitis or "sausage-shaped" finger is a classical feature of seronegative spondyloarthropathies, including psoriatic arthritis. It causes a diffusely swollen digit. The predominant US feature is the presence of flexor tenosynovitis, in up to 94 to 100% of patients (15, 16). Other US findings include tendon thickening, intra-articular synovitis and extensor tenosynovitis. Patients with seronegative spondyloarthropathy have evidence of flexor tenosynovitis without extensor tenosynovitis and synovitis (15). In patients with psoriatic dactylitis, synovitis can be seen in 52% of digits. Other typical manifestations of psoriatic dactylitis are distal interphalangeal (DIP) joint involvement and subcutaneous soft-tissue enlargement. Finally, it seems that US has some limitations in detecting periostitis (16).

In conclusion, US has opened up new horizons in the early recognition of inflammatory joint diseases, especially RA. Sonographic examination of the MCP joints is extremely valuable in detecting synovitis, tenosynovitis and bone erosions before the latter become evident with conventional radiography. By using Doppler sonography with or without sonographic contrast enhancement, it may be possible to monitor disease activity and, therefore, to assess therapeutic response. Also, US can be used to monitor needle position during steroid injections into the joints or tendon sheaths. However, whether MRI or US will have a greater role in the management of patients with early inflammatory arthritis, including RA, remains to be determined.

TRAUMATIC CONDITIONS

Traumatic lesions of the wrist and hand are common and can follow home, professional or sport injuries. A variety of anatomic structures, including bones, joints, muscles and tendons, can be injured. Although differentiation between major or minor lesions relies basically on the clinical examination, imaging modalities have medico-legal value and often play a definite role when physical examination is difficult or nonconcluding (children injuries, presence of multiple lesions or sharp pain limiting an accurate examination, etc). Both MRI and US can evaluate hand and wrist soft tissues. Nevertheless high-resolution US has the advantage of readiness and easy performing. Two factors affect the diagnostic accuracy when performing a US investigation: a good knowledge of the normal US anatomy and of pathological changes and availability of high-quality equipment.

Bone trauma

Key point

Standard radiographs are the mainstay of imaging of all bony trauma and ultrasound, if indicated, must be performed always after X-rays.

Standard radiographs are the mainstay of imaging of all bony trauma and US, if indicated, must be performed always after X-rays. In about 20–25% of patients with a scaphoid fracture the initial radiographs are negative and can lead to

a delayed diagnosis. US has been shown to be able to detect occult bone fractures such as ribs, scaphoid and metatarsal (stress) fractures. The US criteria for the diagnosis of a scaphoid fracture were first based on the increase in the distance between the scaphoid cortex and the radial artery. More recent studies have underlined the usefulness of direct, more reliable, signs such as a break in the hyperechoic line representing the cortex and local haematoma (17). Ultrasound has the advantage over plain radiography in demonstrating cortical breaks and even steps not visible on radiographs if the fracture is not tangential to the beam (Fig. 6.9). Concerning the role of US in the evaluation of scaphoid fractures some points need to be stressed:

- Every effort must be made to obtain good-quality radiographs realised in the proper positions (AP, AP with the fist clenched, AP with medial deviation, strict lateral view).
- If the patient's symptoms persist, another radiograph obtained after two weeks may show the fracture.
- A focal US irregularity of the cortex can represent the normal outline of the scaphoid tuberosity (Fig. 6.10).
- At US a step in the cortex and/or of a local joint effusion are good indicators of a scaphoid lesion. Associated US signs of haemarthroses can suggest CT or MRI for further evaluation.

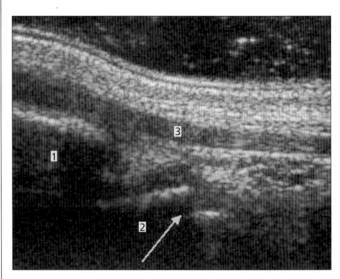

Fig. 6.9 Lateral longitudinal sonogram obtained at the level of the radial styloid (1), external aspect of the scaphoid (2) and extensor pollicis brevis tendon (3). Arrow points to focal interruption of the scaphoid cortex that was not seen in standard radiographs. CT confirmed a fracture of the scaphoid.

US can also detect complications of fractures. In patients with fractures of the distal ephyphisis of the radius or ulna, secondary changes such as tendon, muscle or nervous tears and haematomas, due to local friction related to a callus, can be demonstrated (Fig. 6.11).

Capsulo ligamentous lesions

Wrist

Recently three ligaments have retained the attention of sonologists: the scapholunate and lunotriquetral ligaments and the triangular fibrocartilage complex ligament (TFCC). The TFFC can be assessed by coronal images obtained at the ulnar aspect of the wrist (18). It appears as a triangular structure with the point directed laterally, which presents a mixed echogenicity (Fig. 6.12). Due to its protected position, a traumatic lesion is difficult to detect by US. Moreover we have found accurate measurement of the thickness of the triangular fibrocartilage difficult to obtain. The scapholunate and lunotriquetral ligaments can be examined by axial sonograms obtained with the wrist slightly flexed. The dorsal portion of the scapholunate ligament is almost always detectable as a tick hyperechoic band joining the dorsal scaphoid and the lunate (Fig. 6.13). Dynamic scanning during ulnar and radial deviation does not affect the distance between the two bones (19). Diastasis between the two carpal bones can be affirmed by comparison with the contralateral wrist. We believe that a definite diagnosis of a complete tear can be done only if demonstration of the torn fragments is evident and if unilateral diastasis is found, although this finding may not be present immediately following injury. In conclusion, although US can show the dorsal aspect of the normal scapholunate ligament its place in the work-up of a possible tear is not still determinate, and CT- and MR-arthrography remain the most performing diagnostic tools.

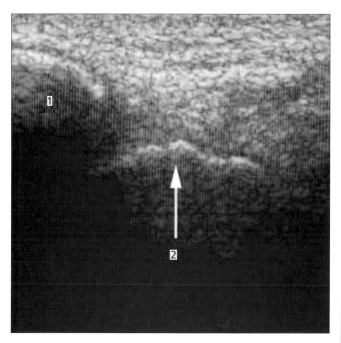

Fig. 6.10 Lateral longitudinal sonogram obtained at the level of the radial styloid (1), external aspect of the scaphoid (2). Arrow points to the scaphoid tuberosity.

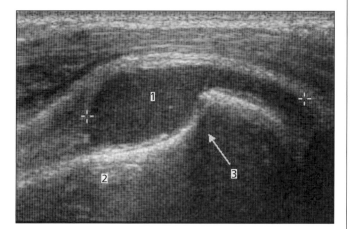

Fig. 6.11 Longitudinal sonogram obtained at the level of the palmar aspect of the radius. A haematoma (1) secondary to exuberant callus formation (3) after a fracture of the distal radius (2) is evident as a hypoanechoic fluid collection located between the radius and the muscle plane.

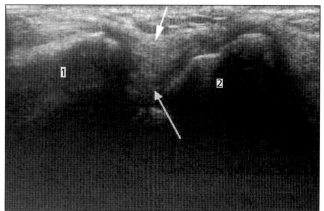

Fig. 6.12 Longitudinal coronal sonogram obtained at the level of the ulnocarpal joint. Between the ulnar head (1) and the triquetrum (2), the triangular fibrocartilage complex ligament appears as a triangular structure with a mixed echogenicity (arrows).

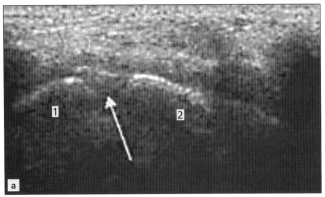

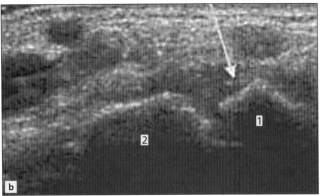

Fig. 6.13 (a) Axial dorsal sonogram obtained over a normal scapholunate ligament. The dorsal portion of the ligament appears as a homogeneous hyperechoic band (arrow) joining the scaphoid (1) and the lunate (2). (b) Axial dorsal sonogram obtained at the same level as that in (a) in a patient who sustained a local injury. Please note the irregular hypoechoic area found at the place of the ligament, which is not still visible. Scaphoid (1), lunate (2).

> **Practical tip**
>
> Due to the protected position of the wrist triangular fibrocartilage, accurate measurement of its thickness and detection of traumatic lesion are difficult to detect by US.

Hand

US of the hand ligaments must be performed with small, high-frequency transducers since capsulo-ligamentous structures are very superficial. MCP and interphalangeal (IP) joints are prone to sprains. There are normally two collateral ligaments, the radial and the ulnar, that limit excursion in the frontal plane. A palmar fibrocartilagineous plaque limits hyperextension. In addition, periarticular tendons seem to play a role in joint stabilisation. Although US can detect the main joint ligaments, others structures such as the lateral bands of the MCP joints are not visible due to their small size.

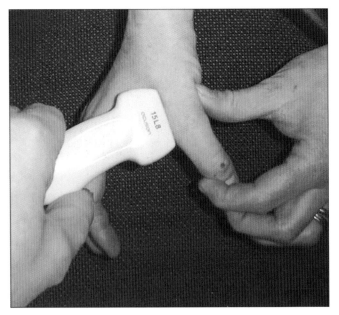

Fig. 6.14 Recommended position of the probe and thumb for longitudinal examination during flexion and cautious valgus stress.

Sprains of the MCP joint of the thumb can be frequently observed after sport injuries as in sky, baseball and contact sports. The most common mechanism is an excessive flexion and valgus stress that leads to distal tear of the ulnar collateral ligament. Standard radiographs must be always obtained to rule out a cortical avulsion of the base of the proximal phalanx. In the case of a Stener lesion (interposition of the adductor aponeurosis between the proximally retracted end of the torn ligament and the distal one), a surgical procedure to avoid decrease in the strength of the thumb pinch that can have severe functional consequences is warranted. US examination must be performed by axial and longitudinal images obtained at rest and during flexion and cautious valgus stress (Fig. 6.14). Differentiation of a sesamoid from a cortical avulsion is easily obtained by demonstration of rounded regular appearance of the sesamoid and by careful interpretation of the standard radiographs. In Stener lesions, the retracted ligament appears as a hypoechoic nodular structure (Figs 6.15a and 6.15b). Axial images obtained at the level of the metacarpal head are very useful in the detection of the displaced ligament. Tears of the radial collateral ligament are by far less common and can be associated with a Stener-like lesion due to interposition of the abductor pollicis aponeurosis. Assessment of

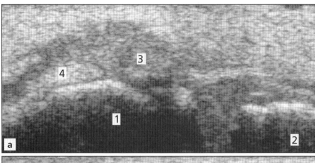

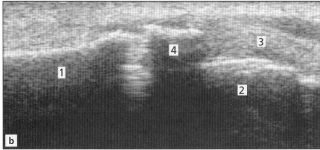

Fig. 6.15 (a) Longitudinal sonogram obtained over the ulnar aspect of the MCP joint of the thumb in a patient with a Stener lesion. The retracted proximal end of the ulnar collateral ligament appears as a hypoechoic mass located at the level of the metacarpal head (3). Aponeurosis of the adductor pollicis (4), metacarpal head (1), proximal phalanx (2). (b) Longitudinal sonogram obtained over the ulnar aspect of the MCP joint of the thumb in a patient with a ligament avulsion. Proximal phalanx (1), metacarpal head (2), normal ulnar collateral ligament (3), cortical avulsion (4).

the collateral ligaments of other MCP joints is difficult due to difficulty to obtain sonograms in the coronal plane. Only the radial collateral ligament of the second MCP and the ulnar collateral ligament of the fifth MCP can be accurately assessed.

> **Practical tip**
>
> US examination of sprains of the MCP joint of the thumb must be performed by axial and longitudinal images obtained at rest and during flexion and cautious valgus stress.

Traumatic lesions of the palmar plate result from hyperextension injuries. At the thumb two possible lesions can be found. Dislocation of the first phalanx with proximal tears of the palmar plate and of the metacarpo glenoid ligament. In more severe sprains rupture of the palmar plate, the metacarpo glenoid ligament as well as of the flexor pollicis brevis can be seen. These traumas deserve high-quality radiographs to detect the position of the bones (particularly sesamoids)

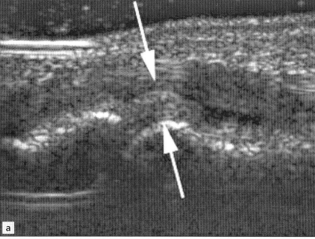

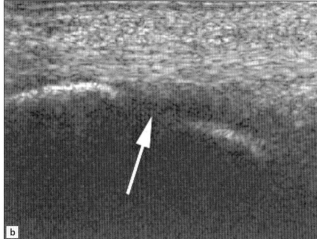

Fig. 6.16 (a) Longitudinal sonogram obtained on the palmar aspect of the proximal interphalangeal joint. Between the arrows is the normal palmar plate. (b) Longitudinal sonogram obtained on the palmar aspect of the proximal interphalangeal joint in a patient with a tear of the palmar plate (arrow).

and cortical chip fractures. US can evaluate palmar plate tears and can localise their site, distal vs proximal, which may have therapeutic consequences since distal lesions are followed by joint instability (Fig. 6.16).

In the sprains of the proximal interphalangeal joints radiographs can show a cortical avulsion, usually at the palmar aspect of the base of the middle phalanx. Torn collateral ligaments appear as hypoechoic and irregular and are associated with a synovial effusion in acute patients.

Tendons disorders

Tendons tears

Flexor tendons. They can tear following a direct or nondirect trauma. Clinical examination usually

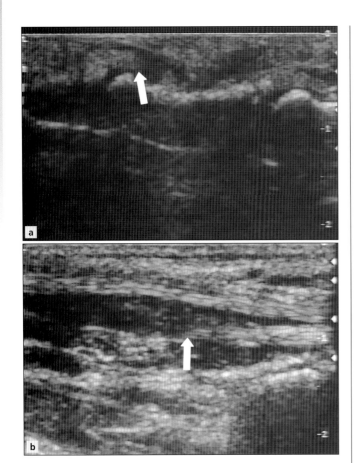

Fig. 6.17 (a) Sagittal sonogram of rupture of distal attachment of flexor digitorum profundus. (b) The ruptured tendon has retracted to the mid-palm.

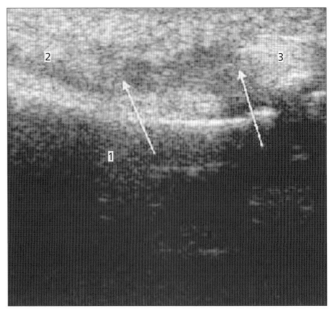

Fig. 6.18 Longitudinal sonogram obtained over the flexor digitorum profundus tendon of the second finger. Middle phalanx (1), retracted tendon (2), distal fibres of the torn tendon (3), fibrous tissue that fills the tendon sheath as a tendon remnant (between arrows). Note the absence of the typical fibrillar echotexture.

allows a definite diagnosis of complete tear. US can be useful in showing the exact site of the tear as well as the retraction of tendon ends. The commonest site of rupture, apart from penetrating trauma, is of the profundus tendon just proximal to its insertion (Fig. 6.17). In a complete tear US shows a complete interruption of tendon fibres and absence of tendon movement at dynamic examination. Attention must be made to avoid mistaking the fibrous tissue that fills the tendon sheath as a tendon remnant (Fig. 6.18). Absence of the typical fibrillar echotexture can help in that differentiation. Proximal scanning shows the retracted tendon, which appears swollen, and irregularly hypoechoic (Fig. 6.19a). Partial tears are more difficult to evaluate and appear as focal hypoechoic areas inside the tendon (Fig. 6.19b). MRI seems to be more accurate in the diagnosis of partial tears.

Extensor tendons. Tears of the extensor tendons at the wrist often result from rheumatoid tenosynovitis. The most commonly affected tendons are the extensor pollicis longus and the extensor digiti minimi, mainly because of their small size and frictions against bone protuberances (Lister tubercle and ulnar head, respectively). Finger extensor tendons are part of the extensor mechanism made by the tendons and the sagittal aponeurosis. MRI allows a better assessment of these tendons and moreover it can depict the paratendinous bands, which are ligamentous bands between the palmar plate and the extensor tendon at the level of the metacarpal head, only shown on axial imaging as well as other joint structures. Distal avulsion of the extensor tendon can be easily detected by US.

Postsurgical appearance. In the postsurgical assessment imaging is required basically in three circumstances:

- Assessment of the healing callus: US is useful in the subacute cases by showing the intratendineous echotexture.
- Clinical suspicion of a new tear.
- Assessment of adherences: although no studies have been published concerning this

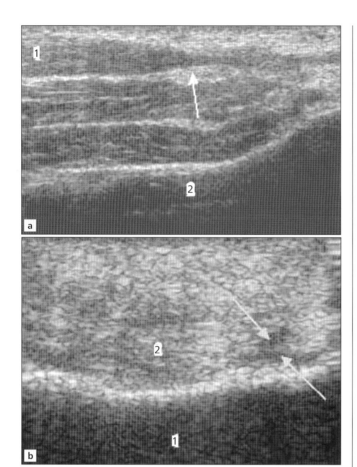

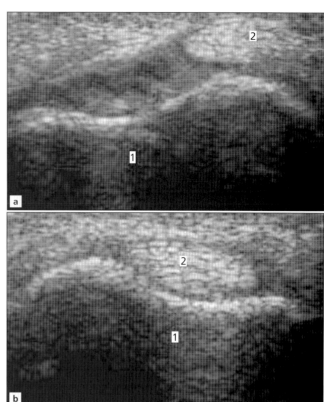

Fig. 6.20 Axial sonogram over the sixth extensor compartment. In (a) the extensor carpi ulnaris (ECU) tendon is dislocated laterally over the dorsal face of the ulna (2). Note the empty groove (1). (b) Contralateral axial sonogram shows the ECU resting within the groove.

Fig. 6.19 Tendon tears. (a) Longitudinal sonogram obtained over the FCR tendon shows a retracted hypoechoic irregular tendon (1) and the complete interruption of the tendon fibres (arrow). Distal radius (2). (b) Longitudinal sonogram obtained over the palmar aspect of the middle phalanx of the second finger shows a focal area (arrows) due to a partial tear of the flexor digitorum profundus tendon. Middle phalanx (1), flexor tendons (2).

topic we believe that US has diagnostic value by demonstrating thickening of the synovial sheath and impingement at the level of the digital pulleys. In addition dynamic examination shows movements of the peritendineous structures during tendon gliding.

Tears of the retinacula

In the majority of cases, tendons do not tear even after a powerful traction, whereas the ligamentous structures that retain them in the proper position (retinacula) can disrupt, leading to tendon instability.

Tears of the extensor carpi ulnaris retinaculum can be observed in sport injuries (tennis) and can be seen in patients suffering from tendinitis or

as an isolated lesion. US can demonstrate the dislocated tendon that can be found medially, close to the extensor digitorum minimi or medial to the ulnar head. Scanning of the fibroosseous compartment shows the empty groove (Fig. 6.20). In subluxation US can demonstrate the relation of the groove and the partially dislocated tendon. In intermittent subluxation the tendon is normally positioned at rest and subluxes during flexion and extension of the wrist. Dynamic US can easily demonstrate during real-time scanning the changes in tendon position that occur with different wrist positions.

Tears of a lateral band of the dorsal aspect of the MCP joint (dorsal sling) can occur following direct trauma, usually following a punch, or be found as the result of chronic local inflammation (as in rheumatoid arthritis). In both circumstances the extensor tendon dislocates in the intermetatarsal space. Attention must be paid during the US examination to both the flexion and extension of the MCP joint since the tendon dislocation, well evident in flexion, can be spontaneously reduced during extension. Performing the examination of the extensor tendons in the routine position (hands resting with the palm on the examination table) can lead to a nondiagnostic examination.

> **Practical tip**
>
> A dynamic examination is necessary to exclude dorsal sling injuries as the extensor tendon may be reduced in extension and displace only in flexion.

Pulley injuries

Two types of pulleys are identified in the fingers. The annular pulleys (A1–A5) form the anterior portion of the osteofibrous digital tunnels in which flexor digitorum tendons are retained. The cruciform pulleys (C1–C3) span from side to side across the volar margin of the phalanges. The annular pulleys prevent palmar tendon dislocation and allow an optimal function of the digits. Functionally, the most important are the A2 which lie in the proximal third of the proximal phalanx and the A4 which cross the middle phalanx. Under normal conditions US demonstration of the A2 DP depends mainly on the quality of the transducer. In sagittal images it appears as a thin hyperechoic line found anteriorly to the flexor tendons at the level of the proximal and middle third of the first phalanx. Ruptures of DP are usually observed at the third and fourth fingers in sports in which strength is applied on flexor tendons (rock climbing, windsurfing) or as a result of a trivial accident (20, 21). US can diagnose DP tears by showing the anterior displacement of the flexor tendons (bowstringing) that are no more retained against the anterior cortex of the phalanx (Fig. 6.21). The most commonly affected pulleys are the A2 and A4 with possible associated involvement of the A3. In forced flexion, the distance between the flexor tendon and underlying phalanx increases if pulley rupture is present. For A2 pulley rupture, a distance of less than 3 mm indicating incomplete rupture with measurements greater than three confirming a complete A2 pulley rupture. The tendon phalanx gap above 5 mm indicates a combined rupture of the A2 and A3 pulleys. Displacement of the tendons following an A4 pulley rupture is less obvious with the

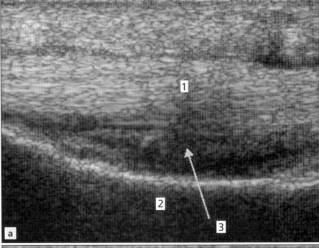

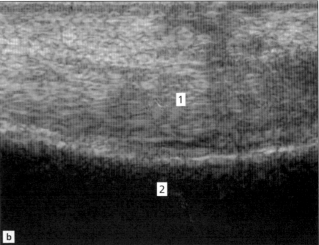

Fig. 6.21 (a) Palmar longitudinal sonogram over the proximal phalanx of the fourth finger. Note the bowstringing of the flexor tendons (1), which are not retained against the bone cortex (2). An effusion inside the tendon sheath appears as a hypoechoic area surrounding the tendon (3). These findings are typical for a complete tear of the A2 digital pulley. (b) Contralateral corresponding sonogram shows the flexor tendons (1) retained against the proximal phalanx (2).

measurement of 2.5 mm indicating a complete rupture. Although many of these lesions are clinically obvious, pain and soft tissue swelling may limit accurate clinical assessment. Furthermore, when injury is confined to a single pulley, the degree of bowstringing may be less clinically obvious. With pulley rupture, usually the bowstringing can be detected at static US performed with the finger extended. Images obtained during resisted flexion show an increase in the bowstringing. Evaluation of the distal A4 DP is more difficult since it must be performed with the finger flexed. Both CT and MRI can detect tendons bowstringing but since DP lesions are usually not associated with other traumatic lesions, we believe that US remains the technique of choice in their evaluation.Tenosynovitis is an important differential diagnosis which can be difficult to distinguish clinically. If these lesions are treated conservatively chronic fibrous tissue can interpose between the tendon and underlying phalanx and result in flexion deformity. Isolated A2 pulley injuries can be treated conservatively but when combined with an A3 injury surgery is recommended.

Collateral ligament injuries in the MCP joints are uncommon. The index finger is the most commonly involved followed by the fifth finger. Radial-sided lesions are significantly more common than ulnar-sided. In the fifth finger displacement of the torn ulnar ligament over the dorsal sling may occur simulating a Stener lesion. Collateral ligament defects are also identified in degenerate joints.

Other lesions

Subcutaneous and muscle haematoma appear on US as fluid collections. A post-traumatic intra-articular effusion can be easily detected in every joint of the hand and wrist by US as a collection filling the joint space and the articular synovial recesses. Abscesses follow penetrating injuries are demonstrated as heterogeneous masses with irregular borders and surrounding hyperaemia. Infective tenosynovitis leads to evident swelling of the thickened sheath by echogenic material, irregular thickening of the tendons and associated contour irregularity. Correlation with the clinical findings can easily lead to a diagnosis of tendon sheath infection.

Foreign bodies (FB) commonly follow open wounds and can be overlooked at the initial clinical evaluation (22). When a FB is suspected, the first imaging modality to be obtained is a standard radiograph since many FB are radioopaque (e.g., metallic fragments). If the radiographs are negative, US can be deployed to detect radiolucent fragments (vegetable and plastic fragments) (Fig. 6.22). US can detect the fragment as a hyperechoic structure with a variable posterior artefact (posterior shadowing or comet-tail artefact), depending on its surface; evaluate its size and relation to adjacent anatomic structures (nerves, vessels); and place a skin mark or eventually allow a US-guided removal.

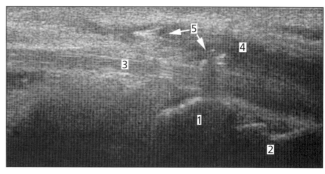

Fig. 6.22 Palmar longitudinal sonogram of the wrist of a patient who sustained a previous (six months) open wound of the left wrist. Normal appearance of the lunate (1), capitate (2) and flexor tendons (3). In a more superficial location, some hyperechoic structures, showing posterior shadowing and surrounded by an ill-defined hypoechoic area, are noted. At surgery several small glass fragments embedded in a perilesional inflammatory area were found.

Differential diagnosis includes granulation or post-traumatic fibrous tissue that appear as focal hyperechoic spots without a definite posterior artefact. Post-traumatic air bubbles in the soft tissue can simulate FB as well. In subacute or chronic cases an inflammatory reaction surrounding the fragment can be detected as a hypoechoic halo. Abscesses caused by a FB have the appearance previously described. Often the hyperechoic fragment can be found inside the abscess.

> **Practical tip**
>
> Ultrasound can detect a foreign body as a hyperechoic structure with a variable posterior artefact (posterior shadowing or comet-tail artefact), depending on its surface; evaluate its size and relation to adjacent anatomic structures (nerves, vessels); and place a skin mark or eventually allow US-guided removal.

ENTRAPMENT NEUROPATHIES

Entrapment neuropathies (EN) refer to disorders in which a nerve undergoes chronic pressure, and secondary dysfunction, by repetitive microtrauma inside a fibrous, osseous or fibroossseus tunnel. The most common ENs of the wrist are the carpal tunnel syndrome (CTS) and Guyon tunnel syndrome.

Carpal tunnel syndrome

The carpal tunnel (CT) is formed posteriorly by the carpal bones and anteriorly by the transverse carpal ligament (TCL), which insert in the scaphoid and trapezium on the radial aspect and into the pisiform and hook of the hamate at the ulnar side. The CT contains eight tendons and the median nerve (MN), which lies just deep to the TCL. Any conditions leading to a local increase in the pressure within the tunnel can lead to compression of the nerve, which, if chronic, results in sensory and motor changes. Regardless of the cause of compression, the MN undergoes morphological changes beginning with oedema and leading ultimately to fibrosis.

The US changes in CTS have been extensively described and can be divided into changes affecting the MN, the retinaculum and the content of the tunnel (23).

MN changes

Size. In CTS, the MN is typically swollen at the proximal portion of the CT and flattened at the distal end. A cross-section area of more than 10 mm^2 is believed to be diagnostic of CTS. Distal flattening of the nerve (evaluated with the flattening ratio that is between the LL and the AP diameter) was also found to be consistent with the diagnosis (Figs 6.23 and 6.24).

MN appearance. The overall echogenicity appears decreased and the internal normal fascicular pattern, due to the internal nervous fascicles, can be less evident. Colour Doppler can show an increase in the flow inside the nerve in more severe cases (Fig. 6.25).

TCL (Flexor retinaculum) changes

The most common finding is volar bulging of the retinaculum, which is secondary to increases in the intracanal pressure. Bulging must be assessed at the distal end of the carpal tunnel. At this level a line joining the tip of the hook of the hamate and the tubercle of the trapezium is made. The largest distance from the retinaculum to the line is measured and reflects the bulging. A value of more then 4 mm is considered abnormal.

Internal content of the CT

The most common cause of CTS is tenosynovitis of the flexor tendons. US detects inflammatory

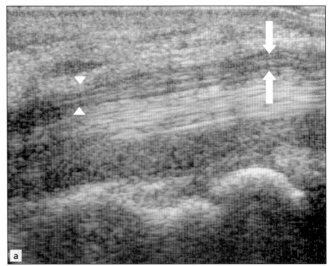

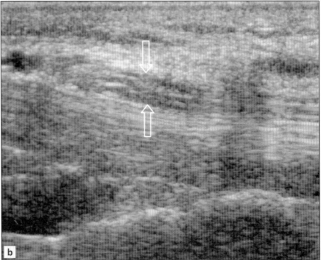

Fig. 6.23 Palmar longitudinal proximal (a) and distal (b) sonograms of a patient presenting with a clinical diagnosis of carpal tunnel syndrome. US shows the median nerve appears swollen proximal to the carpal tunnel (arrows) and distal to it (open arrows). Inside the carpal tunnel the nerve appears thinned (arrowheads).

changes of the tendon sheath as a hypoechoic halo surrounding the tendons, which appear more distinct (Fig. 6.26). Rarely a fluid effusion inside the sheath appears as an anechoic collection. Colour Doppler signals depend on the amount of the hypertrophic pannus and by its biological activity. Acquired focal expansible lesions within the CT can be easily detected. Ganglia are the commonest and present a typical appearance of polycyclic anechoic masses without internal vascular signals. Other solid masses could be a giant cell tumour of the tendon sheath or amyloidal deposit. A congenital lesion can result in compression of the MN. A thrombosed median artery has been described as a cause of CTS. Additionally anomalous

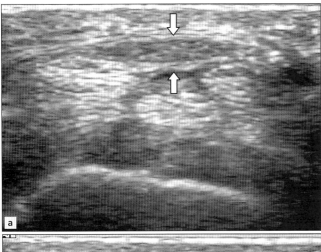

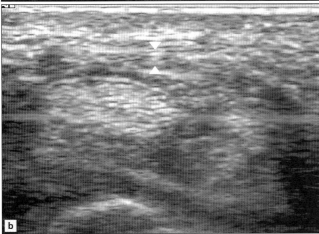

Fig. 6.24 Palmar axial sonograms obtained proximal (a) and inside the carpal tunnel (b) in a patient presenting with a clinical diagnosis of carpal tunnel syndrome. US shows swelling of the median nerve proximally (arrows) and thinning distally (arrowheads).

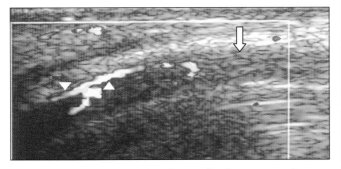

Fig. 6.25 Power Doppler palmar longitudinal sonogram of a patient presenting with a clinical diagnosis of carpal tunnel syndrome. US shows thickening of the MN (arrow) and internal flow signals (arrowheads) consistent with hyperaemia due to neuritis.

muscles inside the tunnel can be demonstrated as solid lesions with typical internal muscle structure that follow tendon gliding at dynamic examination.

Since in the great majority of cases the position of the MN is not affected by tenosynovitis, we

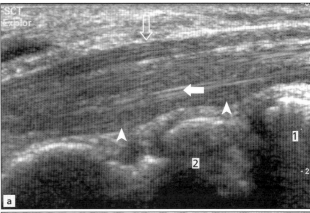

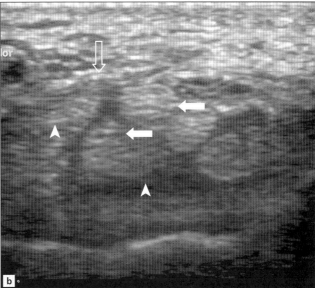

Fig. 6.26 Palmar longitudinal (a) and axial (b) sonograms of a patient presenting with a clinical diagnosis of carpal tunnel syndrome. US shows the flexor tendons (arrows) surrounded by a hypoechoic area (arrowheads) due to tenosynovitis. The median nerve (open arrow) appears normal. Distal radius (1), lunate (2), capitate (3). No focal masses are seen inside the carpal tunnel.

believe that US is not routinely required to guide a carpal tunnel injection. In the rare patient presenting with a localised swelling of the palmar aspect of the wrist US can be useful in exactly localising the MN so as to avoid accidental nerve damage during blinded injection. Rather than injecting during real-time scanning, we prefer to utilise US to mark the skin over the course of the median nerve. Assessment of CTS postsurgical changes is difficult. The flexor retinaculum appears thickened and hypoechoic while the median nerve is located in a more superficial and medial position (Fig. 6.27). Since different surgical procedures can be employed, the sonologist must be aware of which one has been utilised. The finding of a partially

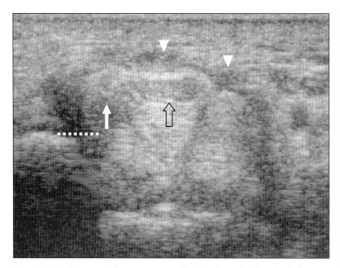

Fig. 6.27 Palmar axial sonograms obtained at the level of the proximal carpal tunnel, in a patient treated surgically for CTS. US shows palmar dislocation (arrow) of the median nerve (open arrow). Please note that the transverse carpal ligament appears irregularly hypoechoic due to postsurgical changes (arrowheads).

sectioned retinaculum does not always mean an inadequate release since in some procedures the retinaculum is partially divided by two parallel sections (distal and proximal). Finding the nerve surrounded by an hypoechoic area can be consistent with postsurgical scarring but this finding must always be correlated with the clinical findings since it can be noted in asymptomatic patients too.

Guyon tunnel syndrome

Located at the medial aspect of the palm, the Guyon tunnel is formed by the TCL, the superficial palmar ligament, the pisiform and the hook of hamate. The tunnel contains the ulnar nerve and the ulnar artery. Both structures divide within the canal into a deep and a superficial branch. The deep ulnar nerve branch is a predominant motor branch while the superficial is mostly sensitive. US can evaluate the normal anatomy of the Guyon tunnel by showing the pulsatile ulnar artery on the lateral aspect and the ulnar nerve. High-resolution transducers can detect the splitting of the nerve into the terminal branches.

In Guyon tunnel syndrome the ulnar nerve can be compressed by a variety of conditions including mass lesions, fracture or chronic external compression such as can occur while biking. Mass lesions causing nerve compression can be detected by US. Three major causes are anomalous muscles located inside the tunnel, thrombosis of the ulnar artery and ganglia. All these lesions can be diagnosed by US. An anomalous muscle appears as a hypoechoic lesion with typical muscle echotexture. As these are common, clinical correlation is important in the diagnosis of the symptomatic lesion. Thrombosis of the ulnar artery appears as an increase in the size of the artery, which appears filled by echogenic material. Colour Doppler shows no internal flow signals. Ganglia appear as small anechoic masses dislocating the ulnar nerve and artery.

TUMOURS AND TUMOUR-LIKE LESIONS

General considerations, technique of examination and guidelines for US report

Mass lesions of the hand and wrist are a very common problem in the daily sonographic practice. When a mass is found at this level the sonologist must evaluate the mass and its relationships with the adjacent structures (24).

Once a mass is located, the first thing to do is to accurately describe its location (subcutaneous tissue, subfascial plane or adherent to bone plane), borders (regular, irregular, dendritic) and internal structure. The distance from the mass and the skin must be measured and reported to allow a base for biopsy or surgical removal. Size must be accurately measured in the three major axes, utilising the electronic calipers. The greater axis must always be related to the main anatomic planes (i.e. major axis of 13 mm in the sagittal plane). Depending on their peculiar composition, masses can be completely anechoic, present a mixed appearance with different amounts of fluid and echogenic material or be echogenic. Completely anechoic lesions usually result from fluid accumulation due to synovial fluid found inside either a joint recess or a synovial tendon sheath. Ganglia can also appear as anechoic lesions but usually present internal septa, which allows for a mixed appearance. Mixed lesions result mainly from ganglia and pseudoaneurysm. Echogenic masses can be hypo-, iso- and hyperechoic, depending on the histologic composition and on the location of the mass.

Lipoma can present different echogenicities. Changes in mass shape and contour when different pressure with the probe is applied must be noted. The examination must be made by applying a minimal amount of pressure since excessive pressure can lead to synovial fluid displacement and tenosynovitis being missed. Once an initial impression is formed, progressively increasing pressure is applied. Using the technique of "ultrasound palpation", ganglia that are filled by thick viscous fluid can be differentiated from synovial-lined lesions that are compressible. Then the positions of the surrounding tendons, fasciae, nerves and vessels in relation to the mass must be accurately described and the distance measured. If the lesion is in contact with a tendon, selective active and passive tendon movement must be made during real-time scanning and movement of the mass with the tendon's motion must be noted. When the mass is located close to a vessel the transducer must be kept immobile and the patient is asked to remain still during real-time scanning to detect Brownian movement in relation to internal very-low-speed blood movement. In masses located near a nerve every effort must be made to detect intralesional or peripheral nerve fascicles since this can allow for a presumptive diagnosis of nerve tumour. A neurogenic tumour typically shows no longitudinal motion in the longitudinal axis of the nerve while it is mobile in the axial

plane. The possibility of evaluating blood perfusion with colour or power Doppler imaging is very useful in differentiating cystic from solid masses. Table 6.1 summarises the lesion criteria that must be analysed and described in the sonographic report.

> **Practical tip**
>
> The initial evaluation of a mass should be undertaken with minimal probe pressure to avoid displacing fluid. Then, gradually increasing and decreasing pressure 'ultrasound palpation' is used to further classify the mass.

The sonographic appearance of the most common masses of the wrist will be briefly described according with their frequency.

Ganglia

Ganglia are the most common expansible lesions of the hand and wrist and a very frequent indication for an US examination (25). They are cystic lesions filled by a variable amount of gelatinous, mucoid, thick fluid. The fluid results from polymerisation of the hyaluronic fluid and has a greyish appearance. A ganglia wall is composed of fibrous tissue and lacks a true synovial lining. The lack of synovial lining and the thick content are the main features that distinguish ganglia from synovial bursa or joint synovial recesses filled by synovial fluid.

Two theories to explain ganglia origin have been proposed. The first refers to ganglia as extrusion of a synovial space that, because of a valve mechanism, leads subsequently to concentration of the internal fluid and loss of the synovial lining. The second theory refers to ganglia as the result of para-articular connective tissue degeneration with secondary myxoid degeneration. Both theories can explain why ganglia may or may not communicate with the joint or tendon sheath cavities.

The most common location is the dorsal aspect of the wrist followed by the palmar aspect and by the palmar aspect of fingers. Clinically ganglia present as painless or slightly painful firm masses. A peculiar ganglia is the so-called "dorsal occult ganglion", which occurs dorsally to the lunate, is clinically occult since its small size prevents its detection at physical examination

Table 6.1

Main characteristics
    Location and depth in respect with the skin
    Size
    Borders
    Internal echogenicity
    Brownian movements
Relations and distance from the adjacent structures
    Tendons
    Fasciae
    Nerves
    Vessels
Dynamic behaviour
    Graded compression
    Tendon movements
    Gliding in respect with nerve
Colour and power Doppler findings
    Avascular
    Avascular with parietal vascularity
    Vascular

and causes pain due to compression on the terminal branches of the sensorial radial nerve. Painful limitation of dorsal or palmar flexion can be an associated finding. A typical finding is that ganglia can intermittently increase and decrease in size. At US ganglia have different appearances, depending on their age and location. Recent lesions appear entirely anechoic due to the presence of very thin or no internal septa; older ganglia present thicker septations that lead to a more echogenic appearance. Some authors also believe that recurrent intralesional haemorrhages with resultant fibrosis can also explain the increased echogenicity. The wall can be eventually demonstrated as a hyperechoic structure.

Dorsal wrist ganglia

These are the most common ganglia. They originate from the dorsal portion of the scapholunate ligament and posterior radiocarpal joint capsule probably as a result of either acute or chronic trauma. Surgical and pathologic studies demonstrated several microcysts inside the posterior capsule of the scapholunate joint that can be responsible for local recurrence if wide excision of the dorsal capsule is not performed during the surgical procedure. Ganglia develop firstly dorsal to the capsule and then extend superficially between the extensor tendons to lie in the subcutaneous tissues. Since this compartment is a low-pressure compartment ganglia can reach a considerable size here. Larger ganglia are typically connected with the capsule and sometimes with the radiocarpal joint space with a tortuous, thin pedicle that sometimes can be detected by US.

The diagnosis of dorsal ganglia is usually made on the basis of physical findings. Nevertheless, US is utilised to confirm the presence of the cystic mass, to localise accurately the relation with the tendons and to evaluate the ganglia size. There is general consensus that only symptomatic ganglia must be treated surgically and no invasive treatment must be performed for cosmetic reasons. Treatment of ganglia relies first on anti-inflammatory drug and physical therapies. Ganglia puncture has been advocated but has a high degree of recurrence. US can guide positioning of the needle tip in the centre of the lesion. A large needle must be utilised because of the thick ganglia content. Aspiration can be facilitated by utilisation of a special handle. Sometimes corticosteroid can be injected inside the lesion in an effort to cause fibrosis of the wall and prevent recurrence.

The US findings of the typical dorsal ganglia include a subcutaneous polycyclic anechoic lesion with internal septations connected to the dorsal capsule through a variable pedicle (Fig. 6.28). Dynamic US in the sagittal plane show no motion of the ganglia with movement of the extensor tendons. Axial images can demonstrate small intermittent radioulnar tilt due to tendon movement. Older lesions frequently appear more echogenic and are more difficult to distinguish from the adjacent structures.

The occult dorsal ganglion appears as a small lesion located just dorsal to the posterior pole of the lunate. Due to its small size the lesion appears mostly hypoechoic. In doubtful cases examining the wrist in a hyperflexed position can increase detectability of the lesion. Local pressure guided by real-time US can demonstrate a correlation with patient symptoms and the lesion demonstrated by US.

> **Practical tip**
>
> In doubtful cases examining the wrist in a hyperflexed position can increase detectability of small, occult dorsal ganglia.

Palmar wrist ganglia

Palmar wrist ganglia are almost always found at the radial aspect of the wrist. They arise from the region of the radioscaphoid or scaphotrapezium joint and dissect proximally. These lesions are usually large and closely related to the radial artery. Clinically they present as painless lumps. Sometimes because of the transmitted pulsatility of the radial artery it's difficult to differentiate palmar ganglia from a pseudoaneurysm on the basis of clinical findings. US demonstrates them as polylobular cystic lesions with a distal pedicle. The connection of the pedicle with the carpal joint is more difficult to assess than with dorsal ganglia. Relations with the radial artery as well as with its palmar branch can be accurately evaluated (Fig. 6.29). On axial images the artery appears as a rounded anechoic structure located palmar and radial to the ganglion. The artery is closely related with the ganglion and

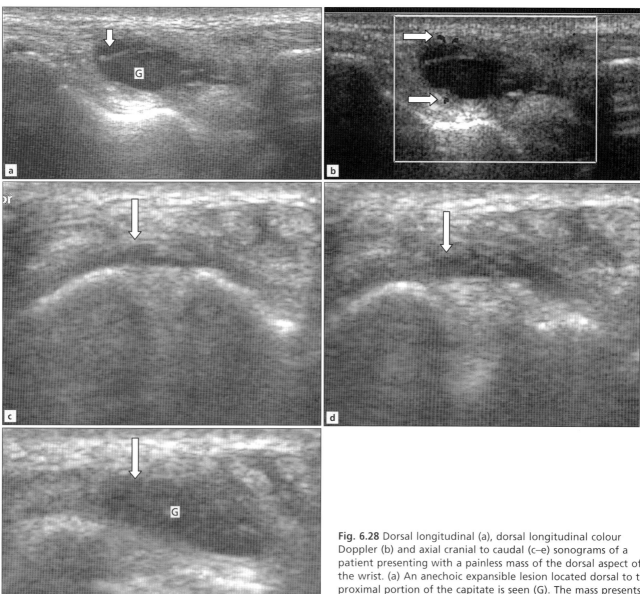

Fig. 6.28 Dorsal longitudinal (a), dorsal longitudinal colour Doppler (b) and axial cranial to caudal (c–e) sonograms of a patient presenting with a painless mass of the dorsal aspect of the wrist. (a) An anechoic expansible lesion located dorsal to the proximal portion of the capitate is seen (G). The mass presents some internal septa (arrow) The appearance is typical for a dorsal ganglion of the wrist. (b) Colour Doppler sonogram shows some flow signals inside the cyst wall (arrows). No internal signals are evident. (c–e) Axial images from cranial to caudal show pedicle of the ganglion arising from the dorsal scapholunate capsule (arrows).

separated from it by a hyperechoic line due to superposition of the arterial and cystic wall. Care must be made not to consider the artery as a lobulation of the cyst particularly if a puncture is considered. Usually this can be easily avoided by scanning on the sagittal plane, increasing pressure of the transducer while scanning in the axial plane, which increases pulsatility of the artery, or utilising colour Doppler imaging. Sagittal sonograms image ganglia as pear-shaped masses. Oblique scans can show the radial artery lying on the palmar cyst wall.

Practical tip

On axial images of palmar ganglia the radial artery appears as a rounded anechoic structure usually located palmar and radial to them. Care must be made not to consider the radial artery as a lobulation of the cyst, particularly if a puncture is considered.

Digital ganglia

Digital ganglia are small cystic lesions found almost always at the base of the fingers. The

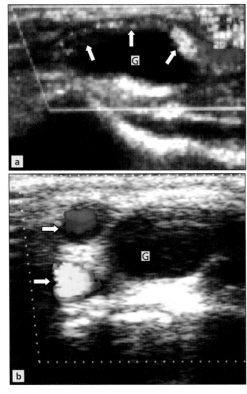

Fig. 6.29 Palmar longitudinal (a) and axial (b) colour Doppler sonograms of two patients with a volar ganglion (G). In (a) the ganglion dislocates the radial artery (arrows), which is closely related to its upper aspect, while in (b) it lies internal to the vessels.

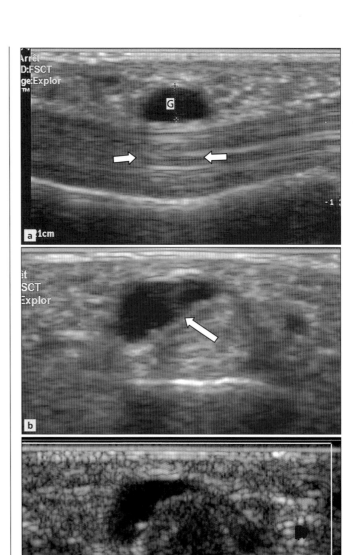

Fig. 6.30 Palmar longitudinal (a), axial (b) and axial colour Doppler sonograms of a patient presenting with a painless mass at the base of the third finger (c). (a) A 2 mm anechoic, expansible lesion located palmar to the flexor tendons is seen (G). The mass presents a definite posterior enhancement (arrows). The appearance is typical for a digital ganglion. (b) Axial sonogram shows the close relation of the ganglion with the A2 digital pulley (arrow). (c) Axial colour Doppler image shows absence of internal flow signals.

fourth finger seems more commonly involved. Clinically they present as very firm masses that can resemble a "bony lesion". They are usually painful particularly when squeezed against the bone surface by an object such as when the patient carries a piece of heavy luggage.

As for the other ganglia the exact pathogenesis is not fully understood. They seem to derive from degeneration of the annular fibrous pulleys. US depicts the digital ganglia as a small (usually 2–5 mm) hypoechoic lesion almost always located palmar to the flexor tendons at the level of the base of the proximal phalanx (Fig. 6.30). Larger lesions can extend on the radial or ulnar side of the tendons. Almost closely related to the flexor digitorum tendons digital ganglia are not connected with the synovial tendon sheath since they originate from the A1 and A2 pulleys. Dynamic examination obtained during movements of the flexor tendons does not result in cystic movements or changes in shape.

Giant tumour of tendon sheath

The nature of a giant tumour of tendon sheath (GTTS) is not yet clearly understood. Some authors consider it a true neoplasm while others think it is a reactive lesion. GTTS are the second most frequent masses of the wrist and hand. They usually arise from a tendon sheath and progressively enlarge, causing pressure erosions on the adjacent bone cortex and tendon displacement. They tend to occur at or distal to the MCP joints, which helps to differentiate them from neurilemomas, which occur more proximally.

US show GTTS as well-defined, solid, hypoechoic paratendineous or para-articular expansible lesions. Colour or power Doppler imaging can show internal flow signals. Erosions on the bone cortex, which are usually well evident at tangential standard radiographs, can be easily detected by US as well. It must be stressed that the sonographic appearance of GTTS is nonspecific since other neoplasms such as tendon fibroma can present in a similar way. The utility of US relies on the confirmation of the solid nature of the mass and in the evaluation of its relationship with the adjacent vessels and nerves in the preoperative planning.

Lipomas

Lipomas of the hand and wrist are usually found at the palm. The diagnosis is clinically suspected in the presence of a soft, painless mass that can get harder with low temperature. US shows lipomas as masses with variable echogenicity that change shape when pressure is applied. When located in subcutaneous fat their borders can be difficult to define since they blend with their surroundings. Lipomas almost always do not show internal flow signals with colour Doppler imaging due to very small internal vessels.

Pseudoaneurysms

Pseudoaneurysms result from traumatic injury to the vessel wall, which allows formation of a blood-filled cavity that can expand and can later be bordered by a fibrous wall. Formation of a thrombus, which completely or partially fills the cavity, is a common finding. Absence of definite elastic fibres in the pseudoaneurysm wall is the histologic hallmark of these lesions and differentiates them from a true aneurysm. Pseudoaneurysms can derives from both arteries and veins. Clinically they present as a soft, compressible mass that, if located superficially,

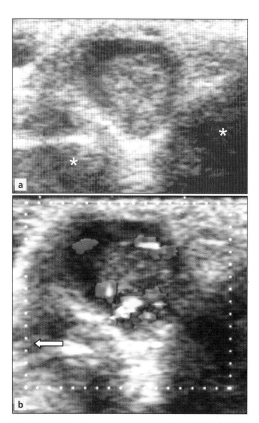

Fig. 6.31 Dorsal axial (a) and axial colour Doppler (b) sonograms of a patient presenting with a painless soft mass of the fourth intermetacarpal space. In (a) a mixed lesion is depicted between the two metacarpals (asterisks). In (b) please note the flow signals partially surrounding the internal echogenic thrombus.

presents a bluish colour. US shows them as masses with internal mixed echogenicity, reflecting the internal constitution (Fig. 6.31). The anechoic portion correlates with the blood-filled cavity while the hypoechoic part refers to the internal thrombus.

Nerve tumours

Nerve tumours can be divided into neurofibromas and neurinomas, depending on their histology. Whereas neurinomas (also known as schwanomas or neurolemoma) arise at the periphery of the nerve and usually grow eccentrically, neurofibromas are embedded inside the nerve and nerve fascicles are seen traversing them. The distinction has practical value since neurinomas can be easily removed surgically whereas removal of a neurofibroma is difficult and frequently leads to sectioning of nerves fascicles if not of the entire nerve, which requires nerve transposition.

Nerve tumours affecting the hand and wrist are mainly located at the wrist and affect the median and ulnar nerve. The US appearance is similar for the two histotypes: a hypoechoic oval or rounded lesion connected to a nerve trunk. However, if the US appearance is not specific, a rounded shape, eccentric position and vascular internal signals are considered findings pointing towards a diagnosis of neurinoma rather then neurofibroma. Demonstration of the nerve entering the lesion at one edge and leaving at the opposite edge is considered as pathognomonic of a nerve tumour. Additionally compression of the mass with the probe can elicit peripheral tingling and confirms the diagnosis of nerve tumour (US Tinel sign). Careful analysis of the mass features and of its relationship with adjacent nerves must always be obtained before obtaining a soft-tissue mass needle biopsy since this can be extremely painful in the case of a neurogenic tumour.

Glomus tumours

Glomus tumours arise from the neuromyoarterial glomus located in the subunguial region of the finger. Typically patients present with awful localised pain that can be elicited by pressure on the nail or by cold exposure. US must be directed on the basis of the clinical symptoms. Glomus tumours appear as a solid hypoechoic mass mostly located under the nail. In larger lesions an erosion of the underlying phalanx can be found. Colour Doppler imaging shows intralesional flow signals related to the high-velocity flow shunt vessels. This finding is fairly specific for the diagnosis.

MISCELLANEOUS CONDITIONS

A variety of other conditions can present as a hand and wrist mass. These include tenosynovitis (particularly extensor tenosynovitis at the hand and de Quervain tenosynovitis), foreign bodies granuloma and soft tissue abscess. These conditions have been described earlier.

REFERENCES

1. Sugimoto H, Takeda A, Hyodoh K. Early-stage rheumatoid arthritis: Prospective study of the effectiveness of MR imaging for diagnosis. Radiology 2000;216:569–75.
2. Boutry N, Lardé A, Lapègue F, Solau-Gervais E, Flipo RM, Cotten A. MR imaging appearance of the hands and feet in patients with early RA. J Rheumatol 2003;30:671–9.
3. Backhaus M, Kamradt T, Sandrock D, Loreck D, Fritz J, Wolf KJ, Raber H, Hamm B, Burmester GR, Bollow M. Arthritis of the finger joints. A comprehensive approach comparing conventional radiography, scintigraphy, ultrasound, and contrast-enhanced magnetic resonance imaging. Arthritis Rheum 1999;42:1232–45.
4. Schmidt WA, Völker L, Zacher J, Schläfke M, Ruhnke M, Ihle-Gromnica E. Colour Doppler ultrasonography to detect pannus in knee joint synovitis. Clin Exp Rheumatol 2000;18:439–44.
5. Walther M, Harms H, Krenn V, Radke S, Faehndrich TP, Gohlke F. Correlation of power Doppler sonography with vascularity of the synovial tissue of the knee joints in patients with osteoarthritis and rheumatoid arthritis. Arthritis Rheum 2001;44:331–8.
6. Steuer A, Bush J, DeSouza NM, Taylor P, Blomley MJ, Cosgrove DO *et al.* Power Doppler ultrasound in early rheumatoid arthritis: A comparative study with contrast-enhanced MRI. Radiology 2001;p 561 (abstract).
7. Szkudlarek M, Court-Payen M, Strandberg C, Klarlund M, Klausen T, Ostergaard M. Power Doppler ultrasonography for assessment of synovitis in the metacarpophalangeal joints of patients with rheumatoid arthritis: A comparison with dynamic resonance imaging. Arthritis Rheum 2001;44:2018–23.
8. Spiegel T, King W, Weiner SR, Paulus HE. Measuring disease activity: Comparison of joint tenderness, swelling, and ultrasonography in rheumatoid arthritis. Arthritis Rheum 1987;30:1283–8.
9. Hau M, Schultz H, Tony HP, Keberle M, Jahns R, Haerten R, Jenett M. Evaluation of pannus and vascularization of the metacarpophalangeal and proximal interphalangeal joints in rheumatoid arthritis by high-resolution ultrasound (multidimensional linear array). Arthritis Rheum 1999;42: 2303–8.
10. Klauser A, Frauscher F, Schirmer M, Halpern E, Pallwein L, Herold M, Helweg G, ZurNedden D. The value of contrast-enhanced color Doppler ultrasound in the detection of vascularization of finger joints in patients with rheumatoid arthritis. Arthritis Rheum 2002;46:647–53.
11. Hau M, Kneitz C, Tony HP, Keberle M, Jahns R, Jenett M. High resolution ultrasound detect a decrease in pannus vascularisation of small finger joints in patients with rheumatoid arthritis receiving treatment with soluble tumour necrosis factor alpha receptor (etanercept). Ann Rheum Dis 2002;61: 55–8.
12. Grassi W, Filippucci E, Farina A, Salaffi F, Cervini C. Ultrasonography in the evaluation of bone erosions. Ann Rheum Dis 2001;60:98–103.
13. Wakefield RJ, Gibbon WW, Conaghan PG, O'Connor P, McGonagle D, Pease C, Green MJ, Veale DJ, Isaacs JD, Emery P. The value of sonography in the detection of bone erosions in patients with rheumatoid arthritis. A comparison with conventional radiography. Arthritis Rheum 2000;43:2762–70.
14. Kotob H, Kamel M. Identification and prevalence of rheumatoid nodules in the finger tendons using high frequency ultrasonography. J Rheumatol 1999;26:1264–8.
15. Olivieri I, Barozzi L, Favaro L, Pierro A, De Matteis M, Borghi C, Padula A, Ferri S, Pavlica P. Dactylitis in patients with seronegative spondyloarthropathy. Assessment by ultrasonography and magnetic resonance imaging. Arthritis Rheum 1996;39:1524–8.

16. Kane D, Greaney T, Bresnihan B, Gibney R, Fitzgerald O. Ultrasonography in the diagnosis and management of psoriatic dactylitis. J Rheumatol 1999;26:1746–51.

17. Hauger O, Bonnefoy O, Moinard M, Bersani D, Diard F. Occult fractures of the waist of the scaphoid: Early diagnosis by high-spatial-resolution sonography. Am J Roentgenol 2002;178(5):1239–45.

18. Chiou H-J, Chang C-Y, Chou Y-H. Triangular fibrocartilage of wrist: Presentation on high resolution ultrasonography. J Ultrasound Med 1998;17:41.

19. Griffith JF, Chan DPN, Ho PC, Zhao L, Hung LK, Metrewell C. Sonography of the normal scapholunate ligament and scapholunate joint space. J Clin Ultrasound 2001;29: 223–9.

20. Klauser A, Frauscher F, Bodner G, Halpern EJ, Schocke MF, Springer P, Gabl M, Judmaier W, Nedden D zur. Finger pulley injuries in extreme rock climbers: Depiction with dynamic US. Radiology 2002;222:755.

21. Martinoli C, Bianchi S, Nebiolo M. Sonographic evaluation of digital annular pulley tears. Skeletal Radiol 2000;29:387.

22. Horton LK, Jacobson JA, Powell A. Sonography and radiography of soft-tissue foreign bodies. Am J Roentgen 2001;176:1155.

23. Buchberger W, Judmaier W, Birbamer G, Lener M, Schmidauer C. Carpal tunnel syndrome: Diagnosis with high-resolution sonography. Am J Roentgen 1992;159:793–8.

24. Bianchi S, Martinoli C, Abdelwahab IF. High resolution ultrasound of the hand and wrist. Review article. Skeletal Radiol 1999;28:121–9.

25. Bianchi S, Abdelwahab IF, Zwass A, Giacomello P. Ultrasonographic evaluation of wrist ganglia. Skeletal Radiol 1994;23:201–3.

Imaging in developmental dysplasia of the hip

7

David J Wilson and Jane Wolstencroft

INTRODUCTION

> **Key point**
>
> Developmental dysplasia of the hip (DDH) occurs in a small but significant number of children.

Developmental dysplasia of the hip (DDH) occurs in a small but significant number of children. It may manifest as an inability to walk by the typical age of around one year. Less severe cases may cause a limp or abnormal gait in childhood. Pain may be the principle complaint when a shallow and mechanically disadvantaged hip develops premature osteoarthritis in young adults. Occasionally the condition is first noticed in middle or later years as an incidental finding. Rarely full dislocation of the hip may present very late. A lifetime of limitation of motion may have been put down to clumsiness or inability at sport.

> **Key point**
>
> There is a window of opportunity within the first 6 months of life to treat DDH.

Early treatment includes double nappies and formal splint therapy (e.g. Von Rosen splint or Pavlik harness) (1, 2). There is a window of opportunity for treatment within the first 6 months of life although splint therapy is only moderately successful. Irreducibility by physical examination and poor coverage on ultrasound examination (Morin < 20%) are factors strongly associated with failure for splint therapy (3). For cases that are overlooked or present later, surgery with derotational osteotomy of the femur or pelvic osteotomies may be required. Those patients who present late with osteoarthritis in a shallow hip may respond to analgesia and anti-inflammatory drugs but many will need surgery such as hip fusion or replacement. In general the earlier the diagnosis is made, the simpler, safer and more effective is the treatment.

DEMOGRAPHICS

The incidence of DDH is reported to be between 1 and 3 cases presenting in the first year per thousand live births. The true incidence of DDH is much higher. Many infants with DDH have few or no symptoms even though the acetabulum is poorly developed. It is only when the mechanical disadvantage leads to premature osteoarthritis that the condition is recognised, usually by plain radiography. There are no precise figures for the overall rate of occurrence but based on the authors' experience it can be estimated to be 15 per thousand live births.

DDH is more common in:

Girls (1 : 9 boys to girls);
In those with other congenital anomalies such a club foot or neuromuscular disorders;
Those with a first degree relative with hip dysplasia;
Infants born by breech delivery; and
Premature birth.

Those infants with at least one risk factor for DDH are three times more likely to have DDH than those who are not at risk (4). The incidence of the disorder may vary with the population. In Crete the incidence is recorded as almost 11 per 1000 newborn infants (5).

Ultrasound screening studies (6) have shown an incidence of:

Graf I: 78.99%;
Graf II: 20.56%; and
Graf III & IV: 0.45%.

In one population study an abnormal ultrasound was seen in 4.7% (7). In 3.36% of cases the hip was shallow (Graf IIA) but 65% of these often become normal within a few weeks.

Those treated with splint therapy are recorded as suffering a low but significant rate (1.06%) of avascular necrosis following splint therapy (7). What cannot be measured is the psychological impact of a period of splint therapy on the child and parents. It seems more than reasonable that treatment should be kept to a minimum.

SCREENING PROTOCOLS

There are three broad strategies in screening for DDH:

(1) Clinical: Clinical examination within the first six weeks of life by Ortolani and Barlow manoeuvres.
(2) Clinical examination plus ultrasound of high-risk infants: This includes those who are abnormal or suspect on clinical examination.
(3) Clinical examination and ultrasound of all infants: This procedure is carried out within the first six weeks of life.

Clinical examination alone is likely to miss 23% of patients in the high-risk group who have an abnormal US. True dislocation is normally detected clinically with good precision but there are occasional oversights. In one study of 9030 infants (8) the sensitivity of clinical and ultrasound examination were independently assessed. As much as 1.4% of hips were considered unstable but only 63% were detected by clinical examination alone. Ultrasound alone overlooked in only 5% of cases.

Careful clinical examination is very reliable at detecting unstable hips (Graf IIC to IV) but poor at detecting shallow acetabula (4).

Strategies where all high-risk infants only are scanned will overlook around 1 : 50 of those with DDH who have no associated risk factors and are abnormal to clinical examination.

Population screening studies are expensive. In addition the low rate of abnormality leads to failures of omission due to a combination of factors: The boredom or fatigue of the examiner, rushed examinations due to large numbers and the natural reluctance associated with making an abnormal diagnosis in an otherwise well infant. Due to a variety of errors, including noncompliance by parents from deprived socio-economic backgrounds, not all infants are screened.

Splint therapy is reported to reduce the incidence of dislocation. There are occasions where a hip reported as having normal depth in early infancy presents with true dislocation by the age of one year. There is debate as to whether dislocation really can occur in hips morphologically normal at birth or whether these are all cases of poor ultrasound technique or misinterpretation of the images.

A review of the literature sponsored by the Canadian Task Force on Preventative Health Care concluded that there is fair evidence to support the use for clinical screening. However, they also felt that there is fair evidence to exclude ultrasound screening for both the whole population and those at high risk. They also felt that there is insufficient evidence to judge the effectiveness of splint therapy but there is good evidence that those with clinically detected DDH should be observed. They could not determine how long this period of observation should be (9). This paper effectively says that the research published to date on US and splint therapy is inadequate to allow firm recommendations.

ULTRASOUND METHODS

Graf

> **Key point**
>
> Graf's method for measuring the shape and size of the acetabulum in young infants requires paying particular attention to the position of the hip, and images must be acquired in a true coronal plane.

Reinhardt Graf, an Austrian orthopaedic surgeon, developed a method for measuring the shape and size of the acetabulum in young infants (10). The technique requires paying particular attention to the position of the hip and images must be acquired in a true coronal plane (Fig. 7.1). The child lies in a foam-padded trough in a lateral position and the hip is flexed to 90°. The ultrasound probe is placed in a coronal plane parallel to the spine. The image should be

centred on the femoral head with the lateral aspect of the ileum in view (Fig. 7.2). Care should be taken to avoid rotation from the coronal plane by a combination of visually observing one's position and maintaining the correct image on the ultrasound screen. A sound knowledge of the normal anatomy is important to achieve

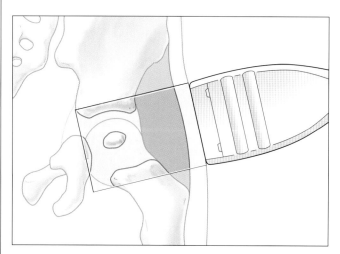

Fig. 7.1 A coronal plane of imaging allows the ultrasound to enter an unossified window in the region of the femoral head via the gluteal muscles, traversing the femoral and entering the triradiate cartilage in the acetabulum.

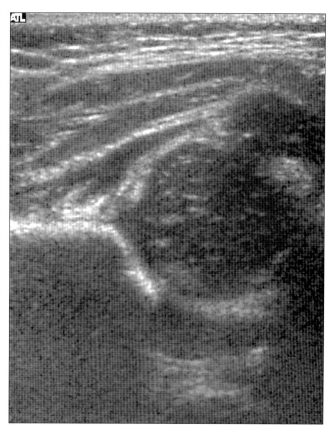

Fig. 7.2 The normal ileum and acetabular roof are seen a "tea spoon" shape. The "egg" of the femoral head sits in the spoon.

this image. Clues that the image is not correctly aligned are that the side of the ileum appears curved and that the triradiate cartilage is not seen at the depth of the acetabulum. Tilting the probe in an anterior or posterior direction may make the acetabulum appear artificially deep or shallow, respectively (Figs 7.3 and 7.4). Describing this process in words is complex, as it is a technique best demonstrated and learnt practically. Supervised training is essential.

> **Practical tip**
>
> While using Graf's method, care should be taken to avoid rotation from the coronal plane by a combination of visually observing one's position and maintaining the correct image on the ultrasound screen.

> **Practical tip**
>
> Clues that the sonogram image is not correctly aligned are that the side of the ileum appears curved and that the triradiate cartilage is not seen at the depth of the acetabulum.

Once the true coronal image is obtained measurements may be taken either on a printed copy or on the screen. Most ultrasound machines will allow the operator to draw lines and measure angles. Some have software specifically designed to measure "Graf" angles but this is not essential. The first line, known as the base line, is drawn along the lateral aspect of the bony outline of the ileum. The second is drawn along the roof of the acetabulum. This roof line is the best fit to the lateral aspect of the acetabular roof. The labrum line is then drawn from the lateral corner of the acetabulum at a tangent to the femoral head along the cartilaginous labrum through its fibrocartilage tip. The angles between the base line and roof line (α) and the base line and the cartilage or labrum line (β) are measured (Fig. 7.5).

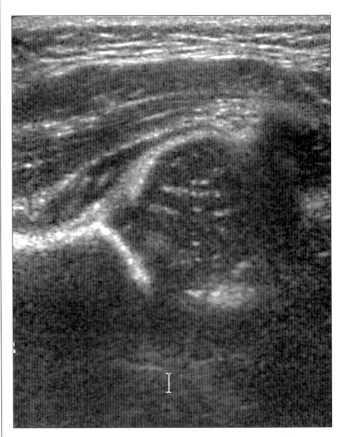

Fig. 7.3 When the probe is too far anterior the "spoon" appears flattened and the echogenic line of the acetabular roof disappears.

Fig. 7.4 When the probe is too far posterior the line of the ileum (handle of the "spoon") appears curled upwards at its lower end.

Practical tip

To measure "Graf" angles, alpha (α) is the angle between the base line (drawn along the lateral aspect of the bony outline of the ileum) and the roof line (drawn as the best fit to the lateral aspect of the acetabular roof); and beta (β) is the angle between the base line and the cartilage or labrum line (drawn from the lateral corner of the acetabulum at a tangent to the femoral head along the cartilaginous labrum through its fibrocartilage tip).

The Graf method has many advocates and in central Europe it is the most commonly used method of measurement. However, there are a number of problems associated with its use. Obtaining a true coronal image requires skill, experience and precision. The division into different diagnostic groups varies with the angles measured and minor inaccuracies or experimental errors alter the recommended treatment. Studies have shown poor reproducibility of placement of the lines and wide interobserver variation especially for the cartilage (labral) line and the resulting β angle.

On the other hand the discipline involved in positioning and measurement probably improves the overall quality of ultrasound studies.

Others

Others techniques of measurement have been described. Morin uses the same coronal image as Graf and the same base line along the ileum. Then two lines are drawn parallel to the base line at a tangent to the femoral head at its most medial and most lateral aspects. By measuring the distance between the base line and the two parallel lines the amount of the femoral head inside the base line may be measured as a proportion of the width of the femoral head (11) (Fig. 7.6). A percentage "cover" is the result. Opinions vary as to what is normal but 52% cover is definitely normal and over 46% is probably adequate (see Fig 7.7).

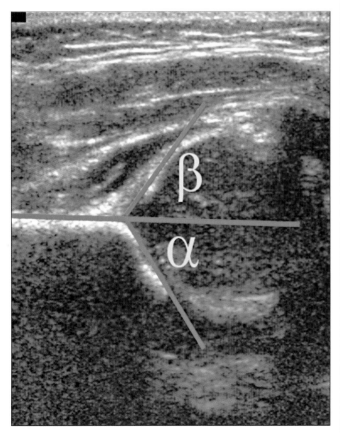

Fig. 7.5 Graf's base line (ileum), roof line (bony acetabulum) and labral line (cartilaginous labrum) describe these two angles. α = roof angle, β = labral angle.

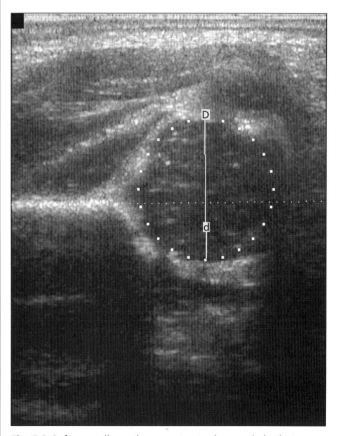

Fig. 7.6 Software allows the operator to draw a circle that can be moved and adjusted to surround the femoral head. A line drawn from the ileum bisects the circle. The head under the base line (d) is taken as a percentage of the diameter of the femoral head (D).

Practical tip

According to Morin's method of measurement, whereby the proportion of the width of the femoral head under the base line (drawn along the lateral aspect of the bony outline of the ileum) is known as the percentage "cover", 52% cover is definitely normal and over 46% is probably adequate.

Some workers have advocated a transverse image of the acetabulum with a qualitative assessment of the acetabular depth. This may be an adjunct in problematic cases.

Frank dislocation is recognised as an absence of the normal congruity of the joint. Ultrasound examination during manipulation will demonstrate whether the hip may be fully reduced and may suggest that there is an obstruction to reduction (Figs 7.8 and 7.9).

Some infants with dysplasia of the hip exhibit a notch in the bony acetabular brim. This may be a sign of a more severe form of dysplasia (Fig. 7.10).

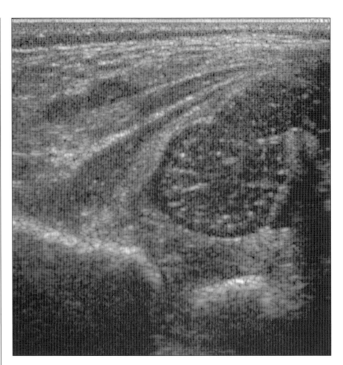

Fig. 7.8 A dislocated femoral head does not fit within the cup or "spoon" of the acetabulum.

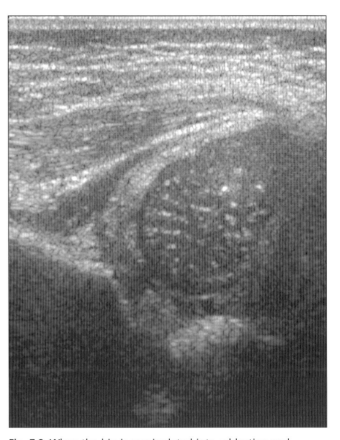

Fig. 7.9 When the hip is manipulated into adduction and external rotation it may reduce from the position seen in Fig. 7.8. In this case there is a block to reduction due to soft-tissue interposition.

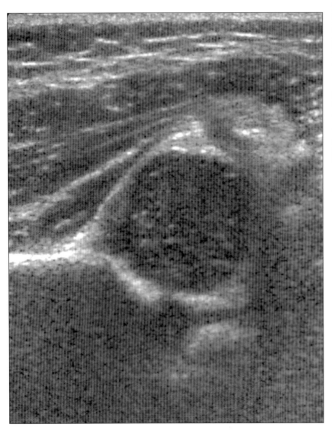

Fig. 7.7 A shallow acetabulum or flat "spoon" may be recognised without recourse to measurement.

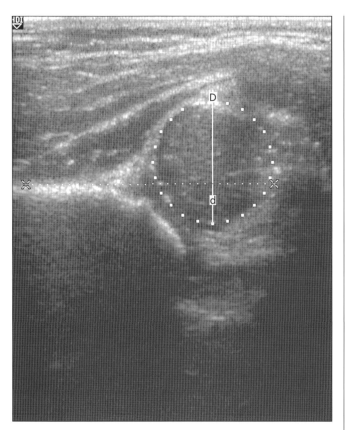

Fig. 7.10 A notch is seen as a kink or indentation in the bony acetabular brim.

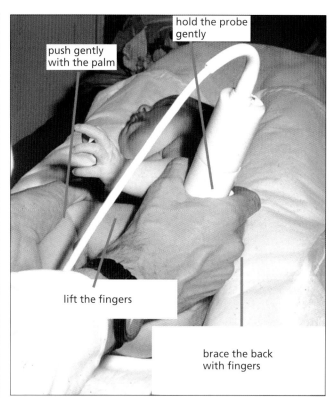

Fig. 7.11 The pressure exerted in the dynamic stress test is mild and should not cause discomfort to the child.

> **Practical tip**
>
> Some infants with dysplasia of the hip exhibit a notch in the bony acetabular brim, which may be a sign of a more severe form of dysplasia.

Dynamic

While shape, depth and alignment of the acetabulum are reproducible and may be compared between patients and serially for each infant there are strong advocates of the dynamic assessment of stability. Subluxation and intermittent dislocation are dynamic events. Ultrasound allows the examination of the hip whilst it is moving and whilst pressure is exerted in a direction that encourages the subluxation. Engesaeter *et al.* showed that the dynamic assessment of the hip was predictive of clinical outcome (12). The methods used vary but most image the hip in the coronal plane and then observe the effect of pressure on the limb in a direction that might push the femoral head out of the joint (Fig. 7.11). The forces used are mild and should not cause discomfort to the infant. The

motion observed will vary but small changes in position (1 to 2 mm) may be studied (Fig. 7.12). Those who use dynamic assessment rely on the change over a few weeks. Dynamically unstable hips that become stable two to three weeks later are regarded as normal. Those that exhibit dynamic motion in excess of 1 mm are observed and if this persists, treatment is commenced.

It is notable that many of the proponents of morphological measurement add dynamic examination while those who previously used dynamic assessment alone now often measure the hip as well.

Careful measurement and treatment based on Graf classification leads to treatment rates that are fairly high. Those who argue for a combination of morphometry, dynamic assessment and early follow-up have lower reported rates of splinting (13).

Pitfalls

Measurements of the hip depend critically on the position of imaging. Figure 7.13 shows the same hip as that in Figure 7.2 with the probe tilted away from the normal coronal plane.

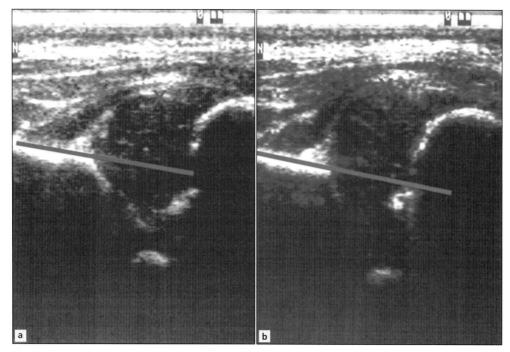

Fig. 7.12 These frames were taken a second apart, (a) before and (b) after pressure was exerted, lifting the femoral head out of the acetabulum.

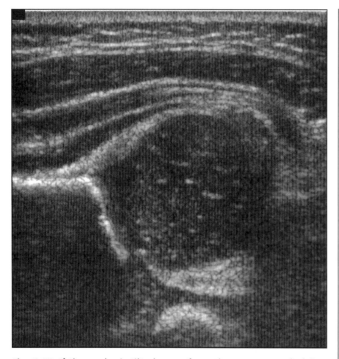

Fig. 7.13 If the probe is tilted away from the true coronal plain it may make the acetabulum artificially deep or shallow.

IMAGING FOR RECOGNISED DYSPLASIA

Follow-up

An early diagnosis of a shallow or unstable hip may be misleading as many children mature very rapidly and within a few weeks the hip may become stable. If the infant is less than six weeks old it is reasonable to delay treatment until a repeat examination is also normal. Most will use an interval of two weeks. Indeed, many prefer not to image the hips until at least four weeks of age to reduce the rate of "false positive" studies. It might be argued that all of these infants stand a risk of the long-term sequelae of premature osteoarthritis but this has not yet been proven by long-term follow-up studies.

When treatment is established, it is usual to review the development of the hips when the infant is three months old. Practice varies between using ultrasound and plain films at this appointment. Certainly by the age of six months ultrasound is becoming more difficult as the advancing bony margins start to obscure the hip. Plain film follow-up at 6 months is standard practice. Severe or worrying cases may also be reimaged at the age of one year. Those who require surgery will be kept under regular review.

The initial plain radiograph should be performed without gonad shielding so that the pubic area and the sacrum are not obscured. Deformities in theses areas will be seen on the first study so subsequent examination should be performed with the shielding in place. Radiation dose should be kept to a minimum and this may be improved by the use of spot film fluoroscopic methods (14).

The plain film should be examined for other deformities. The acetabular angles may be measured by drawing a base line through the triradiate cartilages and then a separate roof line to measure the angle between the base line and this acetabular line (Fig. 7.14). Some experience is required to draw the roof line. Care should be taken not to misinterpret the bony notch that is common as the acetabular margin (15). The mean and standard deviation of these angles vary with side, age, gender and race (16). In general at 6 months of age angles of less than 30 degrees are within two standard deviations of the mean.

Surgery

Following reduction of dislocated hips there are several methods used to ensure the joint is now

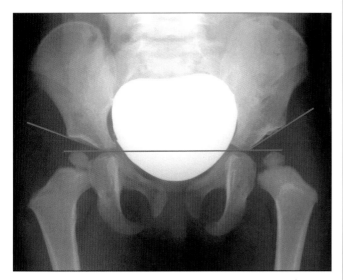

Fig. 7.14 Acetabular angle measurements. A simple protractor or measuring device containing a spirit level or pendulum is an alterative tool.

congruously located. Dislocation often occurs in the anterior–posterior plane so plain films may appear misleadingly normal. Lateral views are impractical as the infant will be in a hip splint or spica. CT and MR both allow an accurate postoperative assessment of the location (17) (Figs 7.15 and 7.16). Clearly MR is preferable for radiation exposure reasons (Figs 7.17 and 7.18). As the child is immobilised in a spica and usually sedated following surgery immobilisation for MR is not a problem (17–22).

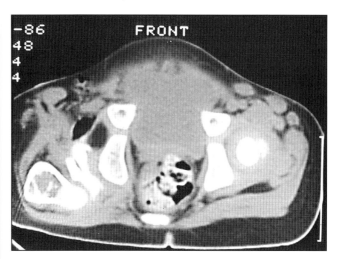

Fig. 7.15 A CT examination after arthrography and an attempted reduction of the dislocation under general anaesthesia. The right hip remains posteriorly dislocated.

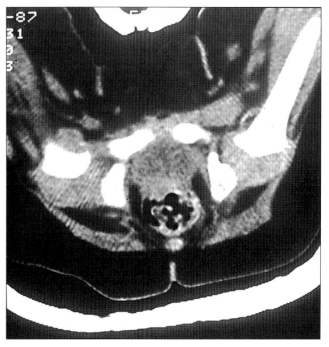

Fig. 7.16 CT of a reduced hip. The infant is in a hip spica.

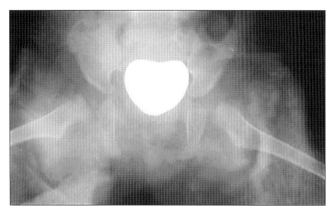

Fig. 7.17 Plain film following operative reduction. The patient then underwent MR examination (Fig. 7.18). Note that the posterior subluxation is not seen in this image.

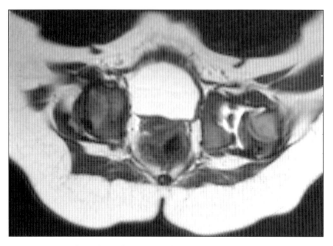

Fig. 7.18 MR has the advantage that there is no ionising radiation. The hips are in a spica, the left hip being subluxated posteriorly. An arthrogram was performed shortly before this study at the time of operative reduction.

Planning surgical osteotomy is complex. The plain film appearances are useful but cross-sectional imaging is more useful in judging shape and alignment. Arthrography is used to assess the best fit of the femoral head and to exclude intra-articular inclusions in many centres (23) but MRI may be as effective (24). Acetabular anteversion varies with each case, although it is increased in some cases there is a wide range and CT is useful for making this measurement and planning effective correctional osteotomies (25). This is one occasion where there is a good role for 3D surface reconstruction from CT data sets (26, 27).

The effect of soft-tissue releases at the time of corrective surgery has to-date been judged empirically. Cross-sectional imaging provides a tool that may produce more accurate outcome measures when muscle and tendon shape and size are measured serially (28).

POPULATION SCREENING

Whether to screen all infants for DDH with ultrasound is an important but currently an unanswerable question. Arguments exist for and against but there are as yet no randomised or controlled studies to prove the case (29).

It is generally accepted that US improves the accuracy of clinical examination alone in the detection of DDH. It is also accepted that early treatment of DDH improves the long-term prognosis. It is intuitive and emotionally attractive to consider that US screening of all infants would give every child the opportunity to benefit from treatment. There is reasonable evidence that a high-risk screening programme (25% of the population) is of benefit.

Against these arguments is the doubt that a population screening process would not have the same accuracy as a high-risk or symptomatic study. Put simply, the diagnostic performance would fall as the rate of normality increases. A greater unknown is the nature of the few cases that evade diagnosis by a high-risk screening process. Are these the same type of case as those detected and treated or are they children who develop subluxation or dislocation later and would be normal to all imaging and clinical examination in the first two to three months of life? This question remains open. There is also, perhaps sadly, the question of cost. Is the expense and diversion of resources worth the benefit? This question can only be answered by studies that determine the clinical benefit of screening, considered within the context of the local and national health service environment, and the answer will vary with the local costs, the background incidence of DDH in that particular population and the precision of the diagnostic methods used (30, 31).

Germany and Austria have undertaken population screening and have encouraged participation by linking the entitlement to child benefit to attendance for screening hip ultrasound. Their experience suggests a very low rate of missed or undetected DDH.

The papers describing these results may be criticised for lack of control groups and there is contradictory evidence to suggest that introducing treatment based on ultrasound grading of hip development has not impacted on the late presentation of DDH (32).

A final unknown is whether early treatment of shallow or unstable acetabula will reduce the severity or incidence of premature osteoarthritis. Experience in Germany and Austria may resolve this matter but with a considerable delay. Certainly this will be after these authors retire from practice!

CONCLUSION

DDH is a serious and crippling disorder. Early diagnosis and treatment leads to improved outcome. Clinical assessment alone is flawed and ultrasound diagnosis aids in detection. Measurement of morphology requires careful attention to technique but does allow decisions with regard to treatment. Many advocate the addition of a dynamic element to the study to discriminate which cases may be left untreated and which require more aggressive management. The ultrasound techniques are demanding and require training and experience. Screening of infants with clinical problems and those at high risk seems wise but the case for whole population examination is not yet proven. There is potential for reducing the incidence and severity of early adult osteoarthritis but further research in this area is required.

Imaging is important in the detection and management of developmental dysplasia of the hip (33–35).

REFERENCES

1. Herring JA. Conservative treatment of congenital dislocation of the hip in the newborn and infant. Clin Orthop 1992;281:41–7.
2. Guille JT, Pizzutillo PD, MacEwen GD. Development dysplasia of the hip from birth to six months. J Am Acad Orthop Surg 2000;8:232–42.
3. Lerman JA, Emans JB, Millis MB, Share J, Zurakowski D, Kasser JR. Early failure of Pavlik harness treatment for developmental hip dysplasia: Clinical and ultrasound predictors. J Pediatr Orthop 2001;21:348–53.
4. Omeroglu H, Koparal S. The role of clinical examination and risk factors in the diagnosis of developmental dysplasia of the hip: A prospective study in 188 referred young infants. Arch Orthop Trauma Surg 2001;121:7–11.
5. Giannakopoulou C, Aligizakis A, Korakaki E, Velivasakis E, Hatzidaki E, Manoura A, et al. Neonatal screening for developmental dysplasia of the hip on the maternity wards in Crete, Greece. Correlation to risk factors. Clin Exper Obstet Gynecol 2002;29:148–52.
6. Bai X, Ji S, Fan G, Yuan Y. [Graf's ultrasound examination method in assessment of dysplasia and congenital dislocation of infant hip]. Zhonghua Wai Ke Za Zhi 2000;38:921–4.
7. Toma P, Valle M, Rossi U, Brunenghi GM. Paediatric hip—Ultrasound screening for developmental dysplasia of the hip: A review. Eur J Ultrasound 2001;14:45–55.
8. Rosenberg N, Bialik V. The effectiveness of combined clinical-sonographic screening in the treatment of neonatal hip instability. Europ J Ultrasound 2002;15:55–60.
9. Patel H, Canadian Task Force on Preventive Health Care. Preventive health care, 2001 update: Screening and management of developmental dysplasia of the hip in newborns. Canad Med Assoc J 2001;164:1669–77.
10. Graf R. [Profile of radiologic-orthopedic requirements in pediatric hip dysplasia, coxitis and epiphyseolysis capitis femoris]. Radiologe 2002;42:467–73.
11. Terjesen T. Ultrasound as the primary imaging method in the diagnosis of hip dysplasia in children aged < 2 years. J Pediatr Orthop B 1996;5:123–8.
12. Engesaeter LB, Wilson DJ, Nag D, Benson MK. Ultrasound and congenital dislocation of the hip. The importance of dynamic assessment. J Bone Joint Surg Br 1990;72:197–201.
13. Taylor GR, Clarke NM. Monitoring the treatment of developmental dysplasia of the hip with the Pavlik harness. The role of ultrasound. J Bone Joint Surg Br 1997;79:719–23.
14. Waugh R, McCallum HM, McCarty M, Montgomery R, Aszkenasy M. Paediatric pelvic imaging: optimisation of dose and technique using digital grid-controlled pulsed fluoroscopy. Pediatr Radiol 2001;31:368–73.
15. Kim HT, Kim JI, Yoo CI. Diagnosing childhood acetabular dysplasia using the lateral margin of the sourcil. J Pediatr Orthop 2000;20:709–17.
16. Caffey J, Ames R, Silverman WA, Ryder CT, Hough G. Contradiction of the congenital dysplasia-predislocation hypothesis of congenital dislocation of the hip through a study of the normal variation in acetabular angles at successive periods in infancy. Paediatrics 1956;17:632–41.
17. Smith BG, Kasser JR, Hey LA, Jaramillo D, Millis MB. Postreduction computed tomography in developmental dislocation of the hip: Part I: Analysis of measurement reliability. J Pediatr Orthop 1997;17:626–30.
18. Stanton RP, Capecci R. Computed tomography for early evaluation of developmental dysplasia of the hip. J Pediatr Orthop 1992;12:727–30.
19. MacDonald J, Barrow S, Carty HM, Taylor JF. Imaging strategies in the first 12 months after reduction of developmental dislocation of the hip. J Pediatr Orthop B 1995;4:95–9.
20. McNally EG, Tasker A, Benson MK. MRI after operative reduction for developmental dysplasia of the hip. J Bone Joint Surg Br 1997;79:724–6.
21. Mandel DM, Loder RT, Hensinger RN. The predictive value of computed tomography in the treatment of developmental dysplasia of the hip. J Pediatr Orthop 1998;18:794–8.
22. Laor T, Roy DR, Mehlman CT. Limited magnetic resonance imaging examination after surgical reduction of developmental dysplasia of the hip. J Pediatr Orthop 2000;20:572–4.
23. Tanaka T, Yoshihashi Y, Miura T. Changes in soft tissue interposition after reduction of developmental dislocation of the hip. J Pediatr Orthop 1994;14:16–23.
24. Aoki K, Mitani S, Asaumi K, Akazawa H, Inoue H. Utility of MRI in detecting obstacles to reduction in developmental dysplasia of the hip: comparison with two-directional arthrography and correlation with intraoperative findings. J Orthop Sci 1999;4:255–63.
25. Kim SS, Frick SL, Wenger DR. Anteversion of the acetabulum in developmental dysplasia of the hip: Analysis with computed tomography. J Pediatr Orthop 1999;19:438–42.

26. Kim HT, Wenger DR. The morphology of residual acetabular deficiency in childhood hip dysplasia: Three-dimensional computed tomographic analysis. J Pediatr Orthop 1997;17:637–47.

27. Dutoit M, Zambelli PY. Simplified 3D-evaluation of periacetabular osteotomy. Acta Orthop Belg 1999;65:288–94.

28. Bassett GS, Engsberg JR, McAlister WH, Gordon JE, Schoenecker PL. Fate of the psoas muscle after open reduction for developmental dislocation of the hip (DDH). J Pediatr Orthop 1999;19:425–32.

29. Kocher MS. Ultrasonographic screening for developmental dysplasia of the hip: An epidemiologic analysis (Part I). Am J Orthop 2000;29:929–33.

30. Rosendahl K, Markestad T, Lie RT, Sudmann E, Geitung JT. Cost-effectiveness of alternative screening strategies for developmental dysplasia of the hip. Arch Pediatr Adolesc Med 1995;149:643–8.

31. Clegg J, Bache CE, Raut VV. Financial justification for routine ultrasound screening of the neonatal hip. J Bone Joint Surg Br 1999;81:852–7.

32. Zenios M, Wilson B, Galasko CS. The effect of selective ultrasound screening on late presenting DDH. J Pediatr Orthop B 2000;9:244–7.

33. Gerscovich EO. A radiologist's guide to the imaging in the diagnosis and treatment of developmental dysplasia of the hip. I. General considerations, physical examination as applied to real-time sonography and radiography. Skeletal Radiol 1997;26: 386–97.

34. Gerscovich EO. A radiologist's guide to the imaging in the diagnosis and treatment of developmental dysplasia of the hip. II. Ultrasonography: anatomy, technique, acetabular angle measurements, acetabular coverage of femoral head, acetabular cartilage thickness, three-dimensional technique, screening of newborns, study of older children. Skeletal Radiol 1997;26: 447–5632.

35. Murray KA, Crim JR. Radiographic imaging for treatment and follow-up of developmental dysplasia of the hip. Semin Ultrasound CT MR 2001;22:306–40.

Ultrasound of the hip

8

Eugene G McNally

IRRITABLE HIP IN CHILDREN

Paediatric indications

> **Key point**
>
> A painful irritable hip is one of the commonest causes of nontraumatic, acute paediatric presentations in orthopaedic practice and ultrasound is an important early diagnostic technique.

The previous chapter dealt with the role of ultrasound in the neonatal hip with particular reference to developmental dysplasia. Ultrasound also has important roles in the older child. A painful irritable hip is one of the commonest causes of nontraumatic, acute paediatric presentations in orthopaedic practice and ultrasound is an important early diagnostic technique. The most common cause is transient synovitis, a disorder incompletely understood but with self-limiting and short-lived symptoms. The aim of early diagnosis is to exclude more serious conditions that, if remained unchecked, can cause serious damage to the developing joint. There are therefore two goals for early imaging: to detect the effusion that is the hallmark of transient synovitis and secondly to guide aspiration and thereby to exclude sepsis. The typical clinical history is of a child aged between 5 and 8 years who has been complaining of hip pain and inability for weightbearing, generally of a few days' duration. On clinical examination the hip is painful with some restriction of range of motion.

> **Key point**
>
> The aim of early diagnosis of an irritable hip is to exclude more serious conditions that, if they remain unchecked, can cause serious damage to the developing joint.

Plain films are of no value in the diagnosis of effusion as they have high false positive and false negative rates. The ultrasound examination takes place with the child supine using an anterior approach. The probe is aligned along the femoral neck by rotating it 45° from the sagittal plane. The standard anatomical section demonstrates the femoral neck as a reflective structure, easily identified by the characteristic appearance to the growth plate and femoral head (Figs 8.1–8.3). Anterior to this the reflective anterior capsule can also be identified and the space between them measured. The undistended capsule is concave upwards, above which lies the iliopsoas muscle, which presents a flat upper border. An effusion has a convex upper border, which helps to differentiate it from either the normal joint or iliopsoas mechanism.

Opinion as to what constitutes an abnormal anterior joint space varies. A figure of 2 mm has been suggested as the upper limit of normal (1, 2). An anterior joint space of up to 5 mm is frequently encountered in asymptomatic older children. Asymmetry is therefore the most helpful sign and a greater than 2 mm difference

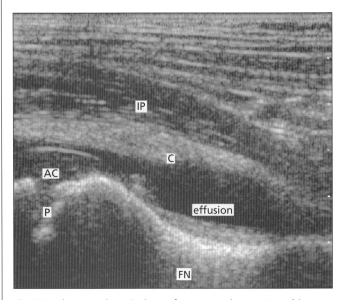

Fig. 8.2 Ultrasound equivalent of anatomy demonstrated in Fig. 8.1. An effusion is clearly demonstrated separating the capsule (C) from the femoral neck (FN). In the young hip the growth plate is easily depicted (P). When the femoral head is fully ossified, articular cartilage (AC) can also be measured with asymmetry between the sides indicative of Perthe's disease. IP = ilipsoas.

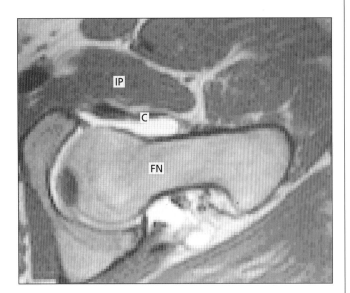

Fig. 8.1 Axial MR arthrogram showing normal anatomical structures. The iliopsoas (IP) overlies the anterior capsule (C). A small quantity of fluid has been introduced into the joint and separates the capsule from the femoral neck (FN).

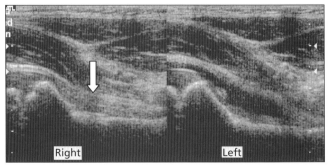

Fig. 8.3 Split screen image comparing the asymptomatic right from the symptomatic and effused left hip. On the right the anterior capsule is concave upwards (arrow) but becomes convex when distended by effusion.

between sides should be regarded as abnormal (3). The absolute measurement is dependent on position as Chan *et al.* found that the maximal distance between the capsule and femoral neck was significantly larger in the extended and abducted hip position than in the neutral hip position (4). Compression of the anterior synovial space may occur if the hip is in the external rotation, and the space may also decompress if the femoral head subluxes as a consequence of the effusion. The subluxed hip can be identified by an increased distance between the acetabular rim and the physis.

Key point

It is not possible to differentiate patients with benign transient synovitis from those with septic arthritis on the basis of clinical and laboratory investigations alone.

The cause of an effusion cannot be determined by its ultrasound appearances, although the largest effusions have been described with benign transient synovitis (2). Differentiating between the more common causes including transient synovitis, Perthe's disease (Fig. 8.4) and septic arthritis can be difficult on clinical grounds. Clinical and laboratory investigations may present a confusing picture, which has lead many to conclude that it is not possible to differentiate patients with benign transient synovitis from those with septic arthritis on the basis of clinical and laboratory investigations alone. Del Becarro *et al.* in a group of 132 children showed that the combination of an erythrocyte sedimentation rate of more than 20 mm per hour and/or a temperature of more than 37.5°C identified 97% of all cases with septic arthritis of the hip (5). A temperature of 37.5°C is relatively common, however; therefore these clinical findings, although sensitive, are nonspecific. There has also been some debate as to whether 97% detection is sufficient given the damage to the growth plate that can occur in those children in whom there is a delayed diagnosis. Kocher and coworkers used four clinical variables to differentiate between septic arthritis and transient synovitis: history of fever, non-weight-bearing, erythrocyte sedimentation rate of at least 40 mm/h, and serum white blood-cell count of more than 12,000 cells/mm^3 (6). The predicted probability of septic arthritis was determined for all combinations of these predictors. The predictive value of one variable alone was very small at 3%. If two positive variables were present the predictive value rose to 40%, considerably less than the 97% reported by the results of Del Becarro *et al.* The presence of three or more variables had a high predictive value of over 90%. Laboratory values in neonates are unreliable (7).

Those who advocate a more conservative approach point to the vast majority of aspirations being sterile and to the risk of inducing septic arthritis as a complication of aspiration. Skinner *et al.* followed 25 patients without aspiration and reported a benign course (8). No cases of septic arthritis were present in the group; therefore it is not possible to say what the false negative rate is in the diagnosis of sepsis. Those in favour of routine aspiration place emphasis on the seriousness of septic arthritis should the diagnosis be delayed and emphasise that the technique is quick with a very low complication profile. There are no reported cases of septic arthritis in the literature arising from diagnostic aspiration. It has been suggested that the trauma of hip aspiration is little more than drawing blood and that it is better to obtain direct evidence of septic arthritis from synovial fluid analysis to indirect evidence from white cell counts or ESR. Bickerstaff, Rydholm and Fink have listed other benefits of direct aspiration including a reduction of intra-articular pressure, which may perhaps reduce the incidence of avascular necrosis, more immediate pain relief and the avoidance of hospital admission (9–11). Although effusions recur following aspiration,

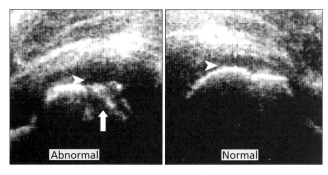

Fig. 8.4 Abnormal ultrasound findings are uncommon in Perthe's disease as the diagnosis is made using plain radiography. Patients will occasionally present with a pain of unknown cause and in these instances fragmentation of the epiphyses (arrow) and thickening of an ossified articular cartilage (arrowheads) in the abnormal compared to the normal side are depicted.

they remain smaller than in unaspirated hips (12). Lee *et al.* have suggested that MRI in the acute phase may have an important role in making this differentiation in a selected group of 22 patients, 8 of them with septic arthritis; characteristic signal abnormalities within the marrow were identified in the patients with septic arthritis as opposed to those with transient synovitis (13). Anecdotal instances of septic arthritis without bone oedema suggest that this sign may be helpful but, like many others, is not completely reliable. Similarly Doppler bloodflow has not been shown to be helpful (14).

> **Practical tip**
>
> Several studies have listed benefits of direct aspiration, including a reduction of intra-articular pressure, which may perhaps reduce the incidence of avascular necrosis, more immediate pain relief and the avoidance of hospital admission.

ASPIRATION TECHNIQUE

In view of the difficulty with differentiating benign from more serous causes of effusion, the protocol in the author's institution is to carry out aspiration in all hips where effusion is demonstrated. The technique for hip aspiration in the child is well described, it is quick and in the vast majority of cases it can be carried out with minimal trauma to the child. Local anaesthetic cream is applied to the skin anterior to the affected hip as soon as the patient presents to hospital. Time spent training the admission nurses in the correct placement of the anaesthetic cream is time well spent. The optimal time between cream placement and the examination depends on the anaesthetic preparation used, but is between 20 and 90 min. Successful aspiration in an accurate and quick fashion depends on accurate identification of the point of maximal anterior capsular distension. This is followed by "blind" aspiration with the confident knowledge of the whereabouts of the effusion (see Chapter 15 and Fig. 15.12).

> **Practical tip**
>
> Time spent training the admission nurses in the correct placement of the anaesthetic cream is time well spent.

Several methods are used in combination to identify the optimal puncture point. They all depend on keeping the probe held vertically over the hip with an angle of 90° to the skin. If the probe is held vertical over the effusion, the aspirating needle can also adopt a vertical approach. The introduction of angles in the determination of the puncture point requires that the same angle be used for aspiration. Replicating angles other than 90° is difficult.

The first method involves marking the central point of each side of the probe when the point of maximal distension has been identified. The intersection of lines joining opposite points identifies the puncture point. A modification of this method used by Berman is to mark the central points of the narrow ends of the probe. The puncture point will lie somewhere along this line. The exact point is determined by moving a small wire, such as a straightened paper clip, and noting where the acoustic shadow crosses the point of maximal joint distension. Another useful technique is to apply a little pressure to the probe once the point of maximal joint distension has been identified. If the probe is quickly removed from the skin, the blanched footplate can be identified and a mark placed at its centre. Combining these techniques means that the aspiration point can be identified with great confidence. The approach to aspiration should be that the probe is not removed until the sonologist is completely confident that the marked point directly overlies the point of greatest joint distension. Once the probe is removed and following a sterile technique, direct puncture with the needle directed at 90° to the skin and without ultrasound guidance will result in aspiration in almost every case. Aspiration should be as complete as possible, as this may result in more rapid resolution of symptoms and a shorter hospital stay (15). There is good correlation between the size of the effusion (9), pain intensity, restriction of movement and intra-articular pressure.

> **Practical tip**
>
> Another useful technique is to apply a little pressure to the probe once the hip's point of maximal joint distension has been identified. If the probe is quickly removed from the skin, the blanched footplate can be identified and a mark placed at its centre.

Transient synovitis

> **Key point**
>
> The diagnosis of transient synovitis is only suggested when other conditions are excluded and signs and symptoms subside without complications.

The diagnosis of transient synovitis is only suggested when other conditions are excluded and signs and symptoms subside without complications (16). Children present with a 1- to 7-day history of pain and limitation of movement. The incidence is approximately 0.2% and up to 25% of those affected will have recurrent episodes (17). A seasonal variation has been reported, with more cases occurring when respiratory tract infection is common, although this has not been the experience in Oxford. Approximately 75% have an effusion, and the condition is more common in boys, with a ratio to girls of 2.5 : 1. There is no side predisposition. Resolution occurs in 75% within two weeks. Persisting effusion is suggestive of another cause, and Perthe's disease should then be considered.

> **Key point**
>
> While resolution occurs within two weeks in 75% of cases, persisting effusion is suggestive of another cause, and Perthe's disease should then be considered.

Septic arthritis

Because of the devastating consequence of bacterial infection within the joint, early diagnosis is mandatory. Typically the effusion is reflective with synovial thickening (18). Particulate matter in the absence of blood should raise suspicion and thickening of the anterior capsule is seen in about 50%. This latter sign also occurs in transient synovitis (19). While the majority of effusions in septic arthritis are reflective, some are echo-free (20). As there are no absolute differences between the clinical presentation or sonographic appearance of a septic effusion and transient synovitis, aspiration has been recommended in all cases. Indeed if septic arthritis is strongly suspected clinically, a negative ultrasound should be followed by MRI.

Perthe's disease

> **Practical tip**
>
> A difference in thickness in the articular cartilage of greater than 3 mm between sides is significant in the diagnosis of Perthe's disease.

The ultrasound findings in Perthe's disease include effusion, thickening of femoral head articular cartilage (21), fragmentation of the epiphysis (Fig. 8.4) and increased femoral anteversion (22). A difference in thickness in the articular cartilage of greater than 3 mm between sides is significant. Cartilage overlying the femoral head only should be included, and it is therefore easier to measure cartilage anteriorly where the femoral head is not covered by acetabulum. The absence of cartilage asymmetry does not exclude the condition, as the disease may be bilateral. An effusion is more common in the early stages of the disease (23). Meyer dysplasia is a condition of unknown aetiology, which is also known as dysplasia epiphysealis capitis femoris. The principal radiological finding is irregularity of the femoral head epiphysis. It is not associated with effusion. Boys are more commonly affected by a factor of 5 and few show symptoms or clinical signs, other than a waddling gait, which is inconsistently found. The postulated pathogenesis is hypoplasia of the proximal femoral epiphyseal cartilage with delayed appearance of single or multiple ossification centres. The process is benign, often bilateral and symmetrical, and the hip always develops normally, so that by age five or six a round epiphysis with a slightly diminished height is seen (24).

Slipped upper femoral epiphysis

Children with slipped upper femoral epiphysis (SUFE) are older than patients with transient synovitis or Perthe's disease: the mean age from several series is 11 years, whereas the mean age in transient synovitis and Perthe's disease is 6.7 years. The ultrasound signs of SUFE include a step in the anterior physeal outline and diminished distance between the anterior acetabular rim and the femoral metaphysis (25, 26). An effusion is seen in about half of the cases and is more likely when the onset is acute. The AP film fails to show displacement in 14% of cases; a frogleg view is necessary to detect these. Ultrasound provides an accurate measurement of the physeal step and the degree of metaphyseal shortening in the acute slip, without the need for ionising radiation (25). In chronic SUFE measurements of the physeal step are unreliable due to metaphyseal remodelling.

> **Practical tip**
>
> In chronic slipped upper femoral epiphysis (SUFE) measurements of the physeal step are unreliable due to metaphyseal remodelling.

The place of MRI in SUFE remains to be established. A T1-weighted image orientated along the femoral neck provides an elegant view of the displacement and the quantity of new bone formation at the site of periosteal stripping. In clear-cut cases MRI probably does not add significantly to the diagnosis but where there is diagnostic difficulty it may have a role.

Miscellaneous

Ultrasound can also be used to assess traumatic separation of the proximal, femoral and humeral epiphysis due to birth injury (27). Sonography has also been used in the assessment of juvenile chronic arthritis (10), particularly in the assessment of the severity of the synovitis prior to synovectomy. In older children with snapping hip, US may show an abnormal jerky movement of the iliotibial band overlying the greater trochanter or gluteus maximus and associated thickening and loss of reflectivity of the iliotibial band (28). Iliopsoas snap can be elicited by initially flexing and externally rotating the hip and then bringing it back to the normal anatomical position. To snap the iliopsoas tendon the patient lies on the unaffected side. The snapping hip is abducted and actively flexed and extended whilst the tendon is observed. A definitive cause will not be found in all cases using ultrasound alone, and many patients require a combination of investigations, with MRI proving particularly efficient (29).

Imaging protocol in children with irritable hip

Plain films are poor at detecting effusions and in children under the age of eight, there is general agreement that ultrasound should be used as the screening method. Over the age of eight radiography should also be employed to detect SUFE. Some centres limit this to a frogleg view only, which is also sufficient for detecting the majority of significant pathologies including Perthe's disease. If an effusion is detected, aspiration provides the most reliable means of excluding sepsis. Following this, if symptoms settle and do not reoccur, then no further imaging is necessary. Patients who fail to settle should be more intensively investigated to exclude Perthe's disease or the uncommon association of osteomyelitis with a sterile effusion.

If no effusion is demonstrated on ultrasound, consideration should be given to other potential causes of pain referred to the hip, such as discitis or other spinal or knee disorder. Clinical hip irritability strongly suggests disease within the hip itself and if symptoms fail to resolve, MRI is indicated.

ULTRASOUND OF THE ADULT HIP

The most common applications for ultrasound in the adult hip are the detection of effusion or synovitis within the hip joint or its adjacent bursae, the assessment of joint replacement and as guidance for the treatment of these findings.

Diagnosis of effusion

The technique for examining the hip has been described elsewhere. Visualisation is rarely as good as in the paediatric hip; nevertheless, the anterior joint space can usually be identified with sufficient clarity to allow accurate measurement (Figs 8.5–8.7). On occasions where the limb is particularly large or swollen, it is appropriate to break the usual golden rule on musculoskeletal imaging and use a lower-frequency curvilinear array probe (Fig. 8.8).

As in children, asymmetry rather than an absolute value is best applied when diagnosing

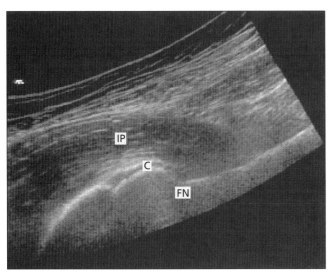

Fig. 8.5 Panoramic view of the adult hip showing the iliopsoas (IP) capsule (C) and femoral neck (FN). The acetabular margin can be depicted. Occasionally good views of the anterior labrum are obtained but ultrasound is unreliable in assessing the pathology within the labrum.

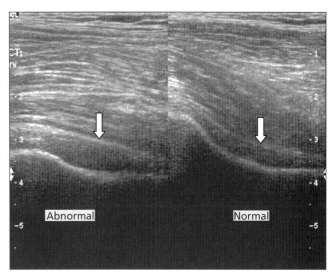

Fig. 8.7 Split screen view comparing asymptomatic and symptomatic hips. The effusion is once again demonstrated by upward convexity of the capsule on the abnormal compared to the normal side (arrows).

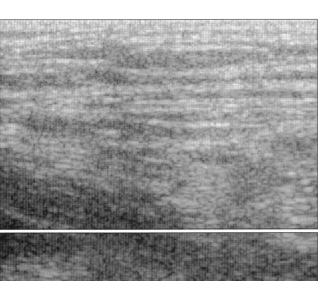

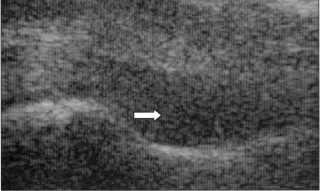

Fig. 8.6 Long-axis view of adult hip showing effusion (arrow).

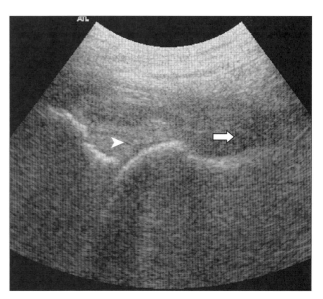

Fig. 8.8 Occasionally in large individuals a curvilinear array probe needs to be used. In this case there is expansion of the joint with a mixture of fluid (arrow) and synovial thickening (arrowhead).

effusion. Unfortunately in many cases, the contralateral hip is not comparable (Fig. 8.7). For example one may wish to assess joint distension in a symptomatic native hip and have an asymptomatic hip implant on the contralateral side (Figs 8.9 and 8.10). An absolute figure of 5 mm along the femoral neck has been suggested by Moss *et al.* (30). The normal distance from the femoral neck to the capsule has been variously reported as 4 to 10 mm. These measurements are really only useful in preoperative patients as postoperatively the size of the pseudocapsule can vary considerably. In the author's experience 5 mm anterior joint space is commonly encountered and is likely to be a sensitive

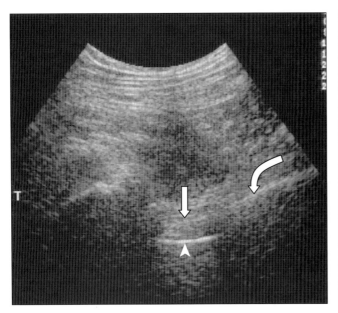

Fig. 8.9 Sagittal image of asymptomatic implanted hip. The easiest landmark to identify is the metallic femoral neck, which is brightly reflective (arrowhead). The reflectivity is different from the bone of the proximal femoral metaphysis (curved arrow), which is also stepped a little anterior from the metalwork. The anterior capsule is depicted by the arrow. Note the normal distance between the arrowhead and arrow representing the pseudocapsule.

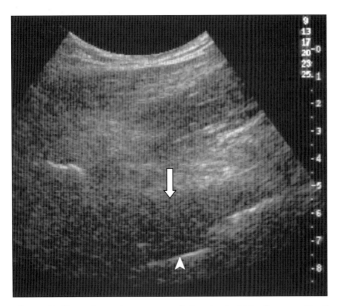

Fig. 8.10 Contralateral symptomatic implanted hip. Same patient as in Fig. 8.9. Note the increased distance between the reflective metalwork (arrowhead) and the anterior capsule (arrow) representing effusion.

but insufficiently specific indicator of disease. A figure of 1 cm is likely to be a better discriminator. This is particularly the case in the postoperative period when disruption of the normal tissue planes can create diagnostic difficulties.

Postoperative complications

In the immediate postoperative period, poorly reflective areas can represent haematoma or sepsis (31), which can be differentiated by US-guided biopsy. Biopsy/aspiration should be limited to patients in whom there is a strong clinical suspicion of sepsis as needling of haematomata is imprudent and may itself induce infection. In the late postoperative period, US can be used to detect effusions and guide biopsies of the pseudocapsule when infection is suspected. Not all effusions signify loosening or infection; some resolve with conservative treatment. Simple aspiration can assist in differentiating septic from aseptic loosening but synovial biopsy is superior. Eisler *et al.* found that the sensitivity of the capsule biopsy cultures was 67%, specificity 68%, positive predictive value 22% and negative predictive value 94%, compared with surgical specimens (32). Conversely, Taylor and Beggs found an accuracy of 95% using fine needle aspiration (33). The optimal technique is to obtain three separate specimens, ideally with a different needle on each occasion. This reduces the possibility of a false negative result.

> **Practical tip**
>
> In the late postoperative period, ultrasound can be used to detect effusions and guide biopsies of the pseudocapsule when infection is suspected.

Other complications following hip replacement include:

Synovial disorders

Ultrasound is not the ideal method of excluding focal diseases of the synovium though they may be encountered during the examination for other reasons. The hip is a common site of involvement of synovial osteochondromatosis and pigmented villonodular synovitis (PVNS). There are no particular ultrasound features of the former entity, although a large synovial mass with isolated joint involvement in the 40-to-60 age group should suggest the diagnosis. Synovial osteochondromatosis is a metaplastic disorder of the synovium whereby prominent synovium villi develop initially cartilaginous and subsequently ossified bodies within them. The ossific and cartilaginous bodies may break off and become loose within the joint. As opposed to PVNS, an ultrasound diagnosis can be suggested when multiple intra-articular loose bodies are detected. A negative ultrasound does not exclude the diagnosis as up to 10% of patients with this condition do not demonstrate calcification within the synovium. Neither diagnosis can be excluded on ultrasound as some areas of the joint cannot be reliably examined. In addition relatively small loose bodies may not cast a sufficiently prominent acoustic shadow to confirm their presence. The differential diagnosis on reflective focii is gas within the joint. Generally moving the hip joint shows a different pattern of response with gas when compared with loose bodies and usually allows them to be reliably distinguished. Using ultrasound to detect the associated effusion has been suggested as a screening test for intra-articular femoral neck fracture when radiographs are negative. Not all fractures are associated with effusion, however.

Bursal disease

Up to 20 different bursae have been described around the hip joint. The most common ones to cause symptoms to bring them to clinical attention are the iliopsoas, trochanteric (Fig. 8.11), subgluteus medius (Fig. 8.12), subgluteus minimus and ischeal bursae (34). The iliopsoas bursa communicates with the hip joint between the iliofemoral and pubofemoral ligaments. It can occasionally extend superiorly into the pelvis and retroperitoneum. Axial imaging with particular attention to the area behind the femoral vessels helps to demonstrate the distended bursa. In the absence of infection, a guided steroid injection may provide relief.

The trochanteric bursa lies deep to the iliotibial tract. Sagittal and axial imaging with the patient in the lateral decubitus position can show the inflamed bursa, which lies on the posterior and posterolateral aspect of the greater trochanter. During the examination, excess pressure should not be applied as it can compress the subtly distended bursa and obscure its detection. Large-volume fluid bursitis is uncommon in this condition other than in postoperative cases. The more common finding is a thin rind of thickened synovium, which can be difficult to differentiate from surrounding tissue. Comparison with the contralateral side can help and suspicion can be confirmed with the clinical finding of local tenderness.

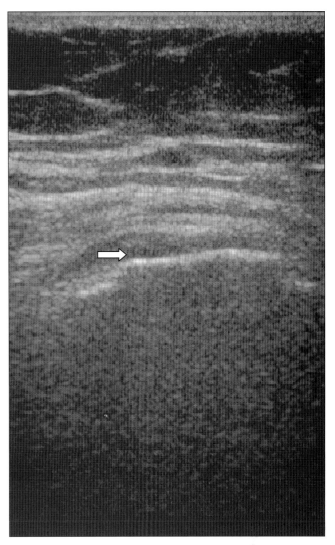

Fig. 8.11 Axial image in the dorsal aspect of the greater trochanter showing a thin rind of poorly reflective tissue representing the minimally distended trochanteric bursa (arrow). Gross distension is uncommon in the presence of trochanteric bursitis and if present usually implies a septic bursitis, bleeding or seroma following a hip implantation.

Trochateric bursitis must be distinguished from subgluteus medius bursitis, which presents a similar clinical picture. The latter is common in the older population where it may be associated with tendinopathy of the gluteus medius tendon. Bursal thickening and focal tenderness occur on the anterolateral aspect of the greater trochanter, helping to distinguish these entities from trochanteric bursitis. There are no studies comparing the respective roles of ultrasound and MRI. The low-grade inflammatory nature of these conditions suggests that fat-suppressed MR imaging would be more sensitive (Figs 8.12 and 8.13), although ultrasound has the advantage of immediate clinical correlation and image-guided therapy. Calcific tendinopathy is not

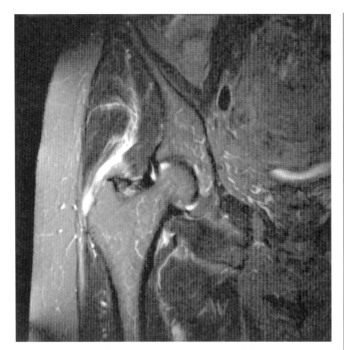

Fig. 8.12 Coronal fat-saturated (STIR) image of the hip demonstrating subgluteus medius bursitis. The gluteus medius bursa lies more laterally and anterior than the trochanteric bursa.

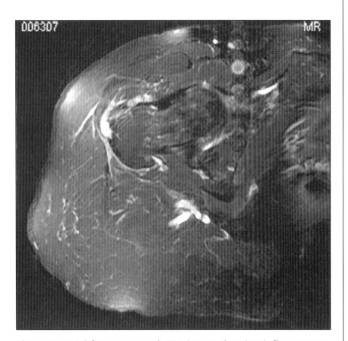

Fig. 8.13 Axial fat-suppressed STIR image showing inflammatory changes surrounding the insertion of the gluteus minimis tendon at its insertion on the anterior aspect of the greater trochanter.

uncommon around the hip and usually affects the gluteus maximus or medius at their insertion into the greater trochanter.

Ischial bursitis is less common than the other bursitises. Clinically pain is felt posteriorly

and may be associated with sciatic symptoms. The bony ischium provides a useful and easily identified ultrasound landmark for the bursa, although the depth of these structures can render them difficult to detect in obese individuals. Care should be taken to accurately identify the sciatic nerve to avoid inadvertent injury during bursal injection.

REFERENCES

1. Adam R, Hendry GM, Moss J, Wild SR, Gillespie I. Arthrosonography of the irritable hip in childhood: A review of 1 year's experience. Br J Radiol 1986;59(699):205–8.
2. Alexander JE, Seibert JJ, Glasier CM, Williamson SL, Aronson J, McCarthy RE, et al. High-resolution hip ultrasound in the limping child. J Clin Ultrasound 1989;17(1):19–24.
3. Terjesen T, Osthus P. Ultrasound in the diagnosis and follow-up of transient synovitis of the hip. J Pediatr Orthop 1991;11(5): 608–13.
4. Chan YL, Cheng JC, Metreweli C. Sonographic evaluation of hip effusion in children. Improved visualization with the hip in extension and abduction. Acta Radiologica 1997;38(5):867–9.
5. Del Beccaro MA, Champoux AN, Bockers T, Mendelman PM. Septic arthritis versus transient synovitis of the hip: The value of screening laboratory tests. Ann Emerg Med 1992;21(12): 1418–22.
6. Kocher MS, Zurakowski D, Kasser JR. Differentiating between septic arthritis and transient synovitis of the hip in children: An evidence-based clinical prediction algorithm. J Bone Joint Surg 1999;81A:1662-70.
7. Klein DM, Barbera C, Gray ST, Spero CR, Perrier G, Teicher JL. Sensitivity of objective parameters in the diagnosis of pediatric septic hips. Clin Orthop Rel Res 1997(338):153–9.
8. Skinner J, Glancy S, Beattie TF, Hendry GM. Transient synovitis: Is there a need to aspirate hip joint effusions? Eur J Emerg Med 2002;9(1):15–8.
9. Bickerstaff DR, Neal LM, Booth AJ, Brennan PO, Bell MJ. Ultrasound examination of the irritable hip. J Bone Jt Surg Ser B 1990;72(4):549–53.
10. Rydholm U, Wingstrand H, Egund N, Elborg R, Forsberg L, Lidgren L. Sonography, arthroscopy, and intracapsular pressure in juvenile chronic arthritis of the hip. Acta Orthop Scand 1986;57(4):295–8.
11. Fink AM, Berman L, Edwards D, Jacobson SK. The irritable hip: Immediate ultrasound guided aspiration and prevention of hospital admission. Arch Dis Child 1995;72(2):110–4.
12. Kesteris U, Wingstrand H, Forsberg L, Egund N. The effect of arthrocentesis in transient synovitis of the hip in the child: a longitudinal sonographic study. J Pediatr Orthop 1996;16(1):24–9.
13. Lee SK, Suh KJ, Kim YW, Ryeom HK, Kim YS, Lee JM, et al. Septic arthritis versus transient synovitis at MR imaging: preliminary assessment with signal intensity alterations in bone marrow. Radiology 1999;211(2):459–65.
14. Fischer SU, Beattie TF. The limping child: epidemiology, assessment and outcome. J Bone Joint Surg Br 1999;81(6): 1029–34.
15. Wilson DJ, Green DJ, MacLarnon JC. Arthrosonography of the painful hip. Clin Radiol 1984;35(1):17–9.
16. Do TT. Transient synovitis as a cause of painful limps in children. Curr Opin Pediatr 2000;12(1):48–51.
17. Alexander JE, Seibert JJ, Aronson J, Williamson SL, Glasier CM, Rodgers AB, et al. A protocol of plain radiographs, hip

ultrasound, and triple phase bone scans in the evaluation of the painful pediatric hip. Clin Pediatr Hagerstown 1988;27(4):175–81.

18. Zieger MM, Dorr U, Schulz RD. Ultrasonography of hip joint effusions. Skeletal Radiol 1987;16(8):607–11.

19. Miralles M, Gonzalez G, Pulpeiro JR, Millan JM, Gordillo I, Serrano C, *et al*. Sonography of the painful hip in children: 500 consecutive cases. Am J Roentgenol 1989;152(3):579–82.

20. Shiv VK, Jain AK, Taneja K, Bhargava SK. Sonography of hip joint in infective arthritis. Canad Assoc Radiol J 1990;41(2): 76–8.

21. Robben SG, Meradji M, Diepstraten AF, Hop WC. US of the painful hip in childhood: Diagnostic value of cartilage thickening and muscle atrophy in the detection of Perthes disease. Radiology 1998;208(1):35–42.

22. Terjesen T. Ultrasonography in the primary evaluation of patients with Perthes disease. J Pediatr Orthop 1993;13(4): 437–43.

23. Wirth T, LeQuesne GW, Paterson DC. Ultrasonography in Legg-Calve-Perthes disease. Pediatr Radiol 1992;22(7): 498–504.

24. Khermosh O, Wientroub S. Dysplasia epiphysealis capitis femoris: Meyer's dysplasia. J Bone Jt Surg Ser B 1991;73(4): 621–5.

25. Kallio PE, Lequesne GW, Paterson DC, Foster BK, Jones JR. Ultrasonography in slipped capital femoral epiphysis. Diagnosis and assessment of severity. J Bone Joint Surg Br 1991;73(6):884–9.

26. Terjesen T. Ultrasonography for diagnosis of slipped capital femoral epiphysis. Comparison with radiography in 9 cases. Acta Orthop Scand 1992;63(6):653–7.

27. Diaz MJ, Hedlund GL. Sonographic diagnosis of traumatic separation of the proximal femoral epiphysis in the neonate. Pediatr Radiol 1991;21(3):238–40.

28. Choi YS, Lee SM, Song BY, Paik SH, Yoon YK. Dynamic sonography of external snapping hip syndrome. J Ultrasound Med 2002;21(7):753–8.

29. Wunderbaldinger P, Bremer C, Matuszewski L, Marten K, Turetschek K, Rand T. Efficient radiological assessment of the internal snapping hip syndrome. Eur Radiol 2001;11(9): 1743–7.

30. Moss SG, Schweitzer ME, Jacobson JA, Brossmann J, Lombardi JV, Dellose SM, *et al*. Hip joint fluid: Detection and distribution at MR imaging and US with cadaveric correlation. Radiology 1998;208(1):43–8.

31. Foldes K, Gaal M, Balint P, Nemenyi K, Kiss C, Balint GP, *et al*. Ultrasonography after hip arthroplasty. Skeletal Radiol 1992;21(5):297–9.

32. Eisler T, Svensson O, Engstrom CF, Reinholt FP, Lundberg C, Wejkner B, *et al*. Ultrasound for diagnosis of infection in revision total hip arthroplasty. J Arthroplasty 2001;16(8):1010–7.

33. Taylor T, Beggs I. Fine needle aspiration in infected hip replacements. Clin Radiol 1995;50:149–52.

34. Meaney JF, Cassar Pullicino VN, Etherington R, Ritchie DA, McCall IW, Whitehouse GH. Ilio-psoas bursa enlargement. Clin Radiol 1992;45(3):161–8.

Ultrasound of knee pathology

9

Lawrence Friedman and Rethy K Chhem

INTRODUCTION

The past decade has seen dramatic advances in musculoskeletal ultrasound (MSUS). This is partly due to significant advantages in technology, with the introduction of high-resolution linear broadband multifrequency transducers, but also as a result of the realisation amongst both imagers and clinicians of the tremendous advantages and usefulness of this modality in evaluating the musculoskeletal system. The most common applications for MSUS of the knee include sport-related injuries, rheumatology, the evaluation of fluid collections and soft-tissue masses (1–5). The specific structures best suited for ultrasound assessment include tendons, muscles and ligaments as well as periarticular soft-tissue masses and fluid collections (6–10). Unlike MRI, ultrasound is able to demonstrate the fibrillar microanatomy of tendons and ligaments, the fascicular pattern of nerves and the pennate structure of muscles (1–5, 8). It must be emphasised that menisci, articular cartilage, bone marrow and the anterior cruciate ligament cannot be accurately assessed by ultrasound and are better evaluated by other imaging modalities, namely magnetic resonance imaging (MRI) (1, 6).

The most important advantage of ultrasound is the ability to dynamically examine, in real time, the exact point of clinical tenderness elicited from the patient and to use the probe as a further important intimate tool in the examination process.

RECENT DEVELOPMENTS

Ultrasound examination of the knee requires a systematic approach. The controlateral knee can easily and effectively be used for comparison (11). A constant interaction between patient and examiner allows for a smooth and better examination. Patient compliance is generally better in response to verbal instructions rather than patient manoeuvring, which can often be painful to the patient after an acute injury. Dynamic assessment includes flexion, extension and rotation of the knee. The free and mobile transducer head becomes an extension of the hand and allows one to interrogate the patient's maximal point of tenderness in all planes. The sonologist is also able to palpate masses and apply graded compression to soft-tissue masses and fluid collections.

For a complete examination of the knee four approaches are employed. These include anterior, posterior, medial and lateral. The examination can be tailored depending on the history and clinical findings. Longitudinal, transverse or oblique scans are obtained, depending on the anatomic orientation or pathology encountered. The structure or disease process is recorded in at least two planes.

ANTERIOR KNEE

Anterior knee pain is one of the most common complaints encountered by the orthopaedist. The causes are numerous and identifying the correct diagnosis can be frustrating to both patient and doctor. Ultrasound provides an excellent non–invasive method in helping to differentiate patellofemoral problems including the common chondromalacia patella, from abnormalities involving the extensor mechanism.

The patient is usually positioned supine or sitting on an examination bed with the knee comfortably partially flexed 15° to 20°, with some support under the knee, usually a pillow or sponge. This eliminates the normal curve of the relaxed quadriceps and patellar tendons and the medial and lateral retinacula. These structures become stretched and parallel to the skin and transducer surface, thereby minimizing artifacts caused by anisotropy. Flexion and extension, however, become important in assessing tears of the extensor mechanism with respect to apposing ends of the torn tendon ends in the case of complete tears. The suprapatellar bursa may contain a small amount of physiological fluid usually no more than 2 mm (6, 12).

Pathology will be discussed under the broad categories related to the extensor mechanism, bursitis and soft-tissue masses.

Extensor mechanism

The ability to assess the tendons of the extensor mechanism of the knee is one of the particular strengths of ultrasound as it is able to accurately evaluate the fibrillary parallel nature of the

normal tendons (8). The normal appearance consists of parallel hyperechoic structures (Fig. 9.1), with the exception of the insertion, which is seen as a hypoechoic area, not to be mistaken as a tear.

Tendinopathy

In tendons without a synovial sheath such as the quadriceps and patellar tendons, tendinopathy may appear as increased tendon size and decreased echogenicity, either focal or generalised (Figs 9.2 and 9.3). Hypoechoic structures can develop between the normal echogenic fibrils and peritendinous fluid may also be present. The appearance represents what is termed tendinosis, a histologic term referring to intrasubstance mucoid degeneration, with the absence of inflammatory cells, when histologically evaluated (8). In chronic stages, calcifications, nodularity and heterogenous echotexture can occur (1, 2, 6, 8). The appearance is thought to represent a precursor in the evolution of progression to a tendon tear. For discussion purposes the above appearance will be referred to as tendinosis, while the presence of additional hyperaemia elicited on power Doppler will be referred to as tendonitis, demonstrating an active inflammatory but not infective process (13). Included under this section will be jumper's knee and Osgood–Schlatter disease.

Jumper's knee. This condition, thought to represent a focal area of tendinosis progressing to a nonhealed partial tear of the proximal patellar tendon, is seen in young adults who participate in sports requiring repetitive extensor mechanism activity such as in kicking or jumping activities and can lead to significant continuing disability. It is thought to represent a reparative process resulting from mucoid degeneration due to repeated tearing of the collagen fibres or poor vascularity of the tendinous insertion of the

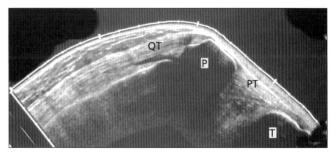

Fig. 9.1 EFOV of extensor mechanism taken with knee in partial extension showing the normal quadriceps tendon (QT), patella (P), patella tendon (PT) and tibia (T).

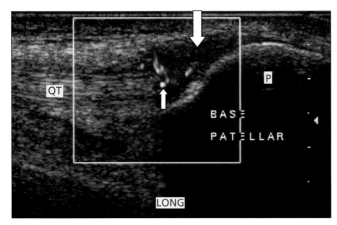

Fig. 9.2 Focal tendinosis in the distal quadriceps tendon seen as a hypoechoic region (large arrow) in the longitudinal plane (LONG). Doppler demonstrates moderate hyperaemia, denoting active inflammation (small arrow). Quadriceps tendon (QT), patella (P). (Printed with permission from Jag Dhanju CCMSU Ultrasound, Toronto, Canada.)

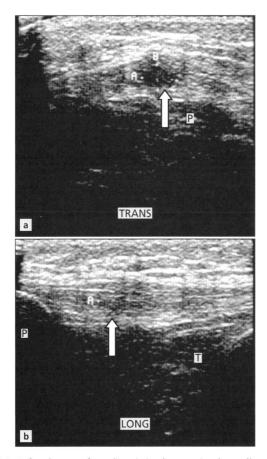

Fig. 9.3 A focal area of tendinosis in the proximal patella tendon seen as a hypoechoic area between the tendon fibrils (arrows) in both the short (TRANS) and longitudinal (LONG) planes. Patella (P), tibia (T). The location in this patient is unusual as tendinosis usually occurs at the proximal and less commonly at the distal end of the patella tendon.

patellar tendon. The proximal and, less commonly, the distal patellar tendon can be affected. Ultrasound usually demonstrates a focal swelling of the posterior aspect of the proximal patellar

tendon associated with a focal anechoic area (Fig. 9.4) (14). Chronic cases develop calcifications (Fig. 9.5) usually close to the cartilaginous insertion (2, 4). Bony spurs may develop at the inferior pole of the patella. Doppler is excellent for assessing the presence and severity of inflammation (Fig. 9.6).

Osgood-Schlatter's disease. This is a chronic stress-related condition of the distal patellar tendon that is common in adolescents and results from an avulsive force upon the tibial apophysis transmitted via the patellar tendon secondary to quadriceps contraction. The process is likely due to repeated microtrauma to the patellar tendon at its site of insertion to the greater tuberosity. Males are affected more commonly than females and there is often a history of involvement with sports. Tenderness over the region is often appreciated clinically, accompanied by soft-tissue swelling. Ultrasound (Fig. 9.7) usually detects swelling of the soft tissues and cartilage of the tibial apophysis, thickening of the distal patellar tendon and distention of the infrapatellar bursa

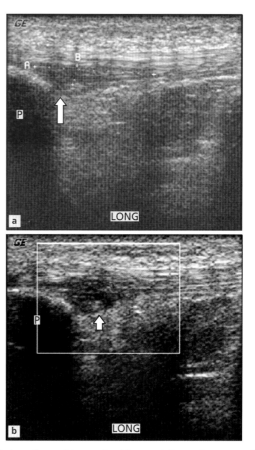

Fig. 9.4 A patient with proximal jumper's knee demonstrating a focal hypoechoic area in the posterior aspect of the proximal patella tendon in the long axis (long arrow) consistent with tendinosis. Note the mild hyperaemia with Doppler (short arrow). Patella (P).

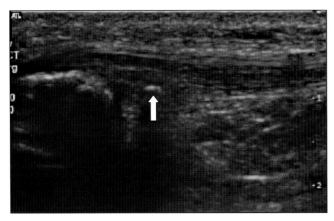

Fig. 9.5 Calcification (arrow) in proximal patellar tendinopathy. (Courtesy Dr EG McNally.)

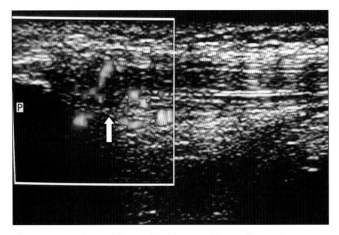

Fig. 9.6 A patient with proximal jumper's knee illustrating marked hyperaemia with power Doppler in the long axis (arrow). Patella (P).

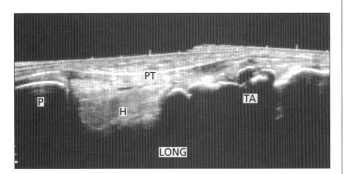

Fig. 9.7 EFOV of a patient with Osgood–Schlatter's disease in the long axis with knee in extension showing irregularity and fragmentation of the distal tibial apophysis. Patella (P); tibial apophysis (TA), patella tendon (PT), Hoffa's fat (H).

(2, 4, 15, 16). Power Doppler can accurately detect inflammation within the tendon or bursa. At a later stage bone fragmentation can occur at the hyperechoic ossification centre (Fig. 9.8). The same appearance can be seen at the distal patella and proximal patella tendon known as Sinding–Larson–Johansen syndrome (14).

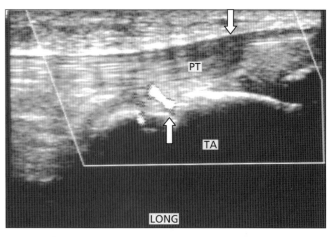

Fig. 9.8 The same patient as that in Fig. 9.6 with a close-up of the distal patella tendon taken in the long axis. Note the hypoechoic swollen distal patella tendon (PT) and the hyperaemia in the retropatella bursal region (arrow). Tibial apophysis (TA).

Partial tears and splitting of the tendon can be seen distally (Fig. 9.9). This can more rarely progress to a full thickness tear.

Tendon tears

Tendon tears, both partial and full thickness, are well suited to ultrasound evaluation. Partial tears present as clefts or relatively well-defined confluent anechoic areas with disruption of the normal fibrillar echotexture. Full thickness tears appear as separated ends of the tendon, tendon retraction, thickened tendon ends and interruption of the regional tendon fibres. Fluid or haematoma may fill the site of the tear and may mask a full thickness tear (6). As a result it may be difficult to visualise the tendon, especially when the haematoma contains echogenic material similar in echogenicity to the tendon itself. Graded careful compression and dynamic assessment of the tendon in flexion and extension will help to differentiate a partial from a full thickness tear.

Patellar tendon. Complete tears of the patellar tendon are the least common cause of extensor mechanism disruption (1). In contrast to quadriceps rupture patients are usually younger, male and typically involved in active sports. The most common site of injury is at the proximal patellar attachment, and patients usually have a history of patellar tendinosis or jumper's knee. Mid-substance tears are less common and usually result from a single severe acute traumatic episode with the knee in flexion. Distal rupture

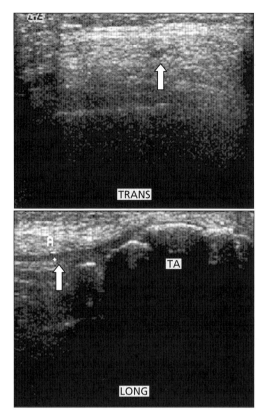

Fig. 9.9 Transeverse (TRANS) and longitudinal (LONG) scans of the distal patella tendon showing the presence of a split in the tendon, one of the known complications of Osgood–Schlatter's disease (arrows). Tibial apophysis (TA).

at the tibial insertion is also uncommon and is usually seen with previous surgery, local steroid injection or Osgood–Schlatter's disease. Acute tears benefit from end-to-end anastomosis while more chronic tears over 6 weeks old require more extensive surgery.

Quadriceps tendon. Quadriceps tendon ruptures result from trauma, are idiopathic or are due to a wide variety of systemic disorders, which include gout, systemic lupus erythematosus, rheumatoid arthritis, diabetes, hyperparathyroidism and chronic renal failure (1). These occur most often at the tendo-osseous junction. The central and anterior segment usually tears first, approximately 2 cm above the upper pole of the patella. Most of the tears are incomplete, usually only involving the rectus femoris tendon. Clinical diagnosis is usually difficult and delay in diagnosis has been reported ranging from 14 days to 1 year after injury. This may complicate repair. Patients give a history of being unable to lift their leg. A suprapatellar defect can be visualised on clinical examination in large tears. Ultrasound can aid in prompt diagnosis (17), as

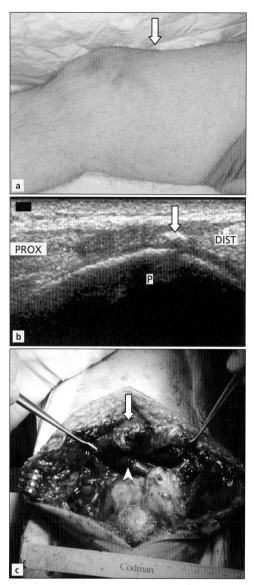

Fig. 9.10 A patient with a complete tear of the quadriceps tendon. The clinical picture (a) shows the concave defect in the suprapatellar region. Ultrasound (b) in the long axis demonstrates the complete tear of the quadriceps tendon with separation of the proximal (PROX) and distal (DIST) end of the torn tendon. Note the avulsed bony fragment off the patella (P) (arrow). Surgical correlation (c) illustrates the torn tendon with separation of the proximal (arrow) and distal tendons (arrowhead).

surgical intervention must occur early in full thickness tears (Fig. 9.10).

> **Key point**
>
> Quadriceps tendon ruptures occur most often at the tendo-osseous junction. The central and anterior segment usually tears first, approximately 2 cm above the upper pole of the patella.

Muscles

The normal muscle bundles are hypoechoic surrounded by perimysium, which is composed of connective tissue, blood vessels, nerves and adipose tissue often referred to as fibroadipose tissue (6). A sheath of dense connective tissue called the epimysium surrounds the entire muscle. A fascial layer may separate single muscles or groups of muscles. The internal structure of a muscle varies on its designated function. Fibres parallel to the long axis are best suited for movement over a long distance. Unipennate, bipennate and circumpennate are better suited for lifting weight over shorter distances. These different patterns can easily be appreciated with ultrasound (Fig. 9.11). In the long axis the pennate pattern is well defined, while in the short axis taken at 90° the appearance resembles that of Van Gogh's "starry sky", due to the hyperechoic septate (that simulate stars) superimposed on the hypoechoic muscle (seen as the night sky).

> **Practical tip**
>
> Dynamic evaluation of muscle injuries during contraction and relaxation is important.

Ultrasound has proven a valuable tool in the assessment of muscle injuries and can accurately diagnose partial (Fig. 9.12) or full thickness tears. Dynamic evaluation during contraction and relaxation is important. Comparison with the other side for altered configuration and asymmetry is helpful. On ultrasound partial tears appear as anechoic clefts or hypoechoic collections within the muscle belly. Partial tears have been graded from I to III, a system helpful in the assessment of healing. Grade I may be normal or contain small haematomas, may be less than 1 cm, and usually heals in 2–3 weeks. Grade II involves less than one-third of the muscle, with

haematomas less than 3 cm, and usually heals in 3–6 weeks. Grade III involves more than one-third of the muscle, with haematomas larger than 3 cm, and usually takes months to heal. It can be difficult to differentiate a high-grade partial tear from a complete tear. In the case of complete tears, the ends of the ruptured muscle are separated, with rounded margins and a loss of regional fibre continuity (18). Clinically complete tears present with a palpable gap in the region of abnormality.

> **Key point**
>
> Partial tears are graded as follows: Grade I may be normal or contain small haematomas, may be less than 1 cm, and usually heals in 2–3 weeks. Grade II involves less than one-third of the muscle, with haematomas less than 3 cm, and usually heals in 3–6 weeks. Grade III involves more than one-third of the muscle, with haematomas larger than 3 cm, and usually takes months to heal.

An important entity to recognise is a pseudotumour of the rectus femoris muscle. This is usually due to a partial tear of this muscle and should not be confused with a true neoplasm. Patients present with a mass that decreases in size with time as apposed to a neoplasm that usually becomes larger. There may or may not be a history of trauma.

> **Practical tip**
>
> An important entity to recognise is a pseudotumour of the rectus femoris muscle, which is usually due to a partial tear of this muscle and should not be confused with a true neoplasm.

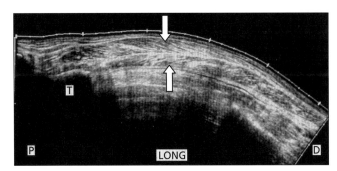

Fig. 9.11 Longitudinal scan (LONG) of the medial gastrocnemius muscle in the calf using the EFOV showing the normal bipennate pattern (arrows). Proximal (P), distal (D), tibia (T).

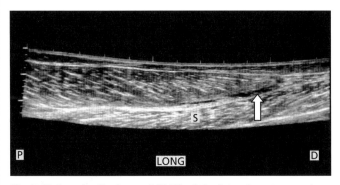

Fig. 9.12 Longitudinal scan (LONG) of the lateral gastrocnemius muscle in the calf using the EFOV demonstrating an aponeurotic tear at the musculo-tendinous junction (arrow). Proximal (P), distal (D), soleus (S).

Bursa

Pathology of the bursae around the knee can be a source of acute and chronic knee pain. Inflammation can result from chronic or acute trauma, haemorrhage, infection and inflammatory or infiltrative disorders. The anatomic bursae related to the anterior aspect of the knee include the prepatellar bursa and superficial and deep infrapatellar bursa. Included in this discussion will be the suprapatellar bursa, considered by many authors to represent a synovial recess, given its continuity with the joint cavity, in most instances. A small amount of fluid in the suprapatellar and infrapatellar bursae is considered normal and should not be reported as bursitis.

The lining of the normal bursa on ultrasound appears hyperechoic, with a slit-like hypoechoic centre. The hypoechoic centre is usually less than 2 mm (6, 19).

Prepatellar bursa

This bursa is located superficial to the distal patella and proximal to one-third of the patellar tendon. Bursitis of the prepatellar bursa is usually occupational and in this case caused by prolonged kneeling (Fig. 9.13). Power Doppler may reveal an inflammatory response. It is important to note that chronic prepatellar bursitis may calcify.

Infrapatellar bursitis

Ultrasound is helpful in differentiating infrapatellar bursitis from patella tendinosis. The presence of a small amount of fluid in the deep infrapatellar bursa is physiological and should not be mistaken as bursitis (Fig. 9.14).

> **Practical tip**
>
> The presence of a small amount of fluid in the deep infrapatellar bursa is physiological and should not be mistaken as bursitis.

Suprapatellar bursitis and synovitis

This bursa develops as a separate synovial space, between the rectus femoris tendon and the femur. From the fifth fetal month, the septum between the bursa and knee joint may perforate. Communication between the bursa and the knee joint is present in 85% of adults. Power Doppler is useful for highlighting the inflammatory process.

Synovial thickening and proliferation can be seen within a bursa, particularly in association with rheumatoid arthritis (Fig. 9.15) and other inflammatory conditions. Echogenic material within may indicate haemorrhage, inflammation or infection. If there is a high clinical suspicion of infection, ultrasound-guided aspiration is a quick, easy and safe method that can be employed for exclusion. Fibrous adhesions may occur in long-standing effusions. Ultrasound can be helpful when clinical differentiation in separating bursitis from tendon problems may be difficult.

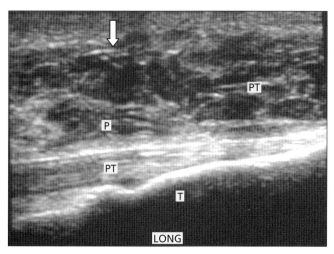

Fig. 9.13 Superficial distal prepatellar bursitis (arrow) in the long axis (LONG) showing thickening of the prepapatellar bursa (P). Distal patella tendon (PT), proximal tibia (T).

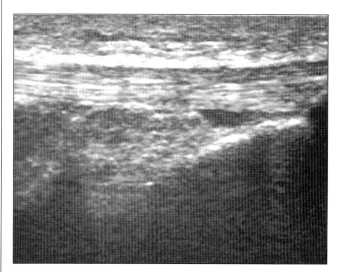

Fig. 9.14 Longitudinal scan of the distal patella tendon with a small amount of fluid in the deep distal infrapatellar bursa. This is normal and should not be mistaken as pathological.

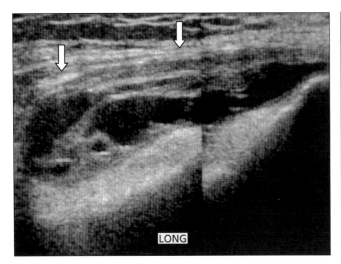

Fig. 9.15 Longitudinal (LONG) scan of the suprapatellar bursa in a patient with rheumatoid arthritis using dual windows to create an extended field of view, showing synovial thickening (arrows).

Cartilage

MRI remains the investigation of choice for chondromalacia and osteochondral pathology. In advanced cases, however, ultrasound can detect cartilage loss or thinning (Fig. 9.16) on the anterior surface of the patella and/or femur (6, 19). Irregularity of the surface, fissuring and rarely defects in the cartilage can be seen.

Chondrocalcinosis affecting the menisci or articular hyaline cartilage can easily be detected using high-frequency probes (Fig. 9.17). Ultrasound may even be more sensitive in the detection of hyaline cartilage calcifications, but less sensitive in the detection of meniscal calcifications, when compared to radiography (3).

Occult fractures and bone

With the development of high-resolution probes ultrasound is proving an excellent method for detecting occult fractures (20, 21). The strong echogenic surface of bone can be used advantageously in order to detect the abnormality. A fracture is seen as a break in the pristine echogenic surface of the bony cortex and may be accompanied by a periosteal reaction and/or hypoechoic haematoma. Doppler can further aid by demonstrating abnormal flow and hyperaemia at the fracture site (Fig. 9.18). Acute fractures including stress fractures can be detected on ultrasound before becoming visible on plain film radiographs (Fig. 9.19). Furthermore there is easy correlation with the patient's point

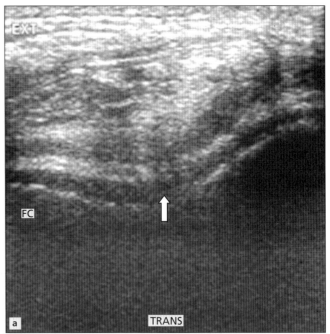

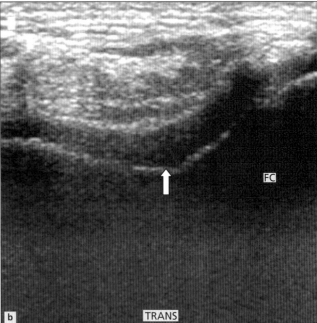

Fig. 9.16 Ultrasound of femoral articular hyaline cartilage in the knee taken in the short axis (TRANS), demonstrating thinning and loss of the cartilage on the right due to degenerative change with normal-appearing cartilage on the left shown for comparison (arrows). Femoral condyle (FC).

of maximum tenderness. Incidental bone lesions, such as enchondromas or bone cysts (Fig. 9.20), can also occasionally be seen (1, 22).

MEDIAL KNEE

The patient lies supine with the knee slightly flexed. The hip is mildly flexed and externally

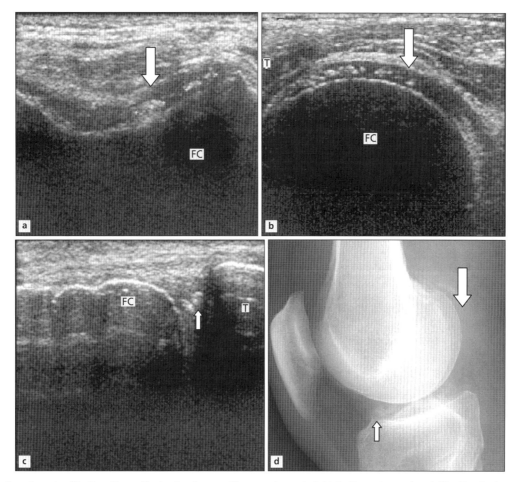

Fig. 9.17 Chondrocalcnosis affecting the articular hyaline cartilage and menisci. Note the echogenic calcification in femoral hyaline cartilage in the axial (a) and longitudinal (b) planes (large arrows). Calcification in the anterior horn of the medial meniscus is shown in (c) (small arrow). The calcifications are verified on plain X-ray (d) by large and small arrows, respectively. Femoral condyle (FC), tibia (T).

rotated. Alternatively, this can be performed with the patient in the lateral decubitus position. In this position, the medial collateral ligament, anterior horn medial meniscus and pes anserine tendon and bursa can be appreciated.

Medial collateral ligament (MCL)

The medial collateral ligament represents the second most commonly encountered injury after the anterior cruciate ligament. The anterior cruciate ligament (ACL) is best addressed using MRI, while MCL injuries are easily and accurately diagnosed with ultrasound and therefore represent the most common ligament injury diagnosed in the authors' practice. It must be remembered that MCL injuries can occur in conjunction with ACL injuries as the third most common group of ligamentous injuries. Injuries to the MCL occur as a result of valgus stress to the knee. The extent of injury to the MCL is usually first evaluated with clinical examination. Isolated tears of this ligament are assessed using a valgus stress technique. Tears of this ligament combined with ACL tears can be tested by valgus stress with external rotation.

On ultrasound the MCL is seen as a structure 8–10 cm in length extending from the medial femoral condyle superiorly to its tibial attachment distally. It has a broad and flat morphology and is composed of superficial and deep layers. The superficial portion appears as a long broad hyperechoic dense fibrillar connective tissue structure. The deep component is composed of the hyperechoic meniscofemoral and meniscotibial ligaments, but can appear more hypoechoic than the superficial layer due to the

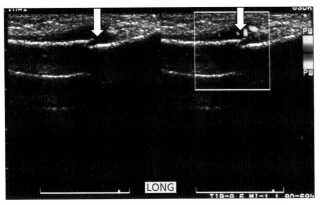

Fig. 9.18 An occult fracture of the distal fibula is seen as a break in the normal echogenic bony surface in the long axis (LONG), accompanied by a periostreal reaction and hypoechoic haematoma (arrow). Note the hyperaemia at the fracture site.

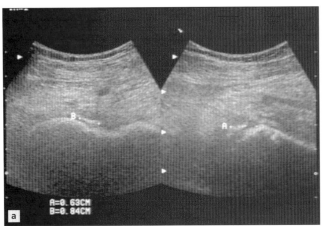

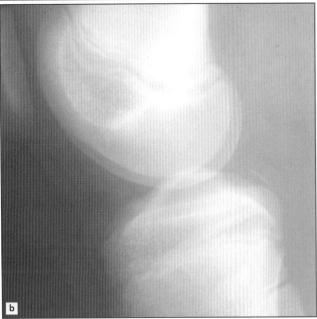

Fig. 9.19 An avulsed bony fragment seen as a hyperechoic linear area adjacent to the posterior aspect of the proximal tibial plateaux on both the short and longitudinal planes. This was initially seen on ultrasound (a) and confirmed with plain film radiographs (b), consistent with a Segond fracture.

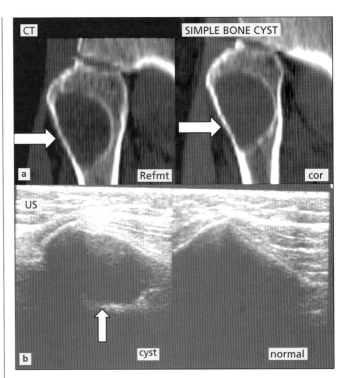

Fig. 9.20 A simple bone cyst was initially diagnosed during routine ultrasound examination of the knee, in the head of the fibula. (b) The cyst is seen bottom left on ultrasound (US) showing posterior wall enhancement compared to the normal right side (arrow). (a) The cyst was confirmed by CT using corresponding coronal (cor) reformatted (Refmt) images (arrows).

orientation of the fibres, which are less parallel to the transducer surface, resulting in anisotropy. A hypoechoic layer of connective tissue separates these layers (6).

The deep component is more commonly torn than the superficial one (19). If the tear is isolated to the deep component, haematoma and/or fluid can displace the superficial layer laterally. Tears of the MCL have a similar appearance on ultrasound as has been described for MRI (23). The ultrasound appearance follows the same principles seen on MRI, including discontinuity of fibres. It is important to make a careful comparison with the normal side for subtle changes in tendon thickness and heterogeneity (11). A grade I tear represents a minimal tear or strain, without clinical instability. It is thought to represent a predominantly periligamentous injury, with microfibre tearing. The ultrasound findings include hypoechoic fluid, due to oedema and haemorrhage parallel to the MCL. A grade II injury represents intrasubstance rupture, with increased instability. Hypoechoic fluid can be identified with associated ligament thickening (Fig. 9.21). A grade III injury represents a complete tear, with significant instability clinically and fibre discontinuity. On ultrasound, hypoechoic fluid and/or haematoma is seen filling the site of the tear, with disruption of both superficial and deep components (Fig. 9.22). In chronic injuries absence or marked thinning of the ligament may be seen. A thick focal area of calcification within the ligament can also indicate a chronic injury (Fig. 9.23) commonly known as Pellegrini–Stiedi syndrome (19). A triad of injury, consisting of torn MCL, medial meniscus tear and ACL rupture and known as O'Donoghue's triad, is often present. This triad at times can also include injury to the femoral attachment of the medial patellofemoral ligament, making it a tetrad (24).

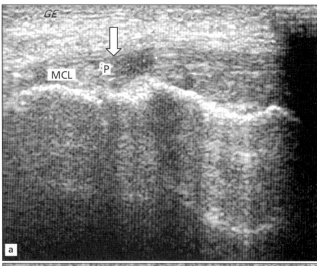

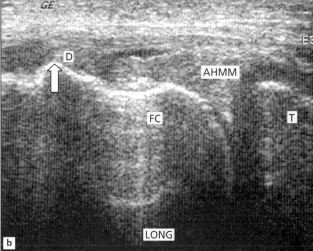

Fig. 9.22 Longitudinal scan (LONG) of the medial collateral ligament (MCL) showing a complete tear of the superior aspect of the MCL seen as a hypoechoic defect between the retracted proximal (P) (top arrow) and distal (D) (bottom arrow) ends of the tendon. Femoral condyle (FC), proximal tibia (T), anterior horn medial meniscus (AHMM).

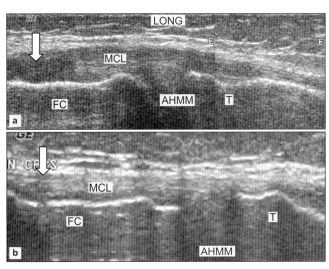

Fig. 9.21 (a) Longitudinal scan of the medial collateral ligament (MCL) demonstrating a partial hypoechoic tear of the superior and deep component of the ligament (arrow). (b) Note the comparative normal MCL (arrow). Femoral condyle (FC), proximal tibia (T), anterior horn medial meniscus (AHMM).

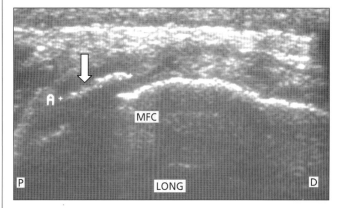

Fig. 9.23 Longitudinal scan (LONG) of the medial collateral ligament illustrating calcification (arrow) consistent with Pellagrini-Stiedi syndrome. Medial femoral condyle (MFC), proximal (P), distal (D).

Medial meniscus

> **Key point**
>
> MRI remains the investigation of choice in evaluating meniscal pathology.

MRI remains the investigation of choice in evaluating meniscal pathology. Ultrasound, however, can elicit meniscal pathology during routine examination of the knee. This requires high-resolution equipment and thorough technique and is more difficult in large and obese patients.

Patients with medial meniscal pathology present with symptoms that vary from a click to locking of the knee and pain overlying the medial joint region. Often point tenderness is elicited when the probe overlies the meniscus in question. The medial meniscus is at least three times more commonly torn than the lateral meniscus (24).

> **Practical tip**
>
> Often point tenderness is elicited when the probe overlies the meniscus in question.

The normal shape and ultrasound appearance of the menisci is of a triangular-shaped hyperechoic structure positioned at the joint space. Artefacts are common (Fig. 9.24) and contralateral comparison is very helpful in

delineating pathology and excluding artefacts. Tears appear as anechoic or hypoechoic linear clefts within the meniscus (Fig. 9.25). Less commonly hyperechoic tears have been described (6). Posterior and peripheral tears are easiest to visualise. Small internal or medial tears can easily be missed, which is part of the limitation of ultrasound in assessing internal derangement. In degeneration, the meniscus can appear swollen and more hypoechoic. Cystic areas can become visible (2). The meniscus often extrudes out of the joint space and can contain small cysts within. Meniscal chondrocalcinosis produces a linear hyperechoic appearance (2, 3). Since the calcifications are small they do not produce posterior acoustic shadowing. Plain film radiographs should be available at the time of the examination and will help to confirm the diagnosis.

> **Practical tip**
>
> Meniscocapsular separation is often seen between the joint capsule and the medial meniscus, particularly with respect to the posterior horn.

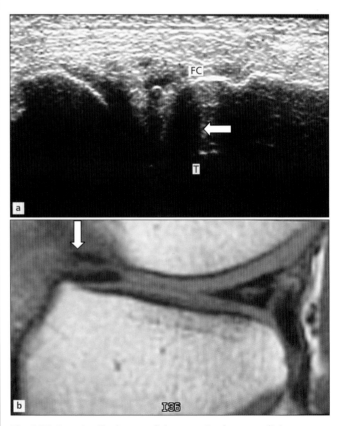

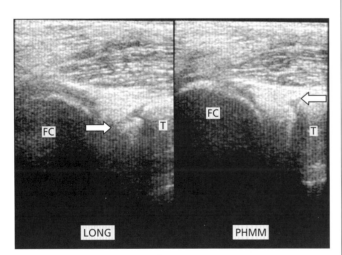

Fig. 9.24 Longitudinal scan of the posterior horn medial meniscus (PHMM) showing a normal hypoechoic oblique cleft not to be mistaken as a tear (arrows). Femoral condyle (FC), tibia (T).

Fig. 9.25 Longitudinal scan of the anterior horn medial meniscus, showing a tear seen as a horizontal hypoechoic cleft (arrow), with corresponding MR (arrow). Proximal tibia (T), medial femoral condule (FC).

Meniscocapsular separation is often seen between the joint capsule and the medial meniscus, particularly with respect to the posterior horn. The area of separation appears as a hypoechoic linear focus between the meniscus and the capsule. This separation can be accentuated by knee flexion and should be assessed in both the short and long axes. This condition must be differentiated from other pathologies, namely, a vertical meniscal tear, the normal recess above or below the peripheral border of the meniscus, a meniscal cyst and bursitis.

Meniscal cysts

Meniscal cysts are encapsulated mass lesions containing synovial-like fluid and can be seen incidentally during imaging or present as a clinically palpable mass. Usually these appear as hypoechoic or partially anechoic structures, adjacent to the meniscus (Fig. 9.26), and may contain debris or septations (25). In long-standing lesions the appearance can become complex, such that they mimic a solid lesion (Fig. 9.27) (26).

These cysts are most often associated with horizontal degenerative tears, but can be associated with other tears. The cyst can also be as a result of primary myxoid degeneration of the meniscus. Bone erosion can occur with large chronic cysts due to the pressure effects (25).

Pes anserine bursa

The pes anserine bursa is located between the conjoined distal tendons of the sartorius, gracilis and semitendinosus muscles and the tibial insertion of the tibial collateral ligament. Clinically patients present with bursitis, resulting in swelling and tenderness inferior to the anteromedial portion of the distal tibia. This condition is commonly observed in athletes and obese people, secondary to arthritis or idiopathically (3). Ultrasound is valuable in separating pes anserine tendinopathy seen as a thickened hypoechoic tendon from bursitis which demonstrates a distended fluid-filled bursa (Fig. 9.28).

LATERAL KNEE

The patient lies supine with the knee flexed and the leg slightly internally rotated. Alternatively, the lateral decubitus position may be employed. The structures seen include the popliteal tendon, iliotibial band, conjoint tendon [biceps femoris tendon and fibular (lateral) collateral ligament], fibular collateral ligament and anterior horn lateral meniscus.

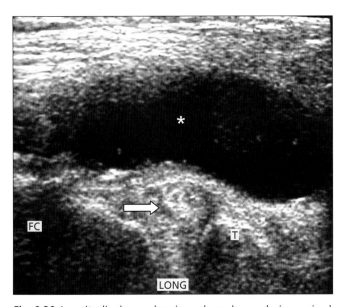

Fig. 9.26 Longitudinal scan showing a large hypoechoic meniscal cyst (asterisk) associated with a tear of the anterior horn medial meniscus seen as a hypoechoic cleft (arrow). Medial femoral condyle (FC), proximal tibia (T).

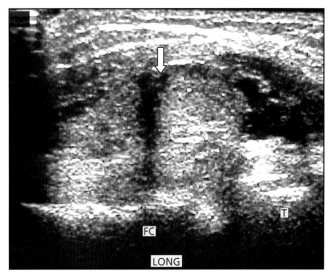

Fig. 9.27 Complex meniscal cyst in long axis resembling a solid mass (arrow). Femoral condyle (FC), proximal tibia (T).

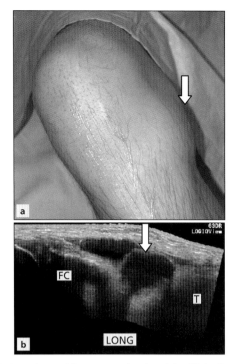

Fig. 9.28 A patient with pes anserine bursitis. Clinically swelling is identified along the superior and medial aspects of the knee (arrow). Ultrasound in the long axis (LONG) illustrates the corresponding hypoechoic distended bursa (arrow). Femoral condyle (FC), proximal tibia (T).

Lateral collateral ligament

The lateral collateral ligament (LCL) is a much thinner structure than the MCL, is approximately 5–7 cm in length and is extracapsular in location. It is a thin band-like structure that is hyperechoic but may appear hypoechoic in its course due to its oblique orientation (19). It runs obliquely, anteriorly and superiorly from the head of the fibula to the lateral femoral condyle. At the head of the fibula it has a conjoined insertion with the biceps femoris tendon that is located more posteriorly. The biceps femoris tendon has a hyperechoic appearance due to its more parallel course to the skin surface and transducer. These structures can therefore be separated by angling the transducer in the correct plane (horizontal to the skin surface for biceps femoris and more obliquely for the LCL). The iliotibial band is a thin hyperechoic structure identified anterior to the LCL, inserting on Gerdy's tubercle on the tibia.

The LCL ligament injury is usually the result of direct varus stress to the knee (24). Injury to the LCL is less common than to the MCL. With a partial tear the ligament is thickened and hypoechoic with loss of definition of the fibrillar pattern (Fig. 9.29). Surrounding fluid may be present. A complete tear of the ligament appears

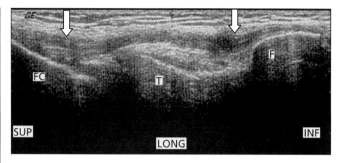

Fig. 9.29 A grade I to II strain of the lateral collateral ligament (LCL) is seen in the long axis (LONG) as a swollen hypoechoic thickened tendon (arrows). Femoral condyle (FC), proximal tibia (T), head of proximal fibula (F), superior (SUP) and inferior (INF).

as complete discontinuity with or without a focal hypoechoic haematoma (1).

Iliotibial band

> **Key point**
>
> Runner's knee, or iliotibial band syndrome, is caused by chronic abrasion of a bursa located between the iliotibial band and the lateral femoral condyle.

The iliotibial band is the very strong, long tendon of the tensor fascia lata muscle. Runner's knee, or iliotibial band syndrome, is caused by chronic abrasion of a bursa located between the iliotibial band and the lateral femoral condyle. This condition is commonly seen in runners who exercise on a banked surface. Ultrasound usually shows an oedematous bursa with or without an effusion. In chronic cases, fusiform thickening to the iliotibial band (Fig. 9.30) and an effusion in the tendon sheath become visible (27).

Biceps femoris

Biceps femoris tendinopathy is seen as diffuse hypoechoic thickening of the tendon. A tear in this tendon is not uncommon and may vary in size from small to a complete rupture. Both tendinosis and rupture usually involve the distal portion of the tendon but can extend proximally to the musculotendinous junction (3).

Lateral meniscus

Tears and cysts have a similar appearance as described earlier in the section "Medial Meniscus". Meniscal cysts are not uncommonly found in the lateral and medial menisci. Clinically, however, these are more obvious laterally. A common pitfall is to diagnose the small hiatus where the popliteal tendon leaves the joint capsule as a cyst. This hiatus commonly fills with fluid when the knee joint contains an effusion.

Popliteus tendon

Popliteus tendinosis is similar in appearance to that of previously described tendons. Popliteus tendon tears are uncommon (Fig. 9.31).

Peroneal nerve

The peroneal nerve is one of the terminal branches of the sciatic nerve. Tumours of the nerve or nerve sheath can occur and can be differentiated from other masses by identifying a normal or thickened nerve entering and or leaving the tumour (Fig. 9.32).

POSTERIOR KNEE

The patient lies supine with both feet hanging over the edge of the bed. In this position, the structures visualised include the popliteal fossa and vessels, the nerves, the medial head of the

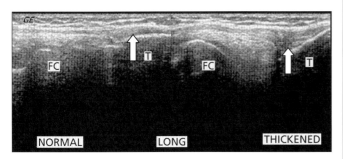

Fig. 9.30 A runner with a chronic thickened iliotibial band seen on the right (arrow) in the long axis (LONG). Note the normal appearance on the left in the comparative knee (arrow). Femoral condyle (FC), proximal tibia (T).

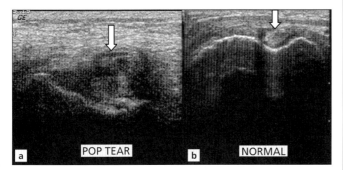

Fig. 9.31 A tear of the popliteus tendon is demonstrated on the left with complete disruption of the normal appearance associated with marked swelling and a hypoechoic defect (arrow). Note the normal echogenic tendon on the right within the popliteus fossa (arrow).

gastrocnemius, semimembranosus and semitendinosus tendons, the posterior cruciate ligament and posterior horns medial and lateral menisci.

Semimembranosus-gastrocnemius bursa

In athletes distension of an otherwise normal semimembranosus-gastrocnemius bursa can commonly occur and is clinically asymptomatic. Enlargement of this bursa is also not uncommonly seen in children presenting as a posterior knee lump. In most patients there is no underlying pathology and most will spontaneously regress. A Baker's cyst represents enlargement of this bursa. To correctly diagnose this entity it is important to identify the neck of the bursa containing fluid between the medial gastrocnemius muscle and semimembranosus tendon. This represents the channel of communication with the joint space, and the route for potential decompression of large intra-articular fluid collections of any aetiology. Baker's cysts most commonly occur at the medial aspect of the popliteal fossa, but can cross the midline and tract superiorly and inferiorly. The shape is variable but usually has a rounded appearance at the cephalad and caudad ends (Fig. 9.33). A pointed end usually represents rupture. Rupture usually occurs inferiorly, although superior rupture has been described (3). A ruptured baker's cyst can mimic deep venous thrombosis (DVT). Both conditions should always be excluded in patients with deep calf pain. Like the suprapatellar bursa a Baker's cyst can undergo various changes, including synovial hypertrophy and act as a reservoir for loose bodies (Fig. 9.34). The cysts can also be complicated by haemorrhaging and calcification (28).

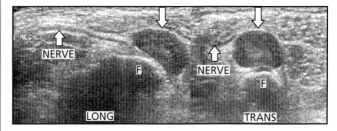

Fig. 9.32 A surgically proven schwannoma of the peroneal nerve seen on ultrasound as a solid eccentric hypoechoic lesion continuous with the peroneal nerve (short arrows) in both the longitudinal (LONG) and transverse (TRANS) planes (arrows), overlying the head of the fibula (F).

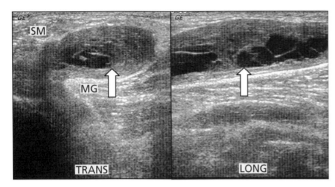

Fig. 9.33 Typical appearance of a Baker's cyst located between the medial head of gastrocnemius (MG) and semimembranosus (SM) with rounded ends (arrow) in both the short (TRANS) and long (LONG) axes. Note a few internal echoes most likely due to haemorrhage.

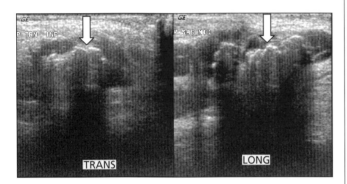

Fig. 9.34 Multiple echogenic loose bodies are identified within a Baker's cyst (arrows), seen in both the short (TRANS) and long (LONG) axes.

Key point

To correctly diagnose a Baker's cyst it is important to identify the neck of the bursa containing fluid between the medial gastrocnemius muscle and semimembranosus tendon.

Key point

A pointed end of a Baker's cyst usually represents rupture.

Posterior cruciate ligament (PCL)

The posterior cruciate ligament is an intracapsular, extrasynovial structure that is regarded to be stronger than the anterior cruciate ligament. Injury to the PCL represents 5 to 20% of all ligament injuries of the knee. In about 25%, such injuries are isolated to the posterior cruciate, which are usually treated conservatively. In instances where the ligament is avulsed from

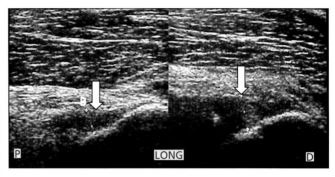

Fig. 9.35 Longitudinal scan (LONG) of the posterior cruciate ligament showing a normal ligament on the left and a thickened ligament due to a partial tear on the right. Proximal (P), distal (D).

its tibial attachment, the bone is reattached surgically. Clinically the quadriceps activation test remains the most popular method for diagnosing a tear.

A number of different mechanisms may be responsible for injuries to the PCL (24). The most common mechanism is a posterior force on an anterior flexed knee, as seen in motor vehicle accidents and typically results in a mid-substance tear of the ligament. A fall on a flexed knee, particularly with the foot in plantar flexion, can result in injury to the PCL. Additional mechanisms relate to hyperflexion, in which a femoral avulsion fracture may occur, and to a posterior force placed on a hyperextended knee, a mechanism that is associated with additional ligamentous and capsular injuries.

On ultrasound the PCL is seen as an oblique (and therefore due to anisotropy) hypoechoic band running from the posterior tibial spine to the lateral margin of the medial femoral condyle (29). Careful comparison with the normal side in cases of suspected injury is important to distinguish between normal and abnormal PCL size. An oedematous ligament has a hypoechoic heterogenous appearance (Fig. 9.35). A complete tear can be seen as discontinuity or absence of the ligament (29, 30).

Anterior cruciate ligament (ACL)

The ACL is an intracapsular extrasynovial structure, which is generally regarded as weaker than the PCL (24). Injuries to the ACL are frequent and may be seen involving other ligamentous structures and adjacent bones. The Segond fracture involving an avulsion cortical injury off the lateral tibial plateau is usually

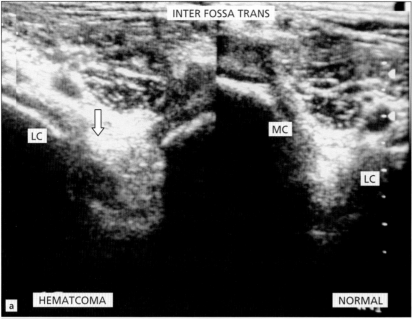

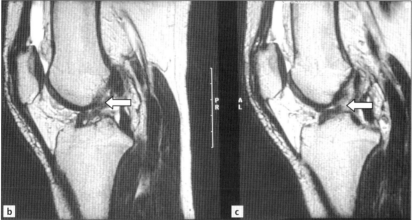

Fig. 9.36 An acute tear of the anterior cruciate ligament. The haematoma adjacent to the medial aspect of the left femoral condyle identified in the intercondylar fossa (inter fossa) (arrow) is an indirect sign of an anterior cruciate ligament tear. Note the corresponding normal intercondylar fossa. An MRI using fast spin echo T2W sequences in the sagittal oblique plane, done within a week, confirms the ACL tear (arrow). Medial femoral condyle (MC) and lateral femoral condyle (LC).

associated with an ACL tear. Ultrasound with careful attention to detail can detect this avulsed bony fragment that can be missed on plain film radiographs if the oblique projections are not obtained.

Many of the ACL injuries are related to sports (24). Deceleration, jumping and cutting are important mechanisms, and the injury may be associated with an audible pop in about 40% of patients (24). The Lachman test, by demonstrating translation of the tibia, allows clinical diagnosis of the ACL.

On ultrasound the ACL can be seen as a hypoechoic linear structure beneath the patella using an oblique sagittal anterior approach with the knee flexed at least 60° (2). This approach is limiting because most patients with an acute injury are unable to adopt this position. In the setting of an acute injury with haemarthrosis a

hypoechoic focal collection along the lateral margin of the femoral intercondylar notch has been reported to have a sensitivity of 91% and a specificity of 100% in the diagnosis of acute rupture of the ACL (31). The hypoechoic collection is thought to represent a haematoma (Fig. 9.36) at the femoral attachment of the ACL (31). Tears at the tibial attachment and chronic tears are not visualised with this method and are best detected by MRI. The sensitivity of this method is best in the first 4 to 5 weeks and decreases with time due to resorption of the haematoma (31).

Popliteal vessels

Although an aneurysm of the popliteal artery is not that common, this diagnosis should always

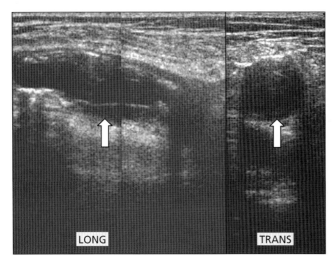

Fig. 9.37 A patient with a popliteal artey aneurysm seen in both the long (LONG) and short (TRANS) axes with a small amount of thrombus (arrows).

be excluded when assessing a popliteal fossa mass (2, 3), especially when a pulsating mass is palpated clinically. An aneurysm is seen as a well-defined cystic mass (Fig. 9.37), with turbulent flow. Pulsed Doppler should be used. The diagnosis can become more problematic when an aneurysm becomes thrombosed. In patients with popliteal pain a DVT of the popliteal vein should be excluded by employing a compression technique as well as colour venous flow. Thrombosis is seen as a popliteal vein that fails to compress and demonstrates absence of normal venous flow on colour Doppler and pulsed Doppler.

MISCELLANOES PATHOLOGY INVOLVING SYNOVIUM, CARTILAGE AND BONE

Arthritis

Routine radiography remains the mainstay in the investigation of arthritis of the knee. Today this can be further supplemented by MRI and ultrasound (1). Findings on ultrasound are, however, not specific for the type of arthritis (1, 32).

Rheumatoid arthritis (RA)

Findings on ultrasound incorporate both intra- and extra-articular pathology (1). The most common intra-articular findings include joint effusion, synovial hypertrophy, synovial cysts, marginal erosions and subchondral cysts. The

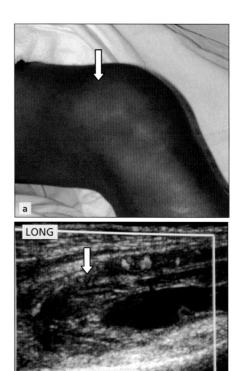

Fig. 9.38 A patient with rheumatoid arthritis showing swelling of the suprapatellar region on clinical examination (small arrow). Ultrasound of the suprapatellar bursa in the long axis (LONG) demonstrates synovial thickening with moderate hyperaemia on Doppler (large arrow).

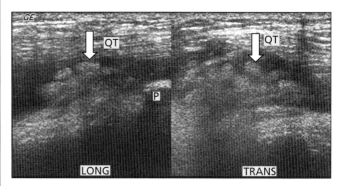

Fig. 9.39 A patient with long-standing rheumatoid arthritis illustrating rice bodies in the suprapatella bursa in both the long (LONG) and short (TRANS) axes (arrows). Patella (P), quadriceps tendon (QT).

degree of synovial inflammation can be assessed by employing colour or power Doppler (Fig. 9.38). Extra-articular findings include tendinosis, tenosynovitis, tendon rupture and bursitis. Small fibrous bodies (rice bodies) related to more chronic rheumatoid arthritis can develop and are usually seen in the fluid-distended suprapatellar bursal region (Fig. 9.39) or within a Baker's cyst associated with RA. It must be noted that at times it can be difficult to differentiate between loose bodies and rice bodies on ultrasound.

Osteoarthritis (OA)

In young patients it is mostly athletes that are referred for ultrasound assessment. Ultrasound is used to focus on synovial thickness, determine synovial fluid volume, determine presence of impingement of plica or synovium, detect osteochondral injury (patellofemoral and tibiofemoral), assess menisci and locate osteochondral loose bodies. In the more elderly ultrasound is used to detect osteochondral defects due to osteonecrosis.

> **Practical tip**
>
> For athletes referred for assessment, ultrasound can be used to focus on synovial thickness, determine synovial fluid volume, determine presence of impingement of plica or synovium, detect osteochondral injury (patellofemoral and tibiofemoral), assess menisci and locate osteochondral loose bodies.

Gout

Ultrasound findings in gout include synovial hypertrophy and joint effusion. In chronic patients bony erosions are visible. Gouty tophi are seldom seen in the knee.

Chondrocalcinosis

Chondrocalcinosis may involve and affect the hyaline cartilage or the menisci. The menisci have been previously discussed. In hyaline cartilage the typical finding on sonography is the presence of hyperechoic linear areas of calcification parallel to the bone surface (Fig. 9.17). This condition may be associated with thinning of the cartilage, joint effusion and synovial proliferation. Ultrasound may be more sensitive than plain film radiographs in the detection of hyaline articular cartilage (3).

Pigmented villonodular synovitis (PVNS)

This condition may present as a focal solitary intra-articular lesion (Fig. 9.40), or when an effusion is present, sonography may demonstrate nodular synovial masses of PVNS.

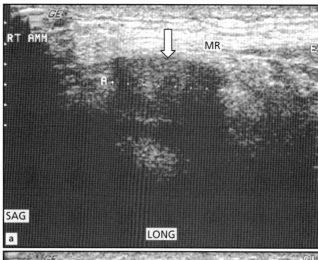

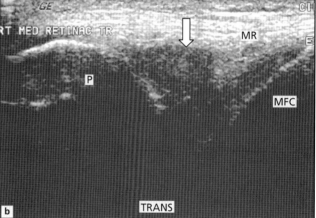

Fig. 9.40 A patient with a surgically proven solitary PVNS located in the anterior and medial recesses of the knee. Ultrasound shows a hypoechoic well-defined lesion beneath the medial retinaculum (MR) and between the patella (P) and medial femoral condyle (MFC) in both the long (LONG) and short (TRANS) axes (arrows). The diagnosis was given as part of the differential diagnosis preoperatively.

Ganglia

> **Key point**
>
> Ganglia are lined by connective tissue, usually contain mucinous fluid, rarely communicate with the joint and may result from myxoid degeneration of the connective tissue. In distinction synovial cysts are lined by synovial cells, contain fluid and may or may not communicate with the joint.

Ganglia are lined by connective tissue, usually contain mucinous fluid and rarely communicate with the joint (3). They may be as a result of myxoid degeneration of the connective tissue. In distinction synovial cysts are lined by synovial cells, contain fluid and, may or may not communicate with the joint. They may originate as herniations of synovium from either the joint or adjacent bursa. The clinical presentation of these two entities is the same and is related to their mass effect.

Ganglia around the knee joint most commonly arise from the superior tibiofibular joint (3) where they can involve or compress muscles, tendons or nerve sheaths. They are mostly asymptomatic, but rarely patients present with ankle drop or weakness due to the ganglia compressing or originating in the peroneal nerve sheath. They are not uncommonly intra-articular arising from the ACL or PCL. These are usually located within the intercondylar fossa adjacent to the cruciate ligaments. Clinically patients may experience knee swelling or restriction of movement associated with pain, due to trapping of the ganglion within the cruciate ligaments. Ganglia may also be seen to be arising from Hoffa's fat pad and surround the patella, presenting as anterior knee swelling or anterior soft-tissue mass (Fig. 9.41).

On ultrasound ganglia present as well-defined often lobulated hypoechoic lesion with or without septations. The lesion may connect to the adjacent tibiofibular joint by a thin stalk within the peroneus longus or tibialis anterior muscle. If clinically warranted the diagnosis can be confirmed by ultrasound-guided aspiration (33). The fluid usually contains thick sticky material with a high concentration of hyaluronic acid.

Bone tumours

These are best assessed by MRI. Ultrasound, however, can be useful in delineating the relationship of the soft-tissue mass or in the case of a cartilage-capped exostosis, or bony lesion, to the neurovascular bundle or adjacent articulating joint (22). Ultrasound can also help direct the biopsy needle away from any adjacent nerves or vessel structures such as the patella (33). Furthermore, ultrasound can help to exclude a DVT, especially in the popliteal vein, as a result of chronic compression.

Loose bodies

Loose bodies appear as echogenic structures of varying size and are usually seen in the most dependent region of an articulate recess (Fig. 9.42) or in a Baker's cyst. They are more readily

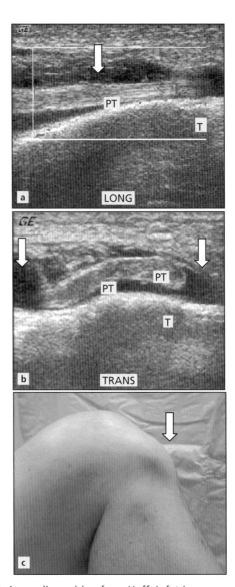

Fig. 9.41 A ganglion arising from Hoffa's fat is seen on ultrasound, surrounding the inferior aspect of the patella in both the (a) long (LONG) and (b) short (TRANS) axes (arrows), presenting clinically (c) as an anterior knee mass (arrow). Patella tendon (PT), proximal tibia (T).

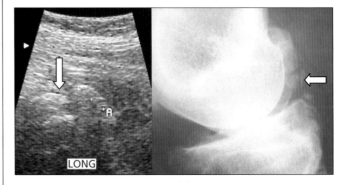

Fig. 9.42 A longitudinal scan (LONG) of the popliteal fossa demonstrating echogenic loose bodies (arrows) with plain film correlation (arrows).

visualised in the presence of a joint effusion in which they are seen as mobile structures separate from the underlying articular bone. The mobility is usually well demonstrated by graded compression. Loose bodies may result from fragmentation of osteophytes in osteoarthritis, an osteochondral fracture or bone and cartilage destruction in a neuropathic joint or associated with synovial osteochondromatosis (34, 35).

POSTOPERATIVE KNEE

The most common indications for assessing the postoperative knee (2) include postoperative haematoma or abscess (Figs 9.43 and 9.44); the

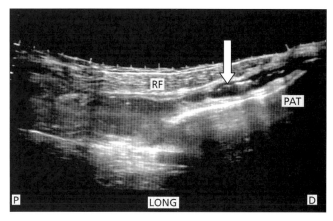

Fig. 9.44 A patient with an abscess localised to vastus intermedius, seen on the EFOV. The abscess is seen as a hypoechoic area with bright internal echoes in the long axis (LONG) due to associated gas collection (arrow). Proximal (P), distal (D), patella (PAT), rectus femoris muscle (RF).

ruling out of postoperative DVT; evaluation of the repaired tendon, ligament or reconstruction; and reaction to foreign body including stitches and hardware. In the case of an excised Baker's cyst, recurrence or leaking from the original stem can be assessed.

PAEDIATRIC KNEE

The paediatric knee presents an ideal site for imaging as the joints are largely composed of cartilage, rather than bone. Cartilage provides a great acoustic window for assessing intra- and extra-articular pathology. It is important not to confuse cartilage with fluid (Fig. 9.45). This is a common pitfall when first evaluating pediatric patients.

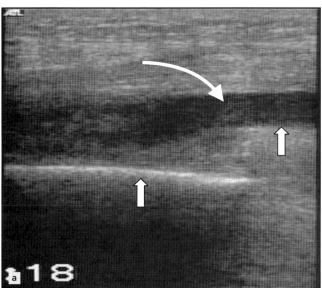

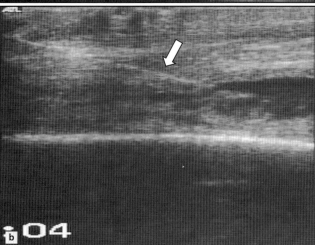

Fig. 9.43 Septic arthritis post total knee replacement. Note in (a) reflective surface of implant on sagittal image (arrow) and effusion with debris (curved arrow) and in (b) needle correctly positioned to aspirate (arrow). The particulate matter within the effusion is better appreciated in (b).

> **Practical tip**
>
> It is important not to confuse cartilage with fluid, which is a common pitfall when first evaluating paediatric patients.

Trauma

Ultrasound is excellent for assessing fractures in the newborn and child when X-rays can be confusing. Salter type I and other subtle fractures can easily be detected on ultrasound. In the older child and adolescents stress fractures can be detected before plain film radiographs become positive.

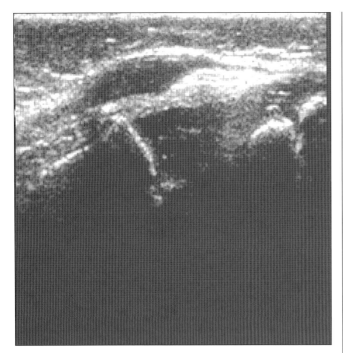

Fig. 9.45 A normal knee in an infant taken in the longitudinal plane. The hypoechoic cartilage in the patella, tibial and femoral epiphyses seen in infants and children should not be mistaken as fluid.

Effusion

Knee effusions are easily detected on ultrasound. If there is any clinical suspicion for infection (Fig. 9.46), the fluid can be accessed using ultrasound guidance.

Cysts

A spontaneous Baker's cyst presenting as a popliteal mass is not an uncommon finding (Fig. 9.47). These are usually not associated with any underlying pathology and usually spontaneously regress without any treatment. Less commonly there is an association with juvenile rheumatoid arthritis (JRA).

Synovitis

Ultrasound is very useful in differentiating synovial thickening related to synovitis from fluid, thereby preventing unnecessary intervention.

Bursitis

As in the adult ultrasound is excellent for evaluating the bursa.

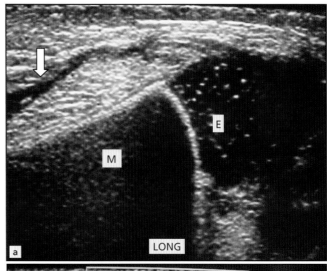

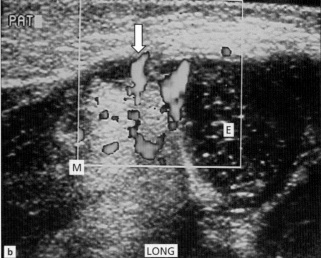

Fig. 9.46 A 3-month-old with a small suprapatellar effusion identified on ultrasound in the long axis (LONG), associated with moderate hyperaemia on Doppler (arrows). On aspiration using ultrasound guidance this proved to be a staphylococcus septic arthritis. Metaphysis (M), epiphysis (E).

Traction apophysitis

Osgood–Schlatter's disease and Sinding–Larsen–Johansson as previously discussed are well delineated with ultrasound.

Tendinopathy

This is similar to findings in the adult.

Discoid meniscus

Ultrasound is able to diagnose a discoid meniscus by careful comparison with the normal side (Fig. 9.48). These occur more commonly laterally and are seen in 1.5 to 4.5% of individuals. They are prone to tear, are associated more commonly with meniscal cysts and present clinically with a snapping knee.

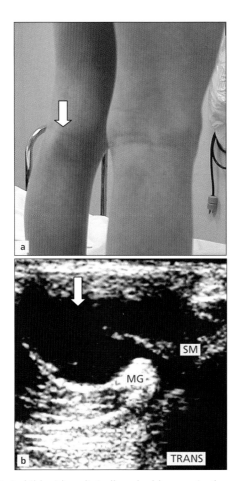

Fig. 9.47 A child with a clinically palpable mass in the popliteal fossa (arrow) was shown to have a Baker's cyst on ultrasound, extending between the medial head of gastrocnemius (MG) and semimembranosus (SM) in the short axis (TRANS) (arrow).

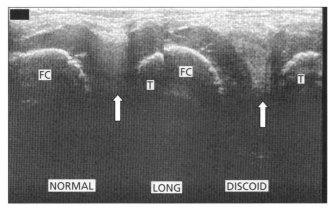

Fig. 9.48 A child presenting with a snapping knee was shown to have an enlarged discoid meniscus (right) (arrow) in the long axis (LONG). The comparative normal meniscus is shown (left) (arrow). Femoral condyle (FC), proximal tibia (T).

REFERENCES

1. Chhem RK, Cardinal E, editors. Guidelines and gamuts in musculoskeletal ultrasound. New York: Wiley; 1999.
2. Grobbelaar N, Bouffard JA. Sonography of the knee: A pictorial review. Semin Ultrasound CT MR 2000;21:231–74.
3. Ptasznik R. Ultrasound in acute and chronic knee injury. Radiol Clin North Am 1999;37:797–830.
4. Bouffard JA, Dhanju J. Ultrasonography of the knee. Semin Musculoskeletal Radiol 1998;2:245–70.
5. Friedman L, Finlay K, Jurriaans E. Ultrasound of the knee. Skeletal Radiol 2001;30:361–77.
6. van Holsbeeck M, Introcaso JH. Musculoskeletal ultrasound. St. Louis: Mosby-Year Book; 2001.
7. Barberie JE, Wong AD, Cooperberg PL, Carson BW. Extended field-of-view sonography in musculoskeletal disorders. Am J Roentgenol 1998;171:751–7.
8. Fornage BD, Rifkin MD. Ultrasound examination of tendons. Radiol Clin North Am 1998;26:87–107.
9. Newman JS, Adler RS, Bude RO, Rubin JM. Detection of soft-tissue hyperemia: Value of power Doppler sonography. Am J Roentgenol 1994;163:385–9.
10. Gibbon WW, Wakefield RJ. Ultrasound in inflammatory disease. Radiol Clin North Am 1999;37:633–51.
11. Lee JI, Song IS, Jung YB, Kim YG, Wang CH, Yu H, et al. Medial collateral ligament injuries of the knee: Ultrasonographic findings. J Ultrasound Med 1996;15:621–5.
12. Brys P, Velghe B, Geusens E, Bellemans J, Lateur L, Baert AL. Ultrasonography of the knee. J Belge Radiol 1996;79:155–9.
13. Weinberg EP, Adams MJ, Hollenberg GM. Color Doppler sonography of patellar tendinosis. Am J Roentgenol 1998;171:743–4.
14. Kalebo P, Sward L, Karlsson J, Peterson L. Ultrasonography in the detection of partial patellar ligament ruptures (jumper's knee). Skeletal Radiol 1991;20:285–9.
15. Lanning P, Heikkinen E. Ultrasonic features of the Osgood-Schlatter lesion. J Pediatr Orthop 1991; 11:538–40.
16. De Flaviis L, Nessi R, Scaglione P, Balconi G, Albisetti W, Derchi LE. Ultrasonic diagnosis of Osgood-Schlatter and Sinding Larson-Johansson disease of the knee. Skeletal Radiol 1989; 18:193–7.
17. Bianchi S, Zwass A, Abdelwahab IF, Banderali A. Diagnosis of tears of the quadriceps tendon of the knee: Value of sonography. Am J Roentgenol 1994;162:1137–40.
18. van Holsbeeck M, Introcaso JH. Musculoskeletal ultrasonography. Radiol Clin North Am 1992; 30:907–25.
19. Strome GM, Bouffard JA, van Holsbeeck M. Knee. Clin Diagn Ultrasound 1995;30:201–19.
20. Craig JG, Jacobson JA, Moed BR. Ultrasound of fracture and bone healing. Radiol Clin North Am 1999;37(4):737–51.
21. Ali S, Friedman L, Finlay K, Jurriaans E, Chhem RK. Ultrasonography of occult fractures: A pictorial essay. Can Assoc Radiol J 2001;52(5):312–21.
22. Sarazin L, Bonaldi VM, Papadatos D, Chhem RK. Correlative imaging and pattern approach in ultrasonography of bone lesions: A pictorial essay. Can Assoc Radiol J 1996;47:423–30.
23. Stoller DW, Cannon WD, Anderson LF. The knee. In: Stoller DW, editor. Magnetic resonance imaging in orthopedics and sports medicine, 2nd ed. New York: Lippincott-Raven; 1997:203–442.
24. Resnick D. Diagnosis of bone and joint disorders, 4th ed. Philadelphia: Saunders; 2002.

25. Rutten MJ, Collins JM, van Kampen A, Jager GJ. Meniscal cysts: Detection with high-resolution sonography. Am J Roentgenol 1998;171:491–6.

26. Seymour R, Lloyd DC. Sonographic appearances of meniscal cysts. J Clin Ultrasound 1998;26:15–20.

27. Bonaldi VM, Chhem RK, Drolet R, Garcia P, Gallix B, Sarazin L. Iliotibial band friction syndrome: Sonographic findings. J Ultrasound Med 1998;17:257–60.

28. Helbich TH, Breitenseher M, Trattnig S, Nehrer S, Erlacher L, Kainberger F. Sonographic variants of popliteal cysts. J Clin Ultrasound 1998;26:171–6.

29. Suzuki S, Kasahara K, Futami T, Iwasaki R, Ueo T, Yamamuro T. Ultrasound diagnosis of pathology of the anterior and posterior ligaments of the knee joint. Arch Orthop Trauma Surg 1991;110:200–3.

30. Wang TG, Wang CL, Hsu TC, Shieh JY, Shau YW, Hsieh FJ. Sonographic evaluation of the posterior cruciate ligament in amputated specimens and normal subjects. J Ultrasound Med 1999;18:647–53.

31. Ptasznik R, Feller J, Bartlett J, Fitt G, Mitchell A, Hennessy O. The value of sonography in the diagnosis of traumatic rupture of the anterior cruciate ligament of the knee. Am J Roentgenol 1995;164:1461–3.

32. Wang SC, Chhem RK, Cardinal E, Cho KH. Joint sonography. Radiol Clin North Am 1999;37:653–68.

33. Fessell DP, Jacobson JA, Craig J, Habra G, Prasad A, Radliff A, et al. Using sonography to reveal and aspirate joint effusions. Am J Roentgenol 2000;174:1353–62.

34. Frankel DA, Bargiela A, Bouffard JA, Craig JG, Shirazi KK, van Holsbeeck MT. Synovial joints: Evaluation of intraarticular bodies with US. Radiology 1998;206:41–4.

35. Bianchi S, Martinoli C. Detection of loose bodies in joints. Radiol Clin North Am 1999;37:679–90.

Ultrasound of the foot and ankle

10

Eugene G McNally

INTRODUCTION

The foot has become one of the most important areas for musculoskeletal ultrasound, rivalling the shoulder for frequency of referral. Most of the structures that surround the foot are superficial and easily accessible to ultrasound diagnosis. Many patients present with symptoms localised to particular areas of the foot and in these instances ultrasound plays an important role in the differential diagnosis. If pain or tenderness is more global, ultrasound is less likely to determine its cause and MRI is more appropriate. Specific areas that are difficult or impossible to examine include the talar dome and the subtalar joints.

The most common focal symptom encountered in the author's practice is posterior hindfoot or heel pain. The principle differential diagnoses here are Achilles tendinopathy and plantar fasciitis, but consideration also must be given to posterior impingement, Sever's disease and fat pad syndrome. Medial-sided symptoms can be due to tibialis posterior tendon disease, tarsal tunnel syndrome and other nerve entrapment syndromes. Laterally peroneal tendinopathy and lateral ligament complex disease are important, along with anterolateral impingement syndromes. Anterior symptoms may relate to anterior or syndesmotic impingement syndrome with anterior tendon disease less common.

POSTERIOR AND HEEL PAD PAIN

Achilles tendon

The techniques used to examine the Achilles tendon have been dealt with elsewhere. The patient is prone with the feet overhanging the end of the couch and the operator sits at the couch end, allowing good access to both the Achilles tendon and plantar fascia. In this position the Achilles tendon can be examined in its full extent from above the musculotendinous junction to its insertion into the os calcis. The width of the

Achilles tendon at its insertion varies from 1.2 to 2.5 cm. Approximately 5–6 cm proximal to the calcaneal insertion the separate tendons of the gastrocnemius and soleus fuse to become one tendon. A further 6–9 cm above this the soleus begins to contribute to the Achilles tendon and rotation of the tendon fibres begins with a 90° medial-to-posterior rotation.

Achilles tendinopathy

One of the most common pathological findings in patients with chronic heel pain is Achilles tendinopathy. Although running is the commonest activity that contributes to overuse Achilles tendinopathy, up to one third of patients do not participate in sports or other vigorous activity. Anatomical factors may be contributory. Most commonly, the tendon is formed with merging of the gastrocnemius and soleus 12 cm above its insertion. Imbalance between the individual contributions of the gastrocnemius and soleus to the achilles tendon can produce abnormal stress within the tendon and result in overuse injury below the normal physiological stress limits. The fibres of the Achilles tendon spiral 90° proximal to distal which increases its ability to elongate. Hyperpronation resulting from the lateral aspect of the heel striking first with a compensatory pronation of the foot may also contribute to tendinopathy. Forefoot varus has been recognised in patients with Achilles tendon problems. Other factors include age, weight, body habitus, vascularity and associated limb torsion and ankle anomalies. Achilles tendinopathy has also been associated with the quinolone antibiotics. Overuse stress of the Achilles tendon may result in either inflammatory changes within the sheath or degeneration of the tendon fibres. Tendinosis and tendinitis are both pathological terms the former implying mucoid degeneration on the latter and inflammatory condition. Unless the histopathological background is understood the term "tendinopathy" is probably most appropriate. Following injury, tendons may heal either by scarring or regeneration. The latter is more physiologically appropriate that may be prevented by the nature of the injury and ongoing overuse. Clinically paratenonopathy and tendinopathy can be distinguished by whether the area of thickening and tenderness moves on dorsal and plantar flexion. Lesions within the tendon will move, however accurate differentiation is difficult. The purpose of ultrasound of the Achilles tendon is to differentiate between paratenopathy, focal or diffuse tendinopathy with or without partial tear or split, complete rupture, insertional tendinopathy, retrocalcaneal bursitis and retro-Achilles bursitis.

The ultrasound appearances of diffuse achilles tendinopathy are a generalised increase in the tendon dimension and decrease in overall reflectivity (Figs 10.1 and 10.2). On axial section, the tendon assumes a more rounded appearance with loss of the normal anterior flat or slightly concave contour.

> **Practical tip**
>
> Paratenonopathy can be quite subtle and on occasion it can be difficult to differentiate the abnormal tendon tissue from abnormal paratenon.

Achilles tendinopathy can be diffuse or focal, acute or chronic. In focal tendinopathy the area of decreased reflectivity involves an area within the tendon, often on the dorsal surface (Figs 10.3 and 10.4). There may be an alteration in the external contour of the tendon with associated thickening

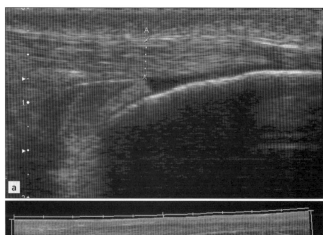

Fig. 10.1 (a) Longitudinal section of normal Achilles tendon. (b) Panoramic view of entire tendon length.

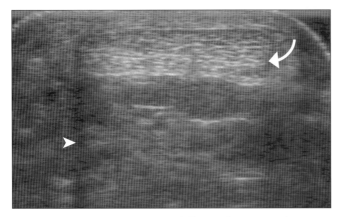

Fig. 10.2 Axial section through Achilles tendon. Note edge artefact (arrowhead). Prominent edge artefact may obscure the tendon margin (curved arrow). In these instances tilting the probe to each side in turn will allow a full examination of the lateral aspect of the tendon.

of the paratenon. Paratenonopathy can be quite subtle and on occasion it can be difficult to differentiate the abnormal tendon tissue from abnormal paratenon (Fig. 10.3). Within the tendon itself, focal tendinopathy may be associated with areas of decreased reflectivity (Figs 10.5 and 10.6). These may represent areas of mucoid degeneration, focal tendon splits or vessels. Colour flow imaging can help with this differential diagnosis (1).

More commonly a greater portion of the tendon is involved, being diffusely swollen and demonstrating more homogenous decreased reflectivity. Rarely a low incorporation of the soleus muscle can mimic tendon thickening due to tendinopathy (2), although the more regular and typical muscle reflectivity of soleus is usually

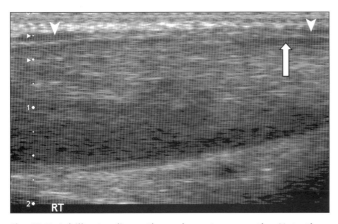

Fig. 10.3 Achilles tendinopathy and paratenonopathy. Note the loss of reflectivity within the posterior aspect of the tendon on this longitudinal section (arrow) in addition to the low attenuation inflammatory changes in the paratenon (arrowheads).

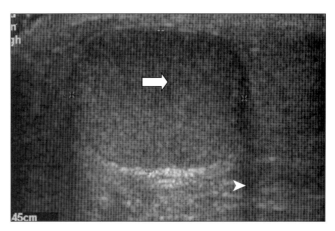

Fig. 10.5 Axial Achilles tendon with diffuse tendinopathy and dorsal fissuring (arrow). The latter is sometimes due to new vessel formation. Note the edge artefact (arrowhead).

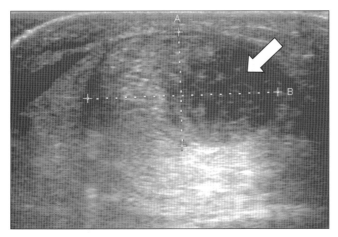

Fig. 10.4 Axial section of Achilles tendon with focal decreased reflectivity on medial aspect of the tendon (arrow).

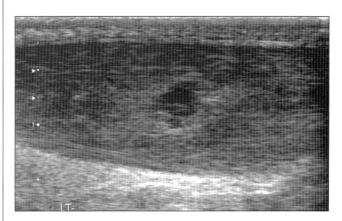

Fig. 10.6 Sagittal section of Achilles tendinopathy with small focal tear.

apparent. Doppler flow studies can demonstrate increased blood flow (Fig. 10.7), particularly on the anterior surface of the tendon, although the significance of the presence and intensity of this phenomenon is unclear. Several vessels can be seen entering the anterior aspect of the tendon. They are usually quite widely spaced. Focal conglomerations particularly in areas where there is more marked tendon degeneration merit particular attention as it may be that these areas act as the initial stress risers for tendon rupture, although evidence for this hypothesis is lacking.

Chronic Achilles tendinopathy has two forms: mechanical and inflammatory. The more common mechanical form affects the proximal two-thirds of the tendon and frequently affects the medial side of the tendon more than the lateral. Although the aetiology remains poorly understood, it is felt to be due to abnormal biomechanics with hyperpronation of the tendon during walking and malrotation between the tibia and hindfoot both implicated. This variety is often bilateral.

The less common inflammatory type of chronic patellar tendinopathy affects the distal third of the tendon close to the insertion into the os calcis. This type may occur secondary to a generalised enthesopathy such as is found in psoriasis (3), Reiter's syndrome or ankylosing spondylitis. In these conditions, plantar fasciitis may also be present and should be specifically sought. Distal third patellar tendinopathy is also more commonly associated with other inflammatory phenomena including pre-Achilles bursitis, retro-Achilles bursitis and insertional tendinosis (4) (Figs 10.8–10.11).

Achilles ultrasound carries a high positive predictive value for tendinopathy, but a negative examination can occur in patients with clinically symptomatic tendinopathy (5). The predictive value on outcome remains unproven, but patients with tendinopathy of the Achilles tendon with normal ultrasound findings have a shorter time to full recovery than those with ultrasound detectable abnormality.

Conversely, ultrasound-detected low reflective areas do not necessarily correspond with symptoms and may be detected in the asymptomatic tendon, though there is an inceased likelihood that the tendon will eventually become symptomatic. The patient may

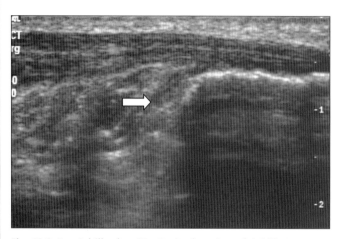

Fig. 10.8 Pre-Achilles bursitis. Sagittal section of Achilles insertion. Pre-Achilles bursitis can sometimes be difficult to detect. In this case subtle fissure is seen within a somewhat heterogeneous Kager's fat triangle (arrow). Dynamic examination with foot movement and alternation probe pressure can help to reveal a more obvious bursitis in these challenging cases.

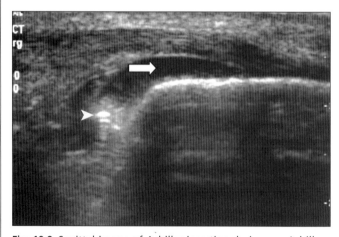

Fig. 10.9 Sagittal image of Achilles insertion during pre-Achilles bursa distension. The bursa is now filled with poorly reflective fluid (arrow). The reflective axial section through the needle with its posterior artefact is easily seen (arrowhead).

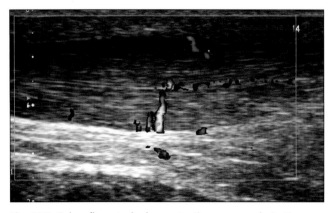

Fig. 10.7 Colourflow study demonstrating neovascularisation within tendinopathic tendon.

also present de novo with rupture as there is a probable association with intratendinous focal abnormality and increased risk of rupture but again this precise relationship has yet to be fully defined. The natural history of Achilles tendinopathy is variable and up to a quarter of patients may ultimately require surgery. Following surgery, recovery to previous activity levels on reduction in pain is the norm, however, many patients will develop tendinopathy in the previously uninvolved contralateral tendon.

Haglunds syndrome

Mechanical factors may also be involved in the aetiology of lower third tendinopathy. In some cases an abnormal spur forms on the posterosuperior margin of the os calcis, which on foot dorsiflexion can impinge the anterior surface of the tendon (Fig. 10.12). This type is referred to as the Haglund syndrome or the pump bump phenomenon (6). The presumed cause is irritation of the posterior os calcis and surrounding structure due to rigid low-backed shoes. Low posterior heel pain is the presenting complaint and a tender swelling may be felt. Treatment is by modification of footwear or the use of an orthosis, aimed at lifting the heel and correcting excessive pronation. Surgical excision is reserved for patients where conservative measures fail.

> **Practical tip**
>
> On MR, the Achilles bursa measures approximately 1 cm in lateral diameter and 7 mm inferosuperior. More than 1 mm of fluid distension is abnormal.

> **Practical tip**
>
> Contrast between synovial thickening and surrounding fat is less than fluid/fat and on occasions careful scrutiny is necessary to detect small bursitides.

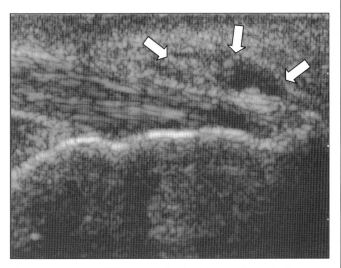

Fig. 10.10 Retro-Achilles bursa. Sagittal image through the Achilles insertion. No distension of the retro-Achilles bursa (arrows).

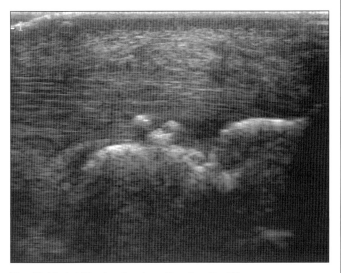

Fig. 10.11 Achilles tendon insertional enthesitis.

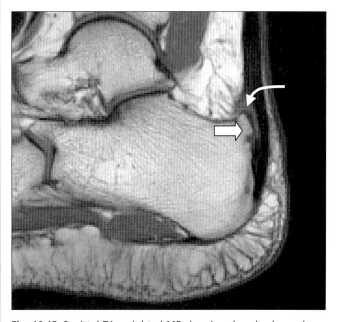

Fig. 10.12 Sagittal T1-weighted MR showing dorsal calcaneal osseus protrusion (bump) with secondary tendinopathy. Note the prominent bony spur on the posterosuperior aspect of the os calcis (arrow) with associated inflammatory changes in the pre-Achilles bursa and anterior aspect of the Achilles tendon (curved arrow).

The normal immediate anterior relation of the Achilles tendon is Kager's fat triangle, and the pre-Achilles bursa lies at the inferior-most tip. On high-quality ultrasound it is normal to identify a small quantity of fluid in this space. On MR, the bursa measures approximately 1 cm in lateral diameter and 7 mm inferosuperior (7). More than 1 mm of fluid distension is abnormal. In addition to fluid distension, synovial thickening of the bursa may occur and in some instances this is the more dominant finding. Contrast between synovial thickening and surrounding fat is less than fluid/fat and on occasions careful scrutiny is necessary to detect small bursitides (Figs 10.8 and 10.9). In acute cases there may also be a large synovial mass with associated increased blood flow evident on Doppler signal. Less commonly, synovial distension of the retro-Achilles space occurs as retro-Achilles bursitis (Fig. 10.10). In both cases, although more usually with pre-Achilles bursitis, chronic changes can result in calcification.

Rare forms of Achilles tendinopathy, including calcific tendinopathy and that related to chronic xanthomatous tendinopathy, which is most usually seen in patients with familial hyperlipidaemia, occur. Also uncommon is ossification, which can also result in fracture (6).

Achilles rupture

> ### Key point
>
> Rupture of the Achilles tendon occurs in one of three places, the commonest being in the mid-portion of the tendon, approximately 5–6 cm above its insertion.

Typically, Achilles tendon rupture occurs in the fourth to fifth decades. Seventy-five percent of cases are associated with racket or bowls sports or other athletic activity. The second peak of injury occurs in the eighth decade and it is much more common in males with the ratio to females of approximately five. Ruptures are said to be more common on the left and an association with blood type "O" have been identified.

There appears to be an increased prevalence of hypoechoic areas in tendons that have ruptured suggesting that there is an association between the two. However, many patients with complete Achilles tendon rupture have had no pre-existing symptoms. Tendon degeneration can occur without symptoms and ultrasound changes can be present without symptoms. Pain in the Achilles region is common amongst elite badminton players reported by thirty percent as being present in the previous five years and ongoing in seventeen percent. Some correlation with the weekly training load was detected.

Rupture of the Achilles tendon occurs in one of three places. The commonest of these is in the mid-portion of the tendon, approximately 5–6 cm above its insertion (8). Rupture of the Achilles tendon in this location is most commonly associated with chronic tendinopathy. Elevated serum lipids may also predispose (9). Patients are typically between 30 and 50 years, the onset is often acute, with racket sports, especially badminton, frequently being implicated. The patient will feel a sharp sensation in the hindfoot and often describe a feeling as though they have just been kicked. It is not unusual for patients to hear a snap as the tendon ruptures. After a short period a characteristic haematoma develops, tracking from the level of rupture inferiorly to form a crescent-shaped bruise on either side of a malleolus.

The second most common site is at the musculotendinous junction. The clinical pattern and onset are similar, although clinical examination can often determine that tenderness is a little more proximal than at the more classical site. In patients with a low soleal incorporation this clinical differentiation is more difficult (Fig. 10.13). The combination of musculotendinous and tendon substance tears account for over 95% of injuries. A dramatic variant of this is an aponeurotic shear injury involving the entire belly (usually medial) of the gastrocnemius (Fig. 10.14) The third and least common type is an avulsion, either from the Achilles tendon insertion itself or as an avulsion fracture (Fig. 10.15). In these cases the underlying bone is often abnormal, predisposing factors include steroid use, diabetes, rheumatoid arthritis, metabolic bone disease and renal failure.

> ### Practical tip
>
> In some cases the gap caused by Achilles rupture can be difficult to see due to the combination of organised haematoma within the gap and poor demarcation of the tendon ends secondary to chronic tendinopathy; dynamic tendon movement is very helpful in confirming the diagnosis.

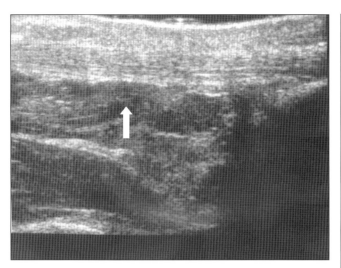

Fig. 10.13 Sagittal view of Achilles tendon with low soleal incorporation. A minor musculotendinous junction tear is present (arrow), which was clinically interpreted as a mid-substance tendon tear due to the location of the tenderness. Note the short distance between the soleal insertion and the os calcis.

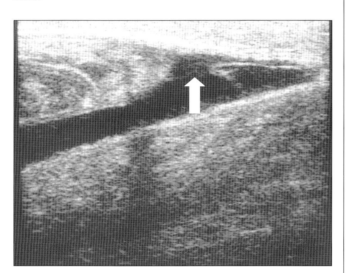

Fig. 10.14 Sagital image of confluence of medial head of gastrocnemius and soleus. The gastrocnemius head has been completely avulsed (arrow) and has retracted. The space between the muscle aponeurosis has filled with fluid, presumably blood.

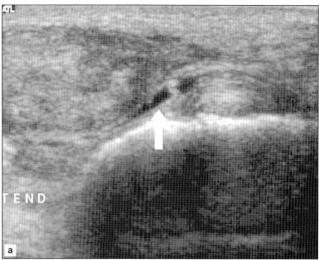

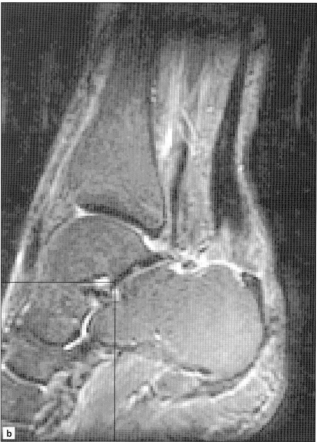

Fig. 10.15 (a) Subtle insertional Achilles tear in patient with Reiter's syndrome (arrow). (b) Sagittal STIR MR correlation in same patient.

The ultrasound diagnosis of acute Achilles rupture is made by demonstrating a full thickness interruption of the normal tendon tissue. The space is usually filled with fluid, haemorrhage (Fig. 10.16) and debris (Fig. 10.17). In some cases the combination of organised haematoma within the gap and poor demarcation of the tendon ends secondary to chronic tendinopathy can make the gap difficult to see. In these instances, dynamic tendon movement is very helpful in confirming the diagnosis (Fig. 10.17b). Gentle dorsal/plantar flexion movements of the patient's foot will show discontinuity of movement between the tendon ends and often will open a gap in the tendon that has previously been difficult to see. The dynamic examination can also be helpful to differentiate between severe partial and complete tears. In a majority of instances where a presumptive diagnosis of a severe partial tear has been made on a static examination, a dynamic study will

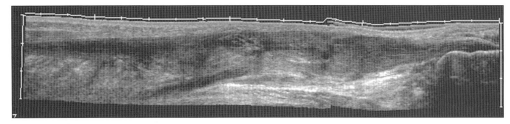

Fig. 10.16 Sagittal image of Achilles rupture filled with reflective haemorrhage.

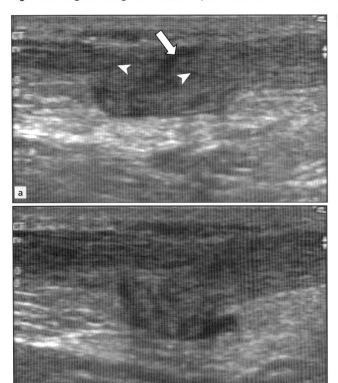

Fig. 10.17 (a) Full thickness Achilles rupture, sagittal image. The tear is obliquely orientated without overlap of the tendon ends (arrowheads). Fluid fills the tendon gap (arrow). (b) Foot now moved into the equinus. Note the obliteration of fluid and the more obvious overlap within the tendon ends. The gap between the tendons is now more difficult to visualise. This case emphasises the importance of dynamic examination, both to confirm the presence of a full thickness tear and also to demonstrate approximation of tendon ends on foot equinus particularly if conservative management is being considered. Gentle dorsal/plantar flexion movements of the patient's foot will show discontinuity of movement between the tendon ends and often will open a gap in the tendon that has previously been difficult to see.

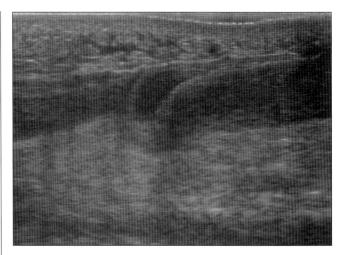

Fig. 10.18 Sagittal image of re-ruptured Achilles tendon following repair. A tense haematoma fills the gap between the tendon ends.

tendon ends is important in treatment planning. Musculotendinous junction tears are generally not treated surgically. Surgical options do exist for ruptures that involve the body of the tendon and these include open or percutaneous techniques (10). Percutaneous suturing is a "blind" technique so it is helpful for the ultrasonologist to mark the location of torn tendon ends on the skin (Fig. 10.19). If conservative treatment is planned the patient will usually be placed in an equinus cast. In these instances it is also useful to repeat the examination following casting to confirm that the gap has not widened. Occasionally the cast can result in pressure on the gastrocnemius muscle, leading to retraction of the proximal tendon end and widening of the gap.

Practical tip

Percutaneous suturing of the Achilles tendon is a "blind" technique so it is helpful for the ultrasonologist to mark the location of tendon ends on the skin. If conservative treatment is planned, the patient will usually be placed in an equinus cast, whereupon it is also useful to repeat the examination following casting to confirm that the gap has not widened.

---

show the rupture to be complete. A poorly reflective line representing an edge artefact arising from the margins of the disrupted tendon has also been described as a useful method for detecting tendon ends. Axial images show a fragmented tendon but usually an intact paratenon (Fig. 10.18).

Differentiation of the precise location of tendon rupture and the size of the gap between

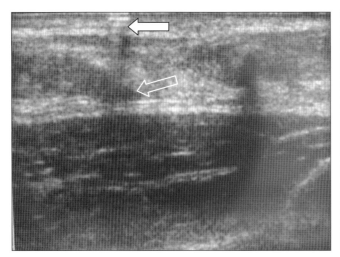

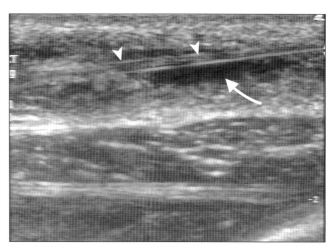

Fig. 10.19 Technique for marking tendon ends. The probe is held over the gap and and an extended paperclip in placed between the probe and skin. The clip is moved up and down until its reverberation shadow (arrow) is cast over the tendon end (open arrow). An indelible mark is placed at the level of the paperclip which is then moved to mark the other tendon end.

Fig. 10.20 Achilles rupture with intact plantaris.

In a proportion of patients an intact plantaris tendon may be identified in association with Achilles tendon rupture (Fig. 10.20). The significance of this in limiting Achilles tendon distraction or its role in surgical decision making is uncertain, but probably not significant.

Plantar fasciitis

Clinically plantar fasciitis presents as pain on the undersurface of the heel. A very common feature is that patients describe it as knife like, generally worse after rest and when exercise is initiated, becoming less painful as the ligament is stretched. Several factors have been implicated in the aetiology of plantar fasciitis, including overuse and muscle imbalance.

Key point

The appearance of a normal plantar fascia is like that of other ligaments: generally reflective with a linear fibrillar structure.

The plantar fascia is best examined with the probe in the sagittal plane. The normal plantar fascia has an appearance typical of other ligaments, it is generally reflective with a linear fibrillar structure. It is normally less than 4 mm thick (10–13). The plantar fascia can be traced from its origin on the undersurface of the os calcis along the entire plantar aspect of the foot,

where it diverges to mingle with the deep fascia underlying the metatarsal heads. The plantar fascia is divided into two principal bundles, medial and lateral. The medial bundle is generally the thicker of the two and is more prone to plantar fasciitis. Fasciitis may be associated with spur formation but most spurs are not associated with symptoms (14).

Key point

The ultrasound appearance of plantar fasciitis includes an increase in calibre greater than 4 mm and a loss of reflectivity of the ligament.

The ultrasound appearance of plantar fasciitis includes an increase in calibre greater than 4 mm and a loss of reflectivity of the ligament (Fig. 10.21). The differential diagnosis on a thickened plantar fascia includes plantar fibromatosis. In this entity, the thickened fascial origin tends to be painless to compression. If this combination is encountered, a careful search for plantar fibromatosis is indicated. In more severe cases abnormal fluid collections can be seen surrounding the plantar fascia and the underlying bone may show an irregular periosteal surface, indicating associated enthesitis.

With continued overuse plantar fasciitis may progress to rupture. In these cases a more acute pain is experienced, which may be accompanied by a snapping sensation and marked swelling. A history of previous steroid injections is reported in up to a third of patients with plantar fascial rupture (15).

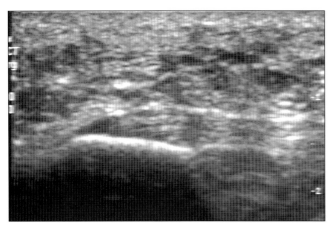

Fig. 10.21 Plantar fasciitis. The plantar fascia measures more than 4 mm and has decreased reflectivity compared with normal.

The management of plantar fasciitis involves a combination of conservative treatment including rest, ice, nonsteroidal anti-inflammatory medication, modification of sports, particularly running on hard surfaces and Achilles stretching exercises. A variety of orthoses including heel and arch support have also been recommended. Hyperpronation of the hind foot has also been implicated and orthoses and shoe support to reverse this have been advised. Guided injections to the perifascial tissues can help reduce the initial symptoms but are rarely effective in isolation.

Sever's disease

In children, calcaneal apophysitis, also known as Sever's disease is a much debated condition. Radiological and ultrasound findings of a multifragmentary calcaneal apophysis is common and does not of itself indicate the presence of disease. The condition is said to occur as a result of chronic traction in the 8- to 12-year-old age group. Predisposing conditions are thought to include a tight Achilles tendon, a valgus hindfoot with varus forefoot and excessive internal femoral rotation. It is generally treated conservatively with a heel raised to shorten the Achilles mechanism and active Achilles tendon stretching.

Less common causes of heel pain include fat pad syndrome, which is thought to be due to repetitive trauma of the heel pad. The differential diagnosis can also be extended to include the sinus tarsi syndrome and calcaneal stress fractures. Painful calcaneal spur syndrome is also a debated entity. Calcaneal periostitis is a similar condition, characterised by pain originating within the medial calcaneal tuberosity. The clinical differential diagnosis is difficult.

MEDIAL HINDFOOT PAIN

Tibialis posterior tendon dysfunction

Tibialis posterior tendon dysfunction (TPTD) is most commonly encountered in middle-aged females. The aetiology is multifactorial with footwear and biomechanical factors both implicated. As with the rotator cuff, intrinsic tendon factors are also important. There is an area of relative hypovascularity within the tendon measuring 14 mm in length, ending approximately 40 mm from its insertion into the navicular. This area appears to correspond with the most common site of tendon rupture. Ultrastructurally the degenerating tendon appears to contain a proportion of Type III collagen higher than normal, presumed to represent attempts at repair. The dominant collagen type remains Type I but the increased proportion of Type III appears to render the tendon less able to respond and resist tension at normal loads. The recent literature emphasises the histological appearances of tibialis posterior tendon disease, which are noninflammatory, representing a tendinosis rather than a tendinitis. In other patients inflammatory changes are more obvious with fluid and tenosynovitis detected on ultrasound, suggestive of a primary inflammatory disorder. Tendinopathy is also more common in patients with known inflammatory conditions such as rheumatoid arthritis. Other medical conditions predispose to TPTD. For example, Holmes and Mann have shown that 60% of patients had one or more of hypertension, obesity, diabetes melitis, previous surgery or trauma to the medial aspect of the foot or steroid exposure (16). Of these the presence of obesity appears to have the greatest correlation with tibialis posterior tendon rupture.

The classification of TPTD described by Johnson and Strom combines symptoms and clinical appearances of the tendon. Type I is pain along the line of the tendon with some swelling. Pes planus has not occurred. Type II is present when there is pes planus but some mobility preserved. Type III is fixed pes planus. Some confusion has arisen with a similar MR classification of tendon disease comprising Types I, II and III. MRI Type I shows a few longitudinal splits without evidence of major degeneration or tendinosis. Type II tendon disease has longitudinal splits and more obvious degeneration. A variable diameter may occur in this group and hypertrophy or atrophy may be noted. Particularly difficult to detect is the atrophic Type II tear where loss of diameter of the tendon compared with flexor digitorum may be the only feature and the tendon may otherwise lack obvious internal degeneration. MRI Type III comprises diffuse swelling of the tendon with a uniform degeneration and scar. The correlation between the two grading systems is not particularly well established although there is some suggestion that MRI has a tendency to overgrade in that the degree of internal tendon derangement as seen on MRI may be associated with a less severe clinical picture than would otherwise be expected.

Key point

The primary role of imaging is to identify patients with tenosynovitis without tendinopathy. In the presence of tenosynovitis and a normal tendon, conservative measures, which may include guided injections, can be considered.

Despite these discrepancies, imaging plays an important role in the preoperative management of patients with tibialis posterior tendon disease. Its primary role is to identify patients with tenosynovitis without tendinopathy. In the presence of tenosynovitis and a normal tendon, conservative measures, which may include guided injections, can be considered. If this fails, surgical tenosynovectomy is carried out. If the tendon is abnormal it is generally felt, though not all agree, that guided injection should be avoided as the deranged tendon may be susceptible to tendon rupture following injections into the tendon sheath. Similarly many surgeons believe that tenosynovectomy alone is inadequate in the management of patients where the underlying tendon is also abnormal and a tendon transfer procedure is often suggested as an adjunct.

Practical tip

There is a possible increased risk of tendon rupture following guided injections into the sheath, if the tibialis posterior tendon itself is abnormal, it is generally felt, though not all agree, that guided injection should be avoided as the deranged tendon may be susceptable to rupture following injections into the sheath.

The tibialis posterior tendon is best examined with the patient in the supine position. Hip flexion and external rotation will place the medial aspect of the hindfoot uppermost, rending it easy to interrogate with the ultrasound probe. As previously defined, careful technique is necessary to ensure that tibialis posterior tendon is correctly differentiated from the adjacent flexor digitorum tendon. Placing the probe in the axial plane along the margin of the medial malleolus followed by small posterior movement with ventral angulation will easily identify the tibialis posterior tendon. Other differentiating features include noting the tibialis posterior is distinctly thicker than flexor digitorum. Tibialis posterior also follows a more parallel course to its insertion into the navicular. Rarely, congenital duplication of tibialis posterior tendon and a common tendon sheath for tibialis posterior and flexor digitorum can occur.

Practical tip

Some features differentiating the tibialis posterior tendon from the flexor digitorum are that it is thicker and runs a more parallel course to its insertion into the navicular.

The normal tendon is approximately 6 mm in diameter although this can vary with the patient's age. A small quantity of fluid may be identified on the deeper surface just below the medial malleolus. Like other tendons, the normal ultrasound appearances are of a generally reflective structure with a typical parallel pattern of tendon fibrils. The tendon is more difficult to examine close to its insertion into the navicular. This is because divergent tendon fibres cause the typical anisotropic loss of reflectivity as they insert into bone. Fortunately, the commonest area for tibialis posterior tendinopathy is adjacent to the medial malleolus rather than closer to its insertion. An exception to this is where there is an accessory os tibiale externum where a painful pseudarthrosis can arise. In these cases the accessory ossicle is apparent on ultrasound. While perilesional inflammatory changes may be apparent, MR is required to demonstrate the pseudarthrosis to best effect and to depict the intraosseus oedema that separates a symptomatic from a nonsymptomatic lesion.

> **Practical tip**
>
> In some cases a small bony spur can be identified in association with the anteromedial aspect of the tibia and this acts as a useful sentinel to the underlying tendinopathy.

The characteristic ultrasound appearances of tibialis posterior tendinopathy are thickening of the tendon, decreased reflectivity, fluid and synovial thickening of the tendon sheath (Figs 10.22–10.25). In some cases a small bony spur can be identified on the anteromedial aspect of the tibia and this acts as a useful sentinel to the underlying tendinopathy (Figs 10.23 and 10.26).

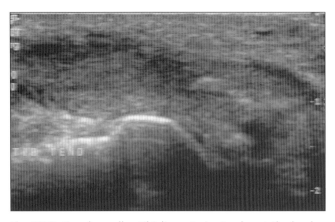

Fig. 10.22 Grossly swollen tibialis posterior tendon at the level of the medial maeolus.

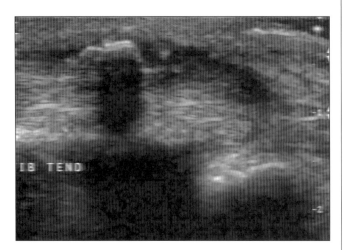

Fig. 10.23 Tibialis posterior tendon with probe angles such that bone is projected superficial to the tendon.

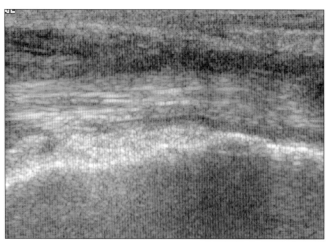

Fig. 10.24 Longitudinal section of tibialis posterior tenosynovitis.

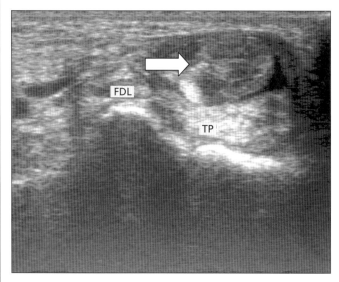

Fig. 10.25 Axial section through tibialis posterior tendon showing marked tenosynovitis with large synovial mass (arrow).

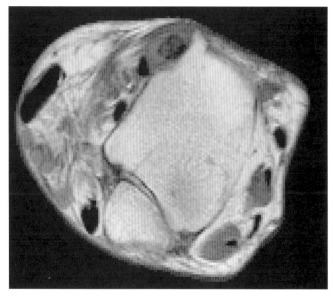

Fig. 10.26 Axial T1-weighted MR section corresponding to Fig. 10.27 but in a different patient. Note the new bone formation on the posteromedial tibia.

Hypertrophic tendinopathy is the commonest variant of this condition, occurring in about 50–60% of patients. In a smaller portion of cases, chronic tendinopathy manifests as a loss of normal tendon volume due to elongation and separation of tendon fibres. Atrophic tendinopathy is more difficult to identify unless the tendon is examined in its entirety and carefully compared both with the adjacent flexor digitorum tendon, which is normally about half its size, and with the contralateral tibialis posterior tendon.

As with the chronic Achilles tendinopathy, focal or diffuse variants can occur. The more common is diffuse tendinopathy, although in the early stages of this process a focal tendinopathy is more characteristic. The earliest lesions can be quite subtle and, in the author's experience, are best appreciated in the axial plane, where a well-demarcated poorly reflective focus can be

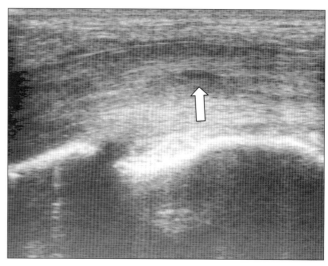

Fig. 10.29 Long axis section of Tib Post tendinopathy with small focal tear.

appreciated within the normally reflective tendon (Figs 10.27–10.29).

Complete rupture of the tibialis posterior tendon generally occurs as a result of chronic tendinopathy. The presence of an os tibiale externum is also more common in patients with tibialis posterior tendon rupture than in the control population (17), although the characteristic site of rupture is in the region of the medial malleolus or just below it. It usually follows a long history of chronic tendinopathy where adhesions that have formed between the tendon and tendon sheath, and also between the tendon sheath and underlying bone. This may cause the tendon to become fixed *in situ* following rupture. In these instances one of the characteristic features of rupture of a tendon, that of tendon retraction, may not be as readily apparent. Following failure of the tibialis posterior tendon, the medial arch of the foot becomes reduced and the arch is preserved only by the calcaneonavicular ligament. When the calcaneonavicular or spring ligament fails in succession, pes planus results.

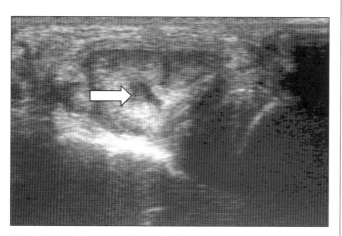

Fig. 10.27 Axial section through tibialis posterior tendon showing tenosynovitis and longitudinal split.

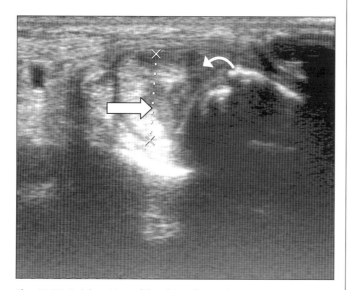

Fig. 10.28 Axial section of focal tendinopathy.

> **Practical tip**
>
> Tendon retraction may be prevented by adhesions that have formed between the tendon, tendon sheath, and underlying bone.

Tarsal tunnel and other nerve entrapment syndromes

A variety of nerve entrapment syndromes have been described in the foot. The most frequently described is tarsal tunnel syndrome. The tibial tunnel is the equivalent of the carpal tunnel in the wrist. The medial-sided tendons, tibialis posterior, flexor digitorum and flexor hallucis in conjunction with the neurovascular bundle, are relatively confined as they pass posterior to the medial malleolus as a consequence of the overlying flexor retinaculum. Increased pressure within this area, which may occur as the consequence of synovitis, ganglion formation or other lesions, leads to compression of the tibial nerve as it passes through the tunnel. Congenital anomalies such as posteromedial coalition (18) or an os sustentaculum, trauma and tight-fitting shoes have also been implicated as causes of this increased pressure. Neural-type pain with tingling or numb sensations occurs in the medial aspect of the foot and extending into the mid- and forefoot is the presenting feature. Focal tenderness and a positive Tinel's sign may also be present. Posterior tibial nerve entrapment may occur more distally in either the medial or lateral branches. Entrapment may occur at the level of the calcaneonavicular joint with sensory signs on the medial plantar aspect of the foot. Lateral plantar nerve entrapment, which may result in sensory disturbance in the fourth or fifth toes, has also been described. The usual site of entrapment is adjacent to the medial calcaneal tuberosity. The differential diagnosis on lateral plantar nerve entrapment is sural nerve entrapment, which can occur as a consequence of recurrent lateral ankle injury with secondary inflammation and perineural fibrosis. The clinical differentiation between sural nerve entrapment and lateral plantar nerve entrapment can be difficult if based on the site of sensory loss but the site of tenderness in sural nerve entrapment is lateral rather than medial.

LATERAL HINDFOOT PAIN

Peroneal tendons

The peroneal tendons are a paired tendons structure that lies in a common sheath on the lateral aspect of the hind foot. As they pass posterior to the lateral malleolus their position is maintained by the presence of a connective tissue band termed the superior peroneal retinaculum. The peroneal tendons are prone to subluxation entrapment, chronic tendinopathy and, rarely, rupture. In many individuals peroneus brevis

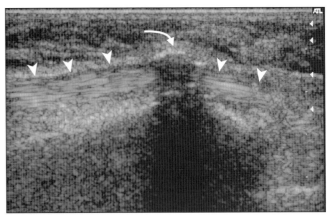

Fig. 10.30 Longitudinal section over lateral malleolus showing subluxed peroneal tendons (arrowheads) secondary to fracture (curved arrow).

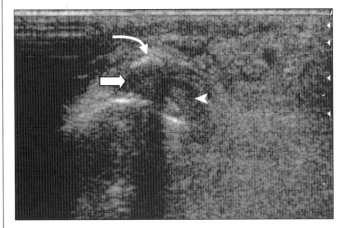

Fig. 10.31 Axial section corresponding to Fig. 10.30. P Longus (arrow), P Brevis (arrowhead) and fracture (curved arrow).

tendon is a rather attenuated structure and can be seen as a small inverted "V" or chevron-shaped structure with peroneus longus nestled into its dorsal aspect. This is a normal appearance to the tendon and should not be misconstrued as an incipient tear.

Peroneal tendon subluxation

Rupture of the superior peroneal retinaculum, with or without associated fracture of the fibula, can result in anterior subluxation of the peroneal tendons on inversion/eversion (Figs 10.30 and 10.31). The presence of a flat posterior aspect to the fibula may also predispose to this. The patient characteristically complains of a painful click and in many individuals the abnormal movement of the tendon can be visualised or at least palpated. As this is largely a clinical diagnosis, imaging is not required although the dynamic role of ultrasound can easily confirm the clinical impression. Occasionally ultrasound can demonstrate whether it is one or both tendons

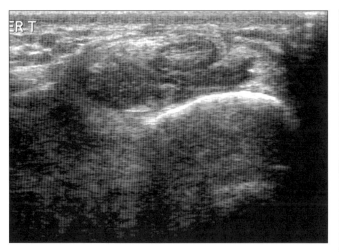

Fig. 10.32 Peroneal tendons have subluxed to lie lateral to the fibular during dynamic scanning.

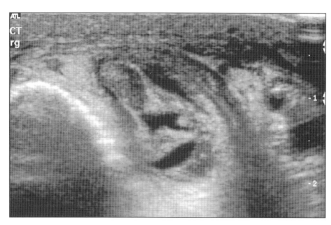

Fig. 10.33 Peroneal tendinopathy and tenosynovitis.

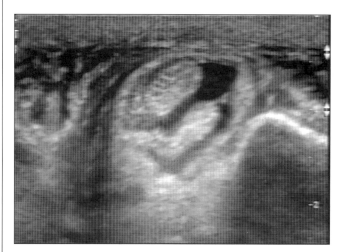

Fig. 10.34 Peroneal tenosynovitis.

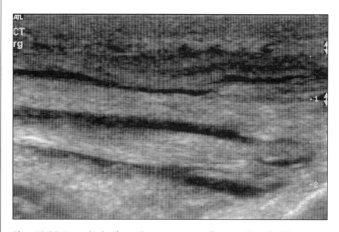

Fig. 10.35 Longituinal section corresponding to Fig. 10.34.

that have subluxed (Fig. 10.32). Diagnosis is followed by operative reduction and repair or reinforcement of the retinaculum.

Peroneal tendon entrapment

Entrapment of the peroneal tendons usually occurs as a consequence of a complex fracture of the os calcis (19). As CT is better at depicting the relationship of the bony fragments, it is the investigation of choice for also demonstrating the associated tendon entrapment. Entrapment may rarely be associated with an enlarged peroneal process of the os calcis (20).

Peroneal tendinopathy

> **Key point**
>
> Peroneus brevis tendinopathy is more common than peroneus longus.

Although less common than chronic tibialis posterior tendinopathy, peroneal tendinopathy represents an important cause of lateral aspect hindfoot pain. The peroneus brevis tendon is more frequently affected. Peroneal tendinopathy manifests as multiple longitudinal splits (21), most commonly within peroneus brevis (22) (Fig. 10.33), coupled with enlargement and thickening of the tendon sheath (23) (Figs 10.34 and 10.35). This characteristic appearance gives rise to the name peroneal split syndrome by which this condition is also known. In some instances a large longitudinal split of peroneus brevis can cause peroneus longus to displace anteriorly, separating the split brevis tendon into two components. The appearance of three tendons within the tendon sheath can be confusing if this phenomenon is not appreciated (24). Peroneus longus tendinopathy also occurs although this is less common (25) and more distal, affecting the tendon at the level of the cuboid notch or at the site of insertion into an os perineum (26). This latter syndrome is more common in diabetics (27). Frank rupture of the peroneal tendons is uncommon.

> **Key point**
>
> Frank rupture of the peroneal tendons is uncommon.

Lateral ligament complex injuries

> **Practical tip**
>
> The lateral ligament complex is examined with the foot in slight plantar flexion and a transverse-orientated probe.

The lateral ligament complex is examined with slight foot plantar flexion and a transverse-orientated probe. The principle ligaments amenable to ultrasound interrogation are the anterior talofibular ligament (ATaFL) and the calcaneofibular ligament (CFL) (28). The anterior talofibular ligament is a small structure running anteriorly between the tibia and the fibula. It generally measures approximately 3 mm in diameter. Anterior talofibular ligament tears are seen as a gross disruption of the normal organised ligamentous structure, which becomes a poorly reflective mass. In patients where there is associated bony avulsion, the diagnosis becomes easier. A clue to the presence of an anterior talofibular ligament tear can be seen on a coronal image of the lateral malleolus where a poorly reflective focus can be seen to lie adjacent to the tip of the malleolus. Using varus stress can increase the sensitivity of the examination (29). Tears of the ATaFL are common and follow most substantial inversion injuries of the ankle (Fig. 10.36). Tenderness is localised to just below and anterior to the lateral malleolus. The clinical features are such that ultrasound is rarely needed to confirm injury. There is no specific treatment for chronic rupture of this ligament if the ankle remains stable.

There are two other components to the lateral ligament complex, the posterior talofibular ligament and the calcaneofibular ligament. The former is a very strong structure and is rarely torn in the absence of frank ankle dislocation. The calcaneofibular ligament is a thicker but a

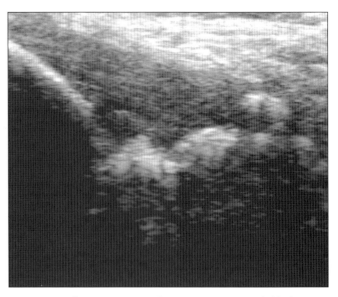

Fig. 10.36 Inflammatory mass from torn anterior talofibular ligament.

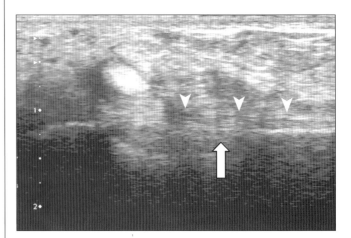

Fig. 10.37 Normal calcaneofibular ligament (arrowheads) separating os calcis (arrow) from peroneal tendons.

defined structure, which can be identified lying between the peroneal tendon sheath and the underlying os calcis (Fig. 10.37). Generally it is thicker and brighter than the anterior talofibular ligament. Rupture of the calcaneofibular ligament confers greater instability on the hindfoot and its presence is often an indication that surgery is required for stabilisation (Fig. 10.38). Osteochondral injuries to the talar dome may also occur following inversion injuries where lateral collateral ligament injuries are suspected. Unfortunately ultrasound is limited in that the entire talar dome cannot be visualised and

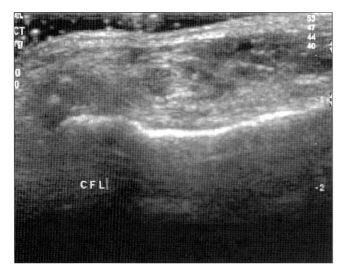

Fig. 10.38 Tilted axial section along calcaneofibular ligament. The ligament itself is intact but is avulsed from the fibula where there is an inflammatory mass.

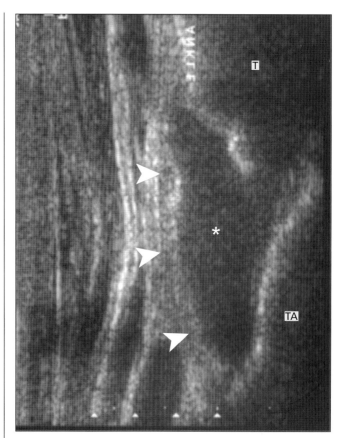

Fig. 10.39 Sagittal section along anterior aspect of ankle joint showing effusion (asterisk) and anterior capsule (arrowheads).

consequently MR is recommended in patients with persistent lateral pain following inversion injury.

ANTERIOR ANKLE PAIN

Tears in the extensor tendons are rare, but are reported in skiers, soccer players and downhill runners. The anterior tibial tendon is the largest and the most commonly injured of the extensor tendons. Anterior ankle pain may also reflect tibio talar joint disease or an ankle impingement syndrome.

Ankle impingement syndromes

Five ankle impingement syndromes are identified. The principal tool in their imaging assessment is MRI (30), although ultrasound plays a more important role in some.

Anterior impingement syndrome

Anterior impingement syndrome is most often described in athletes, particularly sprinters and footballers, and as an occupational hazard amongst those who work on ladders. The diagnosis can usually be made on plain films where a lateral ankle radiograph will demonstrate a characteristic bony spur arising off the anteroinferior margin of the tibia (Fig. 10.39). In many cases this may be associated with a bony divot on the dorsal surface of the talus.

> **Key point**
>
> Diagnosis of anterior impingement syndrome can usually be made on plain films where a lateral ankle radiograph will demonstrate a characteristic bony spur arising off the anteroinferior margin of the tibia.

Ultrasound can readily demonstrate this spur and the associated effusion and synovitis typical of anterior impingement syndrome. The lesion is best diagnosed with the probe in the sagittal plane where the characteristic triangular fat plane that normally fills the space between the tibia and talus is displaced anteriorly and poorly reflective fluid outlines the spur. A rare variant involves a synovial mass without bony involvement and in these instances, ultrasound is pivotal in the presence of normal plain films.

These patients respond well to trimming of the spur (31–33), although it can reoccur, though not necessarily with recurrence of symptoms.

Posterior impingement syndrome

The os trigonum syndrome is due to impingement of the bony and soft-tissue structures between the dorsal aspect of the tibia and talus on plantar flexion. The soft-tissue structures involve connective tissue around the os trigonum, prominent posterior stieda process or occasionally a prominent posterior lip of the tibia (34). An os trigonum is present in up to 10% of the population but of itself is not a cause of symptoms. Posterior impingement syndrome is prominent in patients who consistently hyperplantar flex, such as ballet dancers (35) and gymnasts. Pain generally arises on the posterior and lateral aspect of the ankle joint and palpable swelling may be apparent. Plantar flexion is reduced and causes pain. With more severe involvement of the flexor hallucis longus, pain on flexion of the great toe may be a feature. Posterior tibial nerve irritation may also occur as can inflammation of the posteroinferior tibiofibular ligament, the tibial slip ligament.

Ultrasound can demonstrate a mass deep reflectivity surrounding the os trigonum, which itself may appear irregular. MR is superior in demonstrating the abnormal marrow signal changes that lie within the bone (Fig. 10.40). Posterior impingement syndrome may be associated with flexor hallucis tenosynovitis. Fluid can be identified within the flexor hallucis tendon sheath, although it should be recognised that in a high proportion of normal individuals there is a communication between the tibiotalar joint and the flexor hallucis longus tendon sheath. The identification of small quantities of fluid within the sheath is therefore within normal limits.

Anterolateral impingment syndrome

The anterolateral impingement syndrome is a poorly understood syndrome where a soft-tissue chronic synovial mass is identified at the anterolateral gutter of the ankle. In a tiny proportion of cases this may be associated with the formation of meniscoid-type tissue. The ultrasound appearances of the anterolateral gutter mass have not been fully defined but it

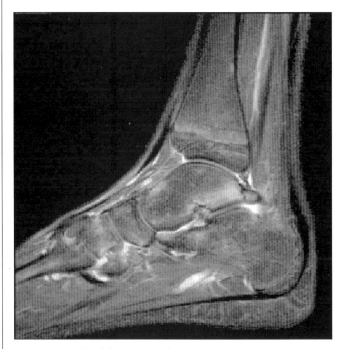

Fig. 10.40 Sagittal fat-saturated STIR image showing inflammatory changes within the os trigonum with soft-tissue inflammatory changes in the surrounding soft tissues typical of os trigonum syndrome.

can be used to detect the presence of an intact anterior talofibular ligament, which makes the diagnosis unlikely. Gadolinium MR arthrography of the tibiotalar joint is superior in its detection and classification of this entity.

> **Practical tip**
>
> Detection by ultrasound of an intact anterior talofibular ligament makes the diagnosis of anterolateral impingement syndrome unlikely.

Anteromedial impingement

This relatively recently described entity is similar to anterolateral impingement. The MR findings include capsular and synovial soft-tissue thickening anterior to the tibiotalar ligaments and associated osseous abnormalities (30). The ultrasound findings have not been described.

Distal tibiofibular impingement

This entity, also called syndesmotic impingement, is characterised by the presence of a synovial mass in the tibiofibular recess of the tibiotalar joint. Generally an arthroscopic diagnosis, the ultrasound appearances in this entity have not been described. The diagnosis is often made arthroscopically when a synovial mass is extruded from the distal tibiofibular joint on squeezing the tibia and fibula. It may be possible to demonstrate this on a dynamic ultrasound examination.

SOFT-TISSUE MASSES OF THE FOOT

The role of ultrasound in the detection and assessment of soft-tissue masses is dealt with elsewhere. Certain soft-tissue lesions are characteristic in the foot and some additional discussion is therefore appropriate. This is particularly true where the mass is located along the plantar surface of the foot, where certain lesions unique to the mid-foot are identified. The most common of these is the plantar fibroma.

Fibroma

> **Key point**
>
> The most characteristic appearance of plantar fibromata on ultrasound is of a moderately well-demarcated, poorly reflective mass superficial to, but intimately related with the plantar fascia, which itself may be distorted or displaced by the lesion.

Plantar fibromatosis, sometimes called Ledderhose disease, affects adults between the ages of 30 and 50 years. They are not uncommonly multiple and bilateral. Like plantar fasciitis they occur more commonly in the medial limb of the plantar fascia. Plantar fibromata can have variable appearances on ultrasound. Most characteristic is a moderately well-demarcated, poorly reflective mass superficial to but intimately related with the plantar fascia (36), which itself may be distorted or displaced by the lesion. In some cases a cicatrised pattern may be identified again centred on the plantar fascia. Lesions can vary considerably is size (Figs 10.41 and 10.42) and may be multiple. There is an association with palmar or plantar contractures. The differential diagnosis of plantar fibroma includes foreign body reaction, implantation and dermoid and subcutaneous fat necrosis. The presence of reflective organic material can assist in the diagnosis of foreign body reaction where a history of puncture injury is not always apparent.

This common entity is to be distinguished from other superficial fibromatous conditions. These include recurring digital fibromas of infancy, which is an uncommon condition. Also

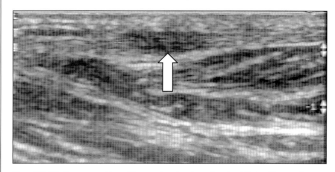

Fig. 10.41 Long section through plantar fascia. Note the rather subtle decreased reflectivity within the fascia of this small plantar fibroma (arrow).

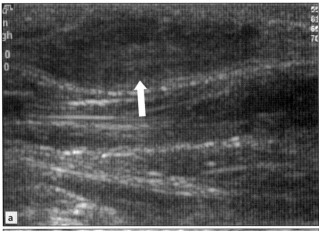

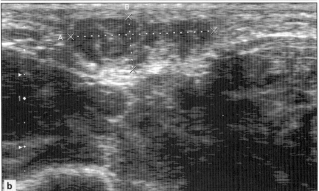

Fig. 10.42 Longitudinal (a, arrow) and axial (b, between markers) images of large lobulated plantar fibroma.

termed Reye tumour, infantile digital fibroma or infantile digital myofibroblastoma, the condition is characterised by multiple painless lesions arising from the distal fingers and toes usually on the dorsolateral aspect. They may be associated with flexion contractures. Older children are most commonly affected by juvenile aponeurotic fibroma, an aggressive fibrous proliferation arising in the aponeurosis of the hands or feet. This lesion may calcify, infiltrate adjacent tissues, and like many others of the fibromatoses has a tendency to recur following incomplete excision. It is twice as common in boys.

The deep fibromatoses are dealt with in Chapter 11.

Morton's neuroma

Another characteristic lesion that occurs only in the forefoot is Morton's neuroma (37). Morton's neuroma is a lesion caused by fibrous degeneration of the plantar digital nerve. In many cases there is an associated intermetatarsal bursitis. It typically occurs in middle-aged

females who complain of pain and parasthesia in the web space. The precise aetiology is unknown although tight footwear have been implicated in its aetiology. Morton's neuromata are most frequently encountered in the third/fourth and second/third web spaces and are rare in the first/second and fourth/fifth.

> **Key point**
>
> Morton's neuromata are most frequently encountered in the third/fourth and second/third web spaces of the foot and are rare in the first/second and fourth/fifth.

> **Practical tip**
>
> Ultrasound examination of the web spaces between the toes is best carried out from the plantar aspect, with the probe initially in the transverse plane at the level of the metatarsal heads. A normal interspace is characterised by reflective material comprising fat and connective tissue. Morton's neuroma is characterized by a poorly defined, poorly reflective mass within the interspace.

Ultrasound examination of the web space is best carried out from the plantar aspect and carries a high accuracy in the detection of neuromata (38, 39). The technique employed by the author is to place the probe initially in the transverse plane at the level of the metatarsal heads and examine each interspace in turn. A normal interspace is characterised by reflective material comprising fat and connective tissue (Fig. 10.43). Morton's neuroma is characterised by a poorly defined, poorly reflective mass within the interspace (Figs 10.44–10.46). Lesions vary in size but Pollack et al. determined that lesions more than 5 mm in size were more likely to cause symptoms (40). In many patients the second/third interspace can be difficult to examine due to approximation of the metatarsal heads and in these instances the diagnosis of Morton's neuroma can be made more difficult.

> **Practical tip**
>
> In some cases a Morton's neuroma becomes more obvious by interdigital palpation with a finger on the dorsal aspect of the foot or by a gentle squeezing of the metatarsal heads.

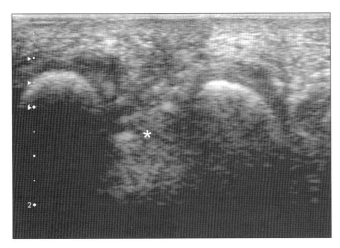

Fig. 10.43 Normal intermetatarsal interspace. Note reflective normal interspace tissue (asterisk)

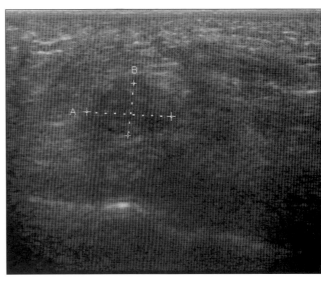

Fig. 10.46 Long-axis sagittal section through Morton's neuroma.

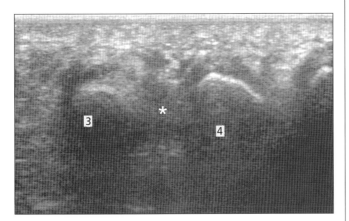

Fig. 10.44 Imaged oriented similar to Fig. 10.43 but with poorly reflective mass within the interspace representing a small neuroma.

In other cases a Morton's neuroma can become more obvious by interdigital palpation with a finger on the dorsal aspect of the foot or by a gentle squeezing of the metatarsal heads (Fig. 10.47). In the latter instance they appear to bulge from between the metatarsal heads on the plantar aspect of the foot and occasionally this can be accompanied by a palpable click, termed a Moulders click (Figs 10.48 and 10.49). Once identified the Morton's neuroma can be injected under ultrasound guidance (Fig. 10.50).

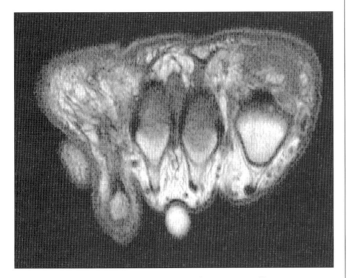

Fig. 10.45 Coronal T1-weighted MRI showing small Morton's neuroma within the third/fourth interspace.

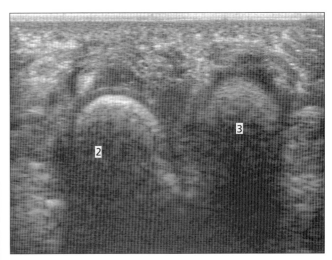

Fig. 10.47 Small hyporeflective Morton's neuroma in the 2nd, 3rd interspace.

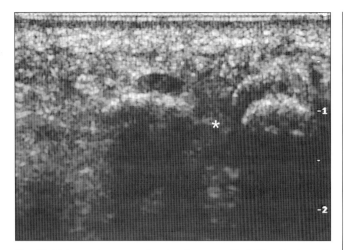

Fig. 10.48 Lateral compression has been applied (Moulder's test) to augment the appearance of this small neuroma. Lying prone and compression in the interspace from above are other manoeuvres that can assist, but are not usually necessary.

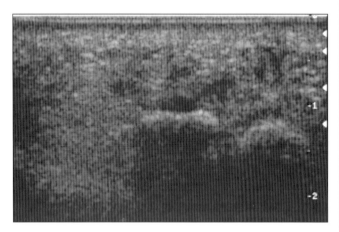

Fig. 10.49 Slightly more heterogenous Morton's neuroma also during Moulder's compression.

Miscellaneous lesions in the foot

> **Practical tip**
>
> Stress and fatigue injuries of the foot and ankle can occur at the medial malleolus, the posterior aspect of the os calcis, the second and third metatarsals and, less commonly, in the bones of the mid-foot.

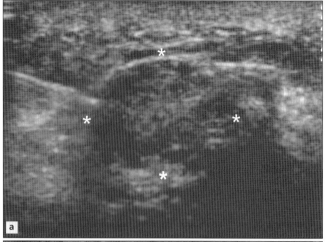

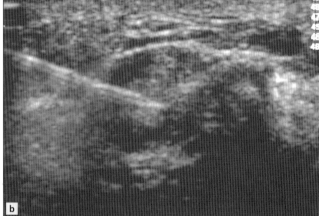

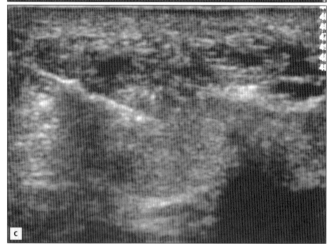

Fig. 10.50 Sagittal image through poorly reflective Morton's neuroma. (a) A needle lies on the edge of the neuroma (between asterisks). (b) The needle has been advanced into the centre of the neuroma and ready to inject. (c) Postinjection, the reflectivity within the neuroma is increased as a result of the corticosteroid.

Although in general ultrasound is unhelpful in the diagnosis of bony disease, it can be a useful adjunct to equivocal plain film radiography in the assessment of stress fracture. Stress and fatigue injuries of the foot and ankle are common. The sites of occurrence include the medial malleolus, the posterior aspect of the os calcis, the second and third metatarsals and, less commonly, in the bones of the mid-foot. Of these, ultrasound is really only useful in the detection of stress fractures of the metatarsals. The commonest location is at the junction of the proximal and middle thirds and careful ultrasound examination in this area can show the periosteal elevation associated with these injuries, even before the plain film becomes abnormal.

Rarer sites of stress fractures include the proximal phalanx of the great toe, which occurs more commonly in patients with hallux valgus. The differential diagnosis here includes sesamoiditis.

Freiberg infraction is a disorder of unknown aetiology affecting the second, occasionally the third, metatarsal head. A combination of trauma and a vascular predisposition is assumed. High-heeled shoes have been implicated as a causative factor. Freiberg infraction is more common in women and most commonly seen in adolescence. Patients may present with pain and limited motion, although symptoms may not begin until degenerative arthrosis has developed.

Turf toe most commonly occurs in football players who play on hard, artificial surfaces and wear lightweight, flexible shoes. Hyperextension injury at the first metatarsophalangeal results in disruption of the volar fibrocartilaginous plantar plate, which extends along the plantar aspect of the toe. The 1st and 2nd rays are the most commonly affected. Increased distance between the sesamoid and the base of the 1st ray can be an additional clue for complete rupture. More severe injuries also involve the intertransverse ligament.

REFERENCES

1. Richards PJ, Dheer AK, McCall IM. Achilles tendon (TA) size and power Doppler ultrasound (PD) changes compared to MRI: A preliminary observational study. Clin Radiol 2001; 56(10):843–50.
2. Mellado J, Rosenberg ZS, Beltran J. Low incorporation of soleus tendon: A potential diagnostic pitfall on MR imaging. Skeletal Radiol 1998;27(4):222–4.
3. Galluzzo E, Lischi DM, Taglione E, Lombardini F, Pasero G, Perri G, et al. Sonographic analysis of the ankle in patients with psoriatic arthritis. Scand J Rheum 2000;29(1):52–5.
4. Olivieri I, Barozzi L, Padula A, De Matteis M, Pierro A, Cantini F, et al. Retrocalcaneal bursitis in spondyloarthropathy: Assessment by ultrasonography and magnetic resonance imaging. J Rheum 1998;25(7):1352–7.
5. Khan KM, Forster BB, Robinson J, Cheong Y, Louis L, Maclean L, Taunton JE. Are ultrasound and magnetic resonance imaging of value in assessment of Achilles tendon disorders? A two year prospective study. Br J Sports Med 2003;37:149–53.
6. Yu JS, Witte D, Resnick D, Pogue W. Ossification of the Achilles tendon: Imaging abnormalities in 12 patients. Skelet Radiol 1994;23(2):127–31.
7. Bottger BA, Schweitzer ME, El-Noueam KI, Desai M. MR imaging of the normal and abnormal retrocalcaneal bursae. Am J Roentgen 1998;170(5):1239–41.
8. Kruger-Franke M, Scherzer S. [Long-term results of surgically treated Achilles tendon ruptures]. Unfallchirurg 1993;96(10):524–8.
9. Mathiak G, Wening JV, Mathiak M, Neville LF, Jungbluth K. Serum cholesterol is elevated in patients with Achilles tendon ruptures. Arch Orthopaed Trauma Surg 1999;119(5–6):280–4.
10. Buchgraber A, Passler HH. Percutaneous repair of Achilles tendon rupture. Immobilization versus functional postoperative treatment. Clin Orthop 1997(341):113–22.
11. Gibbon WW, Long G. Ultrasound of the plantar aponeurosis (fascia). Skeletal Radiol 1999;28(1):21–6.
12. Cardinal E, Chhem RK, Beauregard CG, Aubin B, Pelletier M. Plantar fasciitis: Sonographic evaluation. Radiology 1996; 201(1):257–9.
13. Wall JR, Harkness MA, Crawford A. Ultrasound diagnosis of plantar fasciitis. Foot Ankle 1993;14(8):465–70.
14. LeMelle DP, Kisilewicz P, Janis LR. Chronic plantar fascial inflammation and fibrosis. Clin Podiatr Med Surg 1990; 7(2):385–9.
15. Leach R, Jones R, Silva T. Rupture of the plantar fascia in athletes. J Bone Joint Surg Am 1978;60(4):537–9.
16. Holmes GB, Mann RA. Possible epidemiological factors associated with rupture of the posterior tibial tendon. Foot Ankle 1992;13(2):70–9.
17. Schweitzer ME, Karasick D. MRI of the ankle and hindfoot. Semin Ultrasound CT MR 1994;15(5):410–22.
18. McNally EG. Posteromedial subtalar coalition: Imaging appearances in three cases. Skeletal Radiol 1999;28(12):691–5.
19. Wright DG, Sangeorzan BJ. Calcaneal fracture with peroneal impingement and tendon dysfunction. Foot Ankle Int 1996;17(10):650.
20. Boles MA, Lomasney LM, Demos TC, Sage RA. Enlarged peroneal process with peroneus longus tendon entrapment. Skeletal Radiol 1997;26(5):313–5.
21. Yao L, Tong DJ, Cracchiolo A, Seeger LL. MR findings in peroneal tendonopathy. J Comput Assist Tomogr 1995;19(3): 460–4.
22. Diaz GC, van Holsbeeck M, Jacobson JA. Longitudinal split of the peroneus longus and peroneus brevis tendons with disruption of the superior peroneal retinaculum. J Ultrasound Med 1998;17(8):525–9.
23. Leppilahti J, Flinkkila T, Hyvonen P, Hamalainen M. Longitudinal split of peroneus brevis tendon. A report on two cases. Ann Chir Gynaecol 2000;89(1):61–4.
24. Rosenberg ZS, Beltran J, Cheung YY, Colon E, Herraiz F. MR features of longitudinal tears of the peroneus brevis tendon. Am J Roentgenol 1997;168(1):141–7.
25. Brandes CB, Smith RW. Characterization of patients with primary peroneus longus tendinopathy: a review of twenty-two cases. Foot Ankle Int 2000;21(6):462–8.
26. Sammarco GJ. Peroneus longus tendon tears: Acute and chronic. Foot Ankle Int 1995;16(5):245–53.
27. Truong DT, Dussault RG, Kaplan PA. Fracture of the os peroneum and rupture of the peroneus longus tendon as a complication of diabetic neuropathy. Skeletal Radiol 1995; 24(8):626–8.
28. Milz P, Milz S, Steinborn M, Mittlmeier T, Putz R, Reiser M. Lateral ankle ligaments and tibiofibular syndesmosis. 13-MHz high-frequency sonography and MRI compared in 20 patients. Acta Orthop Scand 1998;69(1):51–5.
29. Gruber G, Nebe M, Bachmann G, Litzlbauer HD. [Ultrasonography as a diagnostic measure in the rupture of fibular ligaments. Comparative study: sonography versus radiological investigations]. Rofo Fortschr Geb Rontgenstr Neuen Bildgeb Verfahr 1998;169(2):152–6.
30. Robinson P, White LM, Salonen DC, Daniels TR, Ogilvie Harris D. Anterolateral ankle impingement: MR arthrographic assessment of the anterolateral recess. Radiology 2001;221(1): 186–90.
31. Branca A, Di Palma L, Bucca C, Visconti CS, Di Mille M. Arthroscopic treatment of anterior ankle impingement. Foot Ankle Int 1997;18(7):418–23.
32. Reynaert P, Gelen G, Geens G. Arthroscopic treatment of anterior impingement of the ankle. Acta Orthop Belg 1994;60(4):384–8.

33. Ogilvie Harris DJ, Mahomed N, Demaziere A. Anterior impingement of the ankle treated by arthroscopic removal of bony spurs. J Bone Joint Surg Ser B 1993;75(3):437–40.

34. Hedrick MR, McBryde AM. Posterior ankle impingement. Foot Ankle Int 1994;15(1):2–8.

35. Wredmark T, Carlstedt CA, Bauer H, Saartok T. Os trigonum syndrome: A clinical entity in ballet dancers. Foot Ankle Int 1991;11(6):404–6.

36. Bedi DG, Davidson DM. Plantar fibromatosis: Most common sonographic appearance and variations. J Clin Ultrasound 2001;29(9):499–505.

37. Morton D. A peculiar and painfull affection of the fourth metatarsophalangeal articulation. Am J Med Sci 1876;71:35.

38. Sobiesk GA, Wertheimer SJ, Schulz R, Dalfovo M. Sonographic evaluation of interdigital neuromas. J Foot Ankle Surg 1997;36(5):364–6.

39. Shapiro PP, Shapiro SL. Sonographic evaluation of interdigital neuromas. Foot Ankle Int 1995;16(10):604–6.

40. Pollak RA, Bellacosa RA, Dornbluth NC, Strash WW, Devall JM. Sonographic analysis of Morton's neuroma. J Foot Surg 1992;31(6):534–7.

Ultrasound of soft-tissue masses

11

Simon J Ostlere

INTRODUCTION

> **Key point**
>
> The vast majority of lesions are benign and in many of these cases malignancy can be excluded from the history and examination without resorting to imaging.

Soft-tissue masses of the musculoskeletal system are extremely common. The vast majority of lesions are benign and in many of these cases malignancy can be excluded from the history and examination without resorting to imaging. Because of the overwhelmingly high ratio of benign to malignant lesions there is often a delay in diagnosing the latter and early imaging is therefore recommended when the nature of a mass is in doubt. Any mass that is steadily increasing in size warrants urgent investigation. When surgery is being considered, imaging can also provide useful information on benign soft-tissue masses with regard to their nature and relation to surrounding structures.

Ultrasound and MRI are the principle techniques for investigating soft-tissue masses. As in other areas of musculoskeletal imaging the two techniques are complementary and both may be employed in any individual case. In most peripheral and superficial lesions ultrasound provides all the information required. Deep, large or diffuse lesions are best initially imaged with MRI. Plain radiograph or CT occasionally gives additional useful information with regard to calcification or subtle involvement of the underlying bone. Ultrasound is the easiest method for guiding percutaneous biopsy.

The clinician referring a patient with a suspected soft-tissue mass is usually asking one or more of the following questions: (a) is there a lesion? (b) where is it? (c) what is it? Ultrasound has been shown to be a highly sensitive technique in the detection of soft-tissue masses. A normal ultrasound examination excludes a soft-tissue mass with a high degree of certainty. Although not often helpful in making a precise diagnosis, ultrasound can readily differentiate solid from cystic lesions. Purely cystic lesions are benign whereas a minority of solid or mixed lesions may turn out to be malignant. Other ultrasound features such as lesion morphology, calcification, compressibility, the presence and type of vascularity and the pattern of internal echoes can all help to narrow the differential diagnosis. MRI will provide additional information with regard to tissue type in lipomatous lesions, fibrous lesions and those containing haemosiderin or other blood products.

Key point

Although not often helpful in making a precise diagnosis, ultrasound can readily differentiate solid from cystic lesions.

Cysts do not require biopsy but are often subjected to therapeutic excision, aspiration or injection. Small superficial solid lesions should be treated by excisional biopsy. Larger or deeper lesions require staging with MRI and, in most cases, preoperative biopsy, which can be performed under ultrasound control.

Although ultrasound is generally nonspecific, a confident diagnosis can commonly be obtained by taking into consideration the clinical features along with the ultrasound appearances. This chapter describes the ultrasound features of the commoner lesions encountered in clinical practice with emphasis on those with more specific ultrasound features.

LIPOMATOUS TUMOURS

Lipomatous tumours range from the benign lipoma to highly maliganant forms of liposarcoma. Well-differentiated liposarcomas do not metastasise but have the potential for local recurrence and rarely dedifferentiation. In general, benign lipoma, its variants and well-differentiated liposarcoma are seen are echogenic lesions on ultrasound in contrast to most other soft-tissue tumours. Although ultrasound may be used to diagnose the simple subcutaneous lipoma, MRI is considered superior for all other

lesions on account of the characteristic signal returned by fat. As deep-seated lipoma cannot be differentiated from liposarcoma, all deep lesions should be imaged by MRI prior to biopsy or surgery.

Lipomas

Lipomas are benign tumours that may occur in almost any part of the body. In the soft tissues they may be divided into superficial and deep lesions.

Superficial lipomas

The majority of lipomas are found in subcutaneous fat. The peak incidence is in the fifth to seventh decade. Lesions predominate in the trunk and proximal part of the limbs, the shoulder girdle region being a particularly common site. An ultrasound request is usually prompted by the patient noticing an increase in the size of a lesion or the discovery of a new lump. Most superficial lipomas have characteristic features on ultrasound and do not require additional imaging or biopsy. A typical subcutaneous lipoma is an elliptical, well-defined, compressible lesion containing short linear reflective striations that run parallel to the skin (Fig. 11.1). The lesion may exhibit acoustic enhancement (1). The reflectivity is variable and depends, in part, on the site of the lesion. Lesions of the head and neck have been described as

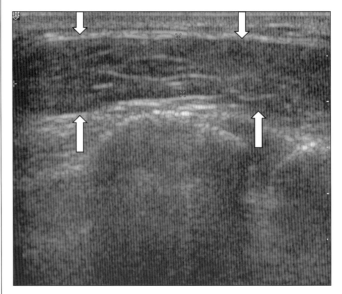

Fig. 11.1 Typical subcutaneous lipoma (arrows). The lesion is hypoechoic and contains linear striations.

being typically hyperechoic, whereas those in the extremities tend to be more variable (2, 3) (Fig. 11.2). Doppler signal is usually not detectable. The lesion occasionally may be almost invisible on ultrasound when the tumour has a similar internal structure as the adjacent subcutaneous fat. A confident diagnosis of a lipoma can be made when there is a palpable superficial mass and no apparent abnormality detected on ultrasound. Although superficial liposarcomas are rare, further imaging and biopsy are required if there are suspicious features such as increased vascularity or rapid growth.

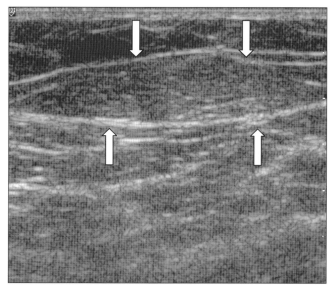

Fig. 11.2 Subcutaneous lipoma. The lesion (arrows) has a typical elliptical shape with multiple striations and is slightly hyperechoic when compared to adjacent fat.

> **Key point**
>
> A typical subcutaneous lipoma is an elliptical, well-defined, compressible lesion containing short linear reflective striations that run parallel to the skin.

Deep lipomas

Deep-seated lipomas are uncommon compared with their superficial counterparts. They tend to present later than superficial lesions and are therefore, on average, larger. Deep lipomas may occur in an intermuscular or intramusculsr position. The shape of the lesion is less predictable as it tends to conform to the surrounding structures. In the author's experience deep lipomas invariably are uniformly hyperechoic relative to muscle (Figs 11.3 and 11.4). Some intramuscular lipoma may have ill-defined borders due to interdigitation of fat with the muscle fibres. This feature is much better demonstrated on MRI and, when present, indicates that the lesion is benign (4). Most deep lesions are best imaged with MRI, ultrasound being reserved for guided biopsy when necessary. Deep-seated lipoma and well-differentiated liposarcoma may have similar ultrasound features and MRI is therefore indicated. Although the detection of nonfatty tissue on MRI implies that the lesion is not a simple lipoma, low-grade liposarcoma may suppress entirely on fat suppression sequences. The presence of thick-enhancing fibrous septa will favour the diagnosis of liposarcoma. Although often performed,

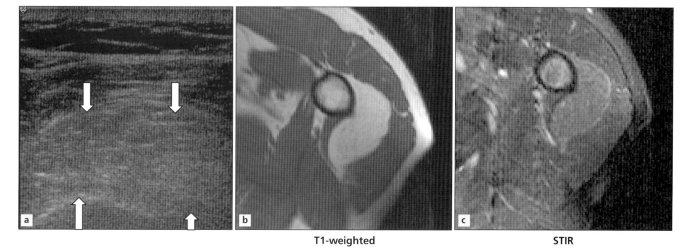

T1-weighted STIR

Fig. 11.3 (a) Deep lipoma. The lipoma is seen as a uniform hyperechoic lesion (arrows) situated deep to muscle. (b,c) T1 and STIR axial images through the upper arm. The lipoma is seen to lie deep within deltoid. The fat suppresses completely on the STIR images. Fine fibrous strands can be seen within the lesion on the T1-weighted image.

percutaneous biopsy in these equivocal cases can be unrewarding as the histological differentiation of low-grade liposarcoma from lipoma may be difficult even with the benefit of the entire resected specimen. In large lipomas ultrasound may detect areas of mineralisation secondary to necrosis, or focal bony hyperostosis if the lesion is lying in a paraosteal position.

Other benign lipomatous tumours

There are several lipoma variants. Angiolipomas are typically small subcutaneous lesions seen in the young adults, are often multiple and do not require imaging.

Fibrolipoma describes a lipoma with abundant fibrous strands. The lesions are hyperechoic lesions that cannot be distinguished from a simple lipoma (Fig. 11.5).

Lipoblastoma is a rare tumour of childhood, usually seen under the age of 3 years. The tumour is typically lobulated, may contain cystic areas and is hypovascular. Fat signal may or may not be seen on MRI or CT (5, 6). On ultrasound the lesion has been described as uniformly echogenic and generally hypovascular although small amounts of flow may be seen on Doppler (7).

Hibernoma is a benign tumour of brown fat. It occurs chiefly in the upper thorax in patients in their fourth and fifth decade. Clinically it behaves in a manner similar to that of simple lipomas. On MR the signal intensity of the lesion is less high on T1-weighted images than that of lipoma reflecting the smaller proportion of fat-containing cells. Hibernoma are more vascular than lipomas and will enhance following contrast. The ultrasound appearances have been described as showing a hyperechoic, vascular mass (8, 9).

Liposarcoma

The term liposarcoma covers a range of tumours with varying histological and imaging features. Liposarcomas often have a nonspecific appearance shared by other soft-tissue sarcomas, although well-differentiated lesions are usually hyperehoic and may mimic a simple lipoma. Occasionally tumours contain foci of calcification or ossification of varying size. The role of ultrasound in these deep-seated lesions is limited as the tissue characteristics and the relationship of the tumour to the surrounding structures is best appreciated on MRI. Ultrasound is an excellent tool for guiding percutaneous biopsy if this is required.

Well-differentiated liposarcoma

This lesion, sometimes termed atypical lipoma, is at the most benign end of the spectrum. The incidence peaks in the sixth and seventh decade and the deep muscles of the proximal portions of the extremities, particularly the thigh, is the most common site. The lesion has no metastatic potential and the prognosis is excellent if excision is complete. Neglected lesions will continue to grow and are at risk of dedifferentiating into a higher grade of sarcoma with high risk of metastases. Unlike other sarcomas an atypical lipoma is typically shown by ultrasound to be a lesion that is hyperechoic relative to adjacent muscle. The tumour may have an identical

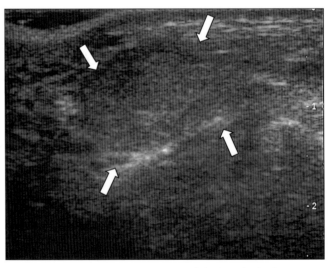

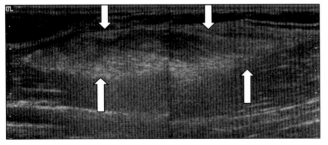

Fig. 11.4 Intramuscular lipoma. The tumour is seen as an elliptical, relatively hyperechoic mass lying within the muscle.

Fig. 11.5 Fibrolipoma of the dorsum of the hand. The lesion (arrows) is echogenic relative to adjacent muscle.

appearance to a deep lipoma (Fig. 11.6). The demonstration of relatively hypoechoic areas and/or internal vascularity on Doppler indicate that the lesion is likely to represent a liposarcoma (Figs 11.7 and 11.8).

> **Key point**
>
> Unlike other sarcomas an atypical lipoma is typically shown by ultrasound to be a lesion that is hyperechoic relative to adjacent muscle.

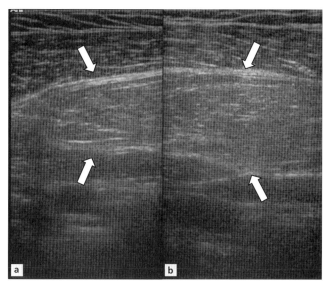

Fig. 11.6 Atypical lipoma of the chest wall. The lesion is uniformly echogenic and cannot be differentiated from a simple lipoma on ultrasound criteria alone.

Myxoid liposarcoma

Myxoid liposarcomas is histologically distinct from low-grade liposarcoma. The lesion contains numerous lipoblasts and small plexiform vessels in a well-vascularised myxomatous stroma that has a variable fat content. The proportion of myxoid material, lipid-containing tumour and more cellular tumour can vary, giving a spectrum of imaging appearances. Some tumours are purely myxoid and give very uniform homogeneous features on imaging. On MRI these lesions are usually returning fairly homogeneous high signal on T2-weighted images and low signal on T1-weighted images, features that, without the benefit of ultrasound or intravenous contrast, could be misinterpreted as representing a cystic lesion. The less-differentiated tumours (merging with round cell liposarcoma) have a more nonspecific appearance on imaging. In most cases of myxoid liposarcoma there is a lipomatous component that can be detected on MRI (10).

High-grade liposarcoma

Higher-grade liposarcomas such as round cell and pleomorphic types have no specific ultrasound features that will differentiate them from other sarcomas. Tumours are often highly heterogeneous on imaging. The lesion may be composed of large areas of tumour of varying histological grade. Referral to the MR images at time of ultrasound-guided biopsy will help ensure that the most aggressive part of the

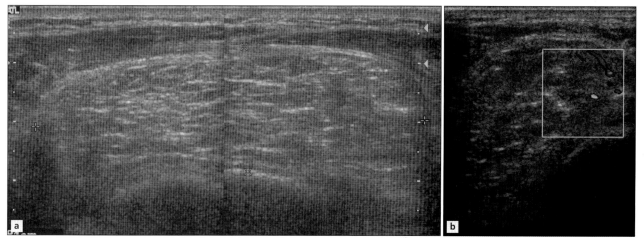

Fig. 11.7 Low-grade liposarcoma. (a) The lesion is seen as a large deep-seated hyperechoic lesion typical of a lipomatous tumour. (b) Some internal vascularity is detected on Doppler, which would be an unusual feature for a simple lipoma.

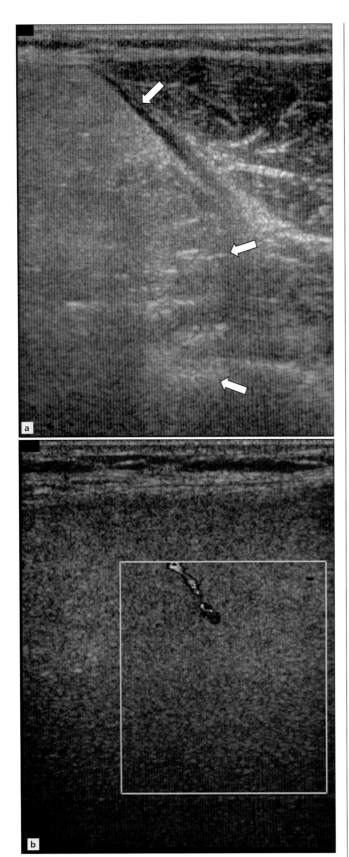

tumour is sampled (Fig. 11.9). Well-differentiated liposarcoma may undergo dedifferentiation to a higher-grade sarcoma. Areas of high-grade sarcoma, usually fibrosarcoma or malignant fibrous histiocytoma, result in a nonspecific heterogenous echo pattern with detectable vascularity on Doppler. On MRI the

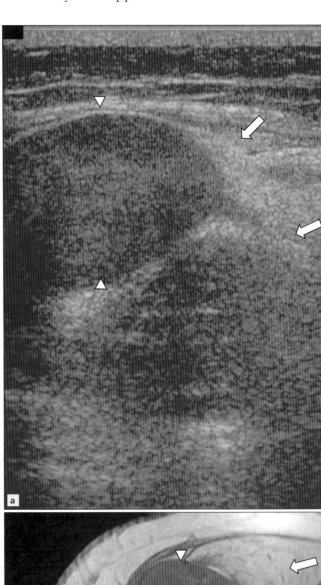

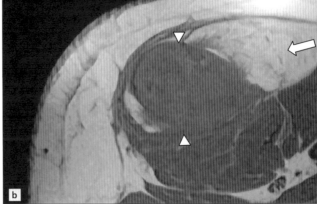

Fig. 11.8 Low-grade liposarcoma of the thigh. (a) This large lesion is uniformly echogenic when compared to the adjacent muscle. (b) There is tumour vascularity, which, along with the size and position of the lesion, indicates that this is a liposarcoma.

Fig. 11.9 High-grade liposarcoma. (a) Ultrasound and (b) T1-weighted MRI. There is a low-grade tumour (arrows), which is uniformly echogenic on ultrasound and returns fat signal on MRI adjacent to a more high-grade tumour (arrowheads), which is hypoechoic on ultrasound and returns low signal on MRI.

dedifferentiated components will be seen as nonfatty signal within the tumour.

MUSCLE TUMOURS

Primary tumours of the muscle are rarely encountered in the musculoskeletal system. Ultrasound features are generally nonspecific. Ultrasound is useful in diagnosing accessory muscles and muscle hernias, both of which may present as a mass.

Smooth muscle tumours

Leiomyomas rarely occur in the musculoskeletal system. They are usually small cutaneous lesions that do not require imaging. Occasionally large and deeper lesions that are hypervascular and often calcify are encountered.

Leiomyosarcoma rarely occur outside the abdominal cavity but may be seen in the subcutaneous tissue or in muscle. They probably arise from vessel walls. Appearance is nonspecific and cannot be differentiated from other aggressive lesions (Fig. 11.10). Central necrosis is a common finding on ultrasound of intra-abdominal lesions (11).

Angioleiomyoma is a relately common superficial painful benign lesion that is very vascular and therefore may be confused with a haemangioma on ultrasound. It occurs primarily in middle age and is twice as common in females (12, 13) (Fig. 11.11).

Striated muscle tumours

Rhabdomyomas are exceedingly rare and in adults occur in the neck region.

Rhabdomyosarcoma is a tumour of childhood and young adults and although not uncommon is rarely seen outside the abdominal cavity and pelvis or head and neck region. Lesions in the extremities are usually intramuscular and occur in adolescence. Ultrasound features described in bladder lesions are similar to other types of sarcoma, showing variable echo pattern and cystic areas presumably representing necrosis (14).

Muscle hernias and accessory muscle

A fascial defect may allow herniation of muscle, which may only be palpable on contraction of the

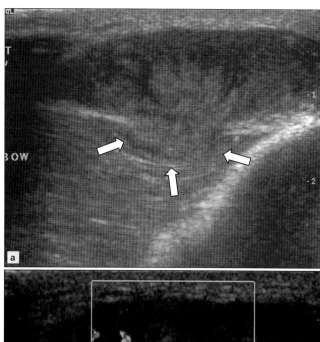
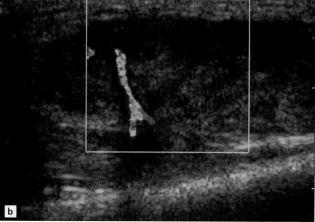

Fig. 11.10 Leiomyosarcoma of the posterior aspect of the elbow. (a) The heterogeneous lesion is centred in the subcutaneous fat. The tumour is seen to invade the adjacent muscle (arrows), demonstrating that this is an aggressive tumour. (b) There are large intralesional vessels seen on colour Doppler imaging.

muscle or, in the lower limb, on standing. The nature of this lesion is easily determined on dynamic scanning (15). The herniated muscle is often hypoechoic, presumably due to minor oedema secondary to recurrent herniation (Fig. 11.12).

Accessory muscle, such as the accessory soleus at the ankle, may present as a mass and/or a neuropathy due to nerve compression. The true nature of the lesion is readily determined by ultrasound (16, 17).

FIBROUS TUMOURS

There are three main types of tumours of fibrous origin: benign focal fibrous tumours, diffuse fibromatous lesions (fibromatoses) and malignant

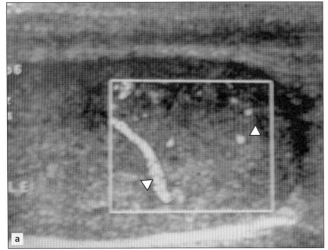

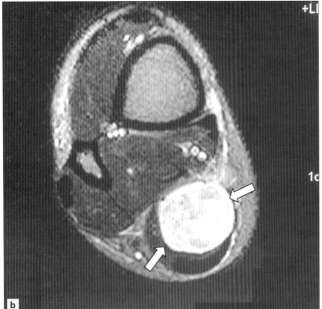

Fig. 11.11 Angioleiomyoma. (a) The lesion is well defined, has a uniform internal structure and contains multiple vessels (arrowheads). (b) T2-weighted MRI shows a well defined lesion within soleus muscle (arrows).

fibrous lesions. In general fibrous lesions are seen as hypoechoic on ultrasound (18).

Benign focal lesions

Fibroma

In the musculoskeletal system fibromas predominately arise from the tendon sheaths of the fingers or thumb. The lesion affects young and middle-aged adults, predominantly men. It is not known whether the lesion represents a neoplasic or reactive process. On ultrasound a fibroma appears as a well-defined hypoechoic mass closely related to the tendon (Fig. 11.13).

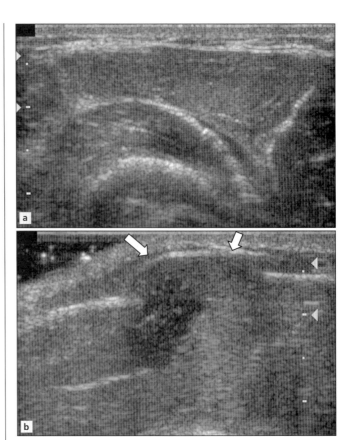

Fig. 11.12 Muscle hernia. (a) At rest, no lesion can be seen. (b) On contracting of the muscle, herniation through the fascia is demonstrated (arrows).

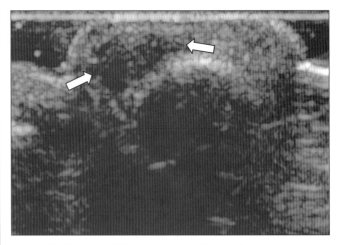

Fig. 11.13 Fibroma of the tendon sheath. The tumour is seen as a small hypoechoic mass (arrows) related to the tendon sheath.

Differentiating fibroma from a giant cell tumour is impossible on ultrasound. On MRI the two lesions may also have similar appearance, as fibrous tissue, seen in fibromas, and haemosiderin, seen in giant cell tumours, are both detected as low signal on T2-weighted images.

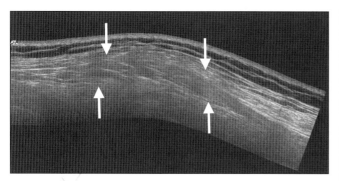

Fig. 11.14 Elastofibroma of the posterior chest wall. The lesion (arrows) is ill-defined and contains multiple striations.

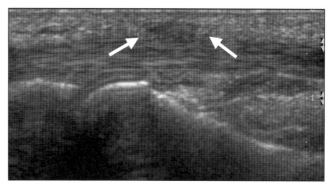

Fig. 11.15 Palmar fibromatosis. A small uniform hypoechoic lesion (arrows) is seen on the plantar surface of the flexor tendon representing the earliest sign of Dupuytren's disease.

Nodular fasciitis

This is a relatively common reactive lesion of unknown aetiology seen predominantly in young adults. The patient presents with a rapidly growing solitary lump and some tenderness. The lesion is usually situated in the subcutaneous tissue but can occur in the intramuscular or intermuscular positions. The lesion involves the upper limb in about half the cases. Although the disease is self-limiting most lesions are excised on account of the alarming growth rate. Histologically the lesion consists of immature fibroblasts in a myxoid matrix (19). In the few reports in the literature the lesions have been described as well defined and of mixed echogenicity. The lesions do not enhance on MR or CT following intravenous contrast (20, 21).

Elastofibroma

> **Key point**
>
> By far the commonest site for an elastofibroma is between the chest wall and the scapula.

Elastofibroma is a benign tumour of unknown aetiology consisting of fibroblasts, collagen and thickened elastic fibres interspersed by fat. It is thought to be a reactive lesion rather than a neoplasm. By far the commonest site is between the chest wall and the scapula. The lesion may be bilateral. On ultrasound the typical features are linear or curvilinear hypoechoic strands against an echogenic background, reflecting the interspersed fatty and fibroelastic components seen on MRI and CT (22) (Fig. 11.14).

Fibromatosis

Palmar and plantar fibromatoses

In these two conditions there is fibrous proliferation of the fascia, resulting in Dupuytren's deformity in the hand and one or more painful nodular lesions in the foot. The condition may be bilateral and the plantar and palmar versions may occur in the same patient, although rarely simultaneously. In the hand the patient may first notice a single nodule in the palm (Fig. 11.15). Progression is slow and unpredictable. Fibrous cords extend from the lesion to the fingers, giving the characteristic feature of Dupuytren's disease. Imaging is rarely required. In the plantar version the patient may present with a lump, pain or both. The nodules are usually solitary and situated either medially or centrally within the fascia (23). Unlike Dupuytren's disease the clinical features are less specific and imaging is useful to confirm the relationship of the lesion to the plantar fascia. On ultrasound a typical plantar fibroma is seen as an elongated hypoechoic, nonvascular lesion with tapered ends, all of which blend into the fascia (Fig. 11.16). A mixed echo pattern can be seen in those lesions larger than 1cm in length (24) (Fig. 11.17). There is usually no flow detected on Doppler (25) but the lesion can be vascular (Fig. 11.18). MRI will confirm the fibrous nature of the lesion, but this is rarely required as the ultrasound appearances are usually specific. Unlike deep fibromatosis the condition is not aggressive, although recurrence following excision is common.

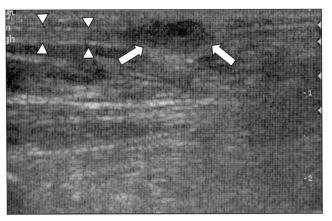

Fig. 11.16 Small plantar fibroma. The lesion (arrows) is hypoechoic and is seen to be in continuity with the plantar fascia (arrowheads).

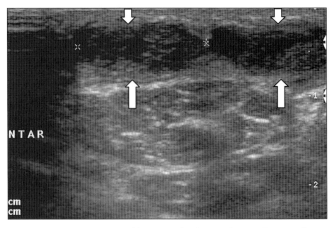

Fig. 11.17 Large plantar fibroma. The lesion (arrows) arises from the fascia and has a heterogeneous echo pattern and a lobulated border. The condition was bilateral in this patient.

Deep fibromatosis (desmoid tumour)

This locally aggressive fibrous lesion of unknown aetiology affects the young adult. The muscles of the shoulder region, trunk and thigh are the commonest sites to be involved. The patient presents with an ill-defined mass. Because of the deep nature of the lesion MRI is often preferred as the primary investigation. Areas of low signal on all sequences reflect the abundant cellular and collagenous fibrous tissue in the lesion although variable amounts of more oedematous, myxoid areas can result in mixed signal intensities. MRI is required to accurately assess the extent of the disease for surgical planning. Ultrasound is less specific, the lesion being seen as a hypoechoic or mildly heterogeneous mass that may appear well defined or ill defined (26) (Fig. 11.19). The lesion may be vascular on Doppler. If percutaneous biopsy is being considered then multiple samples

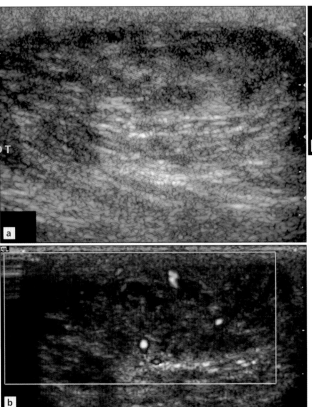

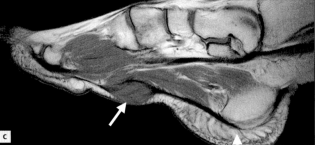

Fig. 11.18 Plantar fibroma. (a) In this case the lesion is heterogeneous. (b) Power Doppler shows that the lesion is highly vascular. (c) T1-weighted sagittal MRI. On MRI the lesion (arrow) is seen to be intimately related to the plantar fascia.

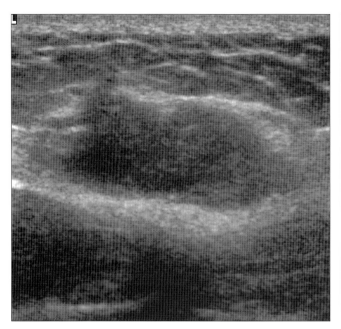

Fig. 11.19 Fibromatosis. The lesion is seen as a hypoechoic mass with irregular outline. This lesion showed no internal vascularity on Doppler.

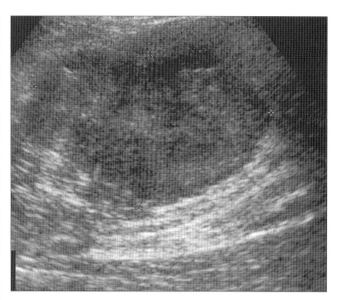

Fig 11.20 Ultrasound of a malignant fibrous histiocytoma of the thigh showing a nonspecific heterogeneous mainly hypoechoic mass.

are required as differentiating fibromatosis from well-differentiated fibrosarcoma may be difficult with a small quantity of material (27).

Malignant fibrous tumours

Fibrosarcomas usually originate from the intermuscular structures and are usually deep-seated lesions of the extremity or trunk, the thigh being the commonest site. The peak incidence is in middle age. Tumours classified as malignant fibrous histiocytoma are now thought to represent a tumour of fibroblastic rather than hisiocytic origin. These lesions predominate in the elderly. The tumour is usually intramuscular but is occasionally seen in the subcutaneous tissue. The thigh is the commonest site followed by the proximal arm. US features of both these malignant tumours are nonspecific and cannot be differentiated from many other types of sarcomas (see below) (Fig. 11.20).

NEURAL TUMOURS

Benign neural tumours

Benign nerve sheath tumour

The two main forms of benign neural tumours are derived from the nerve sheath and are

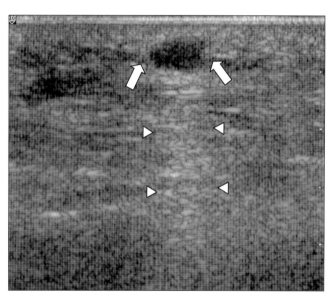

Fig. 11.21 Small neuroma. The lesion (arrows) is uniformly hypoechoic and is causing acoustic enhancement (arrowheads).

termed neurilemoma (benign schwannoma), and neurofibroma. Although benign neural tumours may have a nonspecific appearance on ultrasound, there are often features present that will suggest the diagnosis. Lesions are usually well defined, related to the neurovascular bundle and hypoechoic and may exhibit acoustic enhancement (Fig. 11.21) and variable blood flow on Doppler (Fig. 11.22). In some cases the tumour can clearly be seen to be arising from within a nerve, giving a characteristic appearance (Fig. 11.23). Neurofibromas and neurilemomas

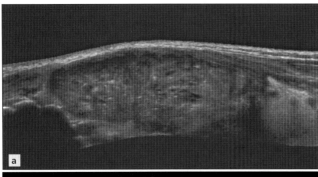

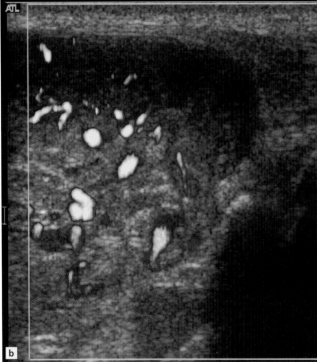

Fig. 11.22 Schwannoma. (a) The lesion is well defined and heterogeneous. (b) On power Doppler the lesion is seen to be highly vascular.

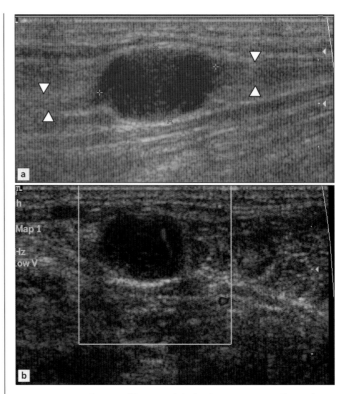

Fig. 11.23 Small neurofibroma. (a) The lesion is typically uniform and hypoechoic and shows acoustic enhancement. It is also clearly seen to be related to the nerve (arrowheads). (b) There is some vascuarity seen within the lesion on power Doppler.

have a similar appearance but can sometimes be differentiated on ultrasound on account of the fact that the former lies centrally and the latter eccentrically in the nerve. Neurofibromas may show a characteristic echogenic ring within the lesion (28) or an echogenic centre (29). Most neurofibromas are solitary. Multiple tumours are the hallmark of neurofibromatosis type 1. Neurilemomas, although rarely multiple, may also be seen in neurofibromatosis. Neurilemomas, when long standing, can cavitate and calcify, features that can readily be detected on ultrasound. Plexiform neurofibroma is a diffuse abnormality of the nerve only seen in neurofibromatosis. The entire nerve is replaced by tortuous mass of expanded nerve fascicles. On ultrasound the nerve is seen to have a nodular appearance with multiple echogenic foci (30).

Nonneoplastic neuromas

Traumatic neuromas represent disorganised neural bundles that grow from the end of a severed nerve. These are commonly seen following amputations. On ultrasound they are hypoechoic lesions seen to arise from the free end of the nerve (Fig. 11.24). Lesions are usually well demarcated, have a bulbous end and can be seen to arise from the nerve sheath. Asymptomatic lesions do occur, making it difficult sometimes to differentiate them from other causes of postamputation pain. On MRI they have a heterogenous signal often with a ringlike pattern on axial T2-weighted images.

> **Key point**
>
> Nonneoplastic neuromas are usually well demarcated, have a bulbous end and can be seen to arise from the nerve sheath. Asymptomatic lesions do occur, making it difficult sometimes to differentiate them from other causes of postamputation pain. On MR they have a heterogenous signal often with a ringlike pattern on axial T2-weighted images.

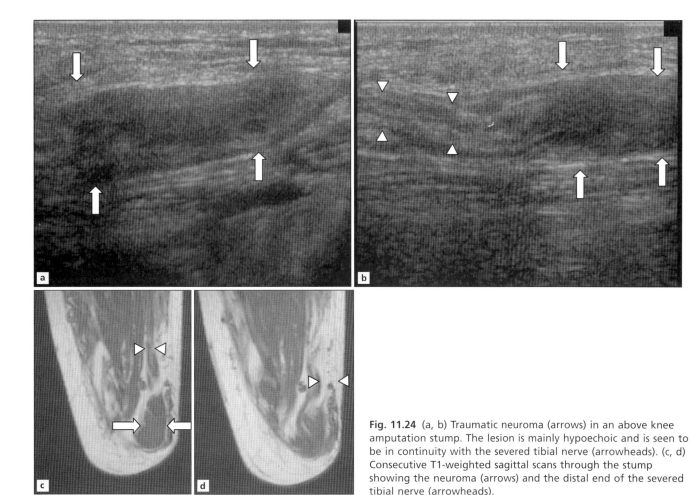

Fig. 11.24 (a, b) Traumatic neuroma (arrows) in an above knee amputation stump. The lesion is mainly hypoechoic and is seen to be in continuity with the severed tibial nerve (arrowheads). (c, d) Consecutive T1-weighted sagittal scans through the stump showing the neuroma (arrows) and the distal end of the severed tibial nerve (arrowheads).

Morton's neuroma is a common reactive lesion that develops due to mucinous degeneration and fibrous proliferation around interdigital nerves of the foot at the level or just distal to the metatarsal head. They are most commonly found at the interspace between the third and fourth digits and are commoner in females. The lesions are seen as well-defined hypoechoic round or disc like lesions lying between the bones and extending into the plantar soft tissue. They are often related with a bursitis of the intermetatarsal bursa. On ultrasound the lesions are best seen in the sagittal plane with the probe on the plantar surface of the foot with pressure being applied on the dorsal aspect of the web space. Lesions usually measure between a half and one centimetre in diameter, and are hypoechoic and hypovascular (Fig. 11.25). Occasionally the digital nerve can be seen in continuity with the lesion (31, 32). Ultrasound-guided steroid injection can be helpful, providing a long-term relief in approximately one-third of the patients. Although it has not been proven whether ultrasound-

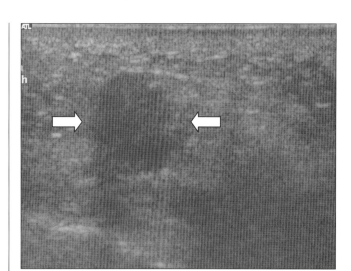

Fig. 11.25 Morton's neuroma. Sagital scan between the metatarsal heads. The neuroma is seen as a hypoechoic, disc-shaped lesion (arrows).

guided injection provides any advantage over blind injection it is easy and convenient to perform following diagnosis. Injecting the lesion with alcohol as a sclerosing agent has also been shown to be effective.

Malignant neural tumours

Malignant peripheral nerve sheath tumours (PNSTs) arise de novo from normal nerves or from malignant transformation of a benign nerve sheath tumour. Half the cases are associated with neurofibromatosis type 1. The lesions do not have any specific features although they are generally larger than neuromas, have a heterogeneous echo pattern and have increased vascularity (Fig. 11.26). As with their benign counterpart, continuity of the tumour with the nerve may be demonstrated. Malignant PNSTs are most common in major nerve trunks including the sciatic, brachial and sacral plexus. Calcification is uncommon and mild when it occurs.

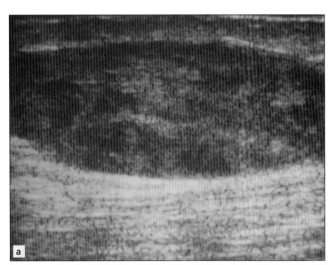

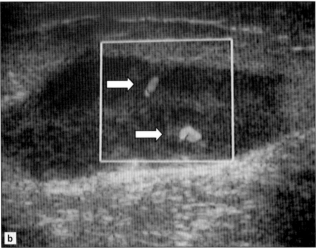

Fig. 11.26 Malignant nerve sheath tumour. (a) The mass is heterogeneous. (b) The lesion is seen to be vascular on colour flow Doppler (arrows).

> **Key point**
>
> Malignant peripheral nerve sheath tumours are most common in major nerve trunks including the sciatic, brachial and sacral plexus. Calcification is uncommon and minor when it occurs.

VASCULAR TUMOURS

Benign tumours

Haemangiomas

Haemangiomas are common benign soft-tissue lesions that may occur in the skin, subcutaneous tissue or muscle. Dermal lesions do not require imaging. The lesions are probably congenital and have little growth potential. Histologically they may contain numerous capillaries, dilated vessels or a combination of both. The lesions may contain fat, which surrounds the vessels. The clinical history may be characteristic with a soft-tissue mass that fluctuates in size. There may be a bluish tinge to the overlying skin in superficial lesions. Patients, who are usually children or young adults, present with a mass that may be painful. Ultrasound appearances are variable. When the lesion consists only of small vessels it may be well defined, uniform, and often echogenic (33) (Fig. 11.27). In other cases ultrasound will show a mixed echo pattern with cystic serpiginous spaces representing dilated vessels (Fig. 11.28). Pheboliths, when present, will be seen as echogenic foci within the lesion (34). Colour flow Doppler is usually positive although slow flow may not be undetected in some cavernous lesions (35). The lesions are often compressible as blood is expelled from dilated vessels. On releasing the pressure colour flow Doppler will be seen to be positive as the vessels refill (Fig. 11.29). With typical clinical features where a lesion is seen to comprise entirely of vessels, a confident diagnosis of haemangioma can be made on ultrasound. However, other highly vascular lesions may mimic haemangioma and MRI should be performed if the diagnosis is in doubt. MRI features, particularly the presence of intralesional fat, may be sufficiently specific to avoid biopsy. Plain films are also useful as phleboliths and deformity or involvement of the adjacent bones may be seen. Analysis of the Doppler signal can be helpful in differentiating

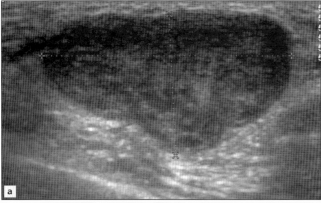

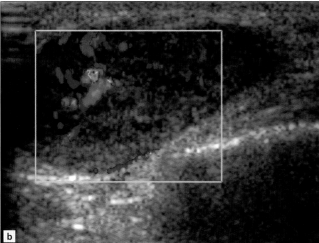

Fig. 11.27 Haemangioma. (a) The lesion is uniform and has an echogenicity similar to muscle. (b) The lesion is highly vascular on Doppler.

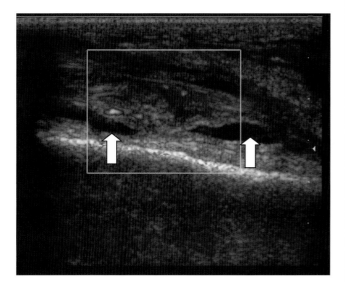

Fig. 11.28 Haemangioma. The lesion is mainly echogenic and is vascular on Doppler. The lesion also contains larger dilated vascular channels (arrows).

haemangiomas from other vascular tumours as the vessel density and peak arterial shift have been shown to be greater in the former in most cases (36, 37). However, in practice, if there is any doubt as to the nature of the lesion, one should proceed to MRI and, if necessary, percutaneous biopsy.

> **Practical tip**
>
> Colour flow Doppler of haemangiomas is usually positive although slow flow may not be undetected in some cavernous lesions. The lesions are often compressible as blood is expelled from dilated vessels. On releasing the pressure colour flow Doppler will be seen to be positive as the vessels refill.

Glomus tumour

Glomus tumour is a small painful vascular lesion composed of cells found in the glomus body. The subungual position at the hand is the commonest site although they may be found in the muscles or subcutaneous fat in the trunk or extremities (38, 39). On ultrasound, glomus tumours are small (<1 cm) hypoechoic, vascular lesions (Fig. 11.30). Deep lesions may not be detected on palpation and the ultrasound operator may have to rely on the fact that the lesion is exquisitely tender to localise the lesion (Fig. 11.31).

Intermediate malignant vascular tumours

Haemangioendotheliomas (36) are rare vascular tumours of intermediate malignancy. There are several histological types, the two commonest being epithelioid and spindle cell haemangioendotheliomas. Epithelioid haemangioendotheliomas are solid tumours found in a deep or superficial location in adults. They are slowly progressive and although about a third of treated cases have metastases only half of these die from their disease. Spindle cell haemangioendotheliomas are superficial tumours of the extremity consisting of cavernous channels, which tend to be locally multifocal but do not metastasise but may recur locally.

Haemangiopericytoma is a tumour of adult life and presents as a slow-growing, painless mass usually in the lower extremity. The lesion is well defined and highly vascular. On ultrasound the lesion is seen as a hypoechoic mass, which may

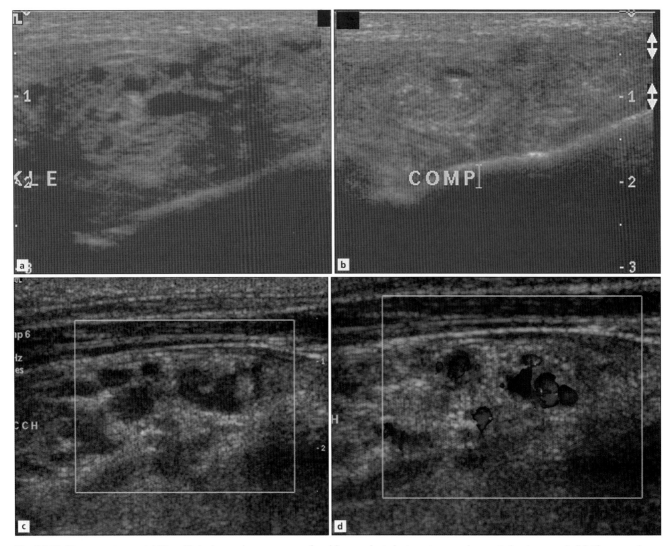

Fig. 11.29 Haemangioma. (a) The dilated vessels are seen as focal hypoechoic lesions in an echogenic background. (b) The vascular channels disappear on compression. (c) Minimal flow seen on Dopper on static imaging. (d) On release of compression positive flow can be seen as the vessels fill with blood.

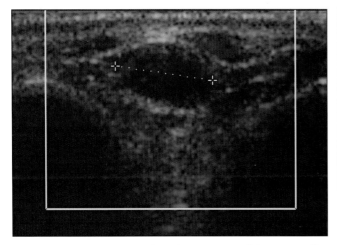

Fig. 11.30 Glomus tumour of the hand. The small lesion is well defined and shows some vascularity on power Doppler.

show acoustic enhancement (40). On Doppler the lesion is highly vascular and spectral analysis may show intratumoral arteriovenous shunting (41) (Fig. 11.32). Metastases occur in the minority of patients.

Malignant vascular tumours

Angiosarcomas are rare tumours that can occur in the deep soft tissues. More often they are cutaneous lesions of the head and neck that do not require imaging. Deep lesions may be related to previous insult such as a foreign body or radiation. The tumour consists of multiple vascular channels lined by malignant endothelial cells and may contain thrombus. The tumour is highly haemorrhagic and may be confused with a chronic haematoma.

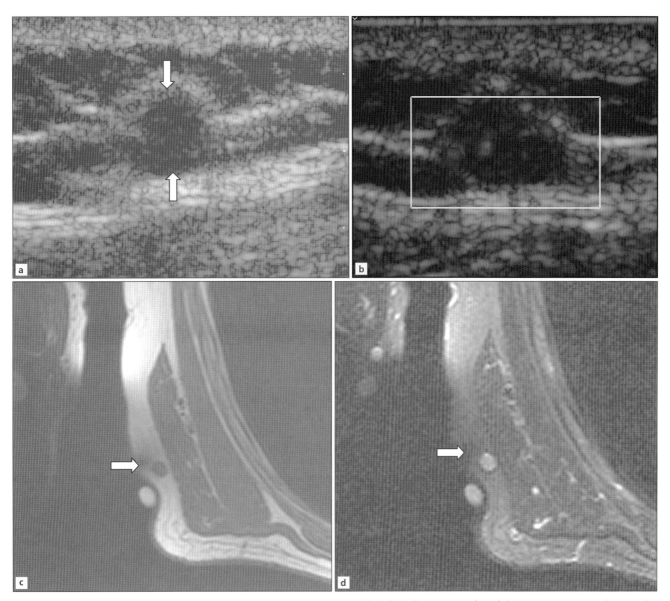

Fig. 11.31 Glomus tumour. (a) The small round lesion (arrows) is situated in the subcutaneous fat of the posterior upper thorax. The lesion is almost invisible on ultrasound. (b) The lesion is seen to be vascular on power Doppler. (c) T1-weighted image of the posterolateral thorax showing a glomus tumour in the subcutaneous fat (arrow). (d) The lesion returns high signal on the STIR image (arrow).

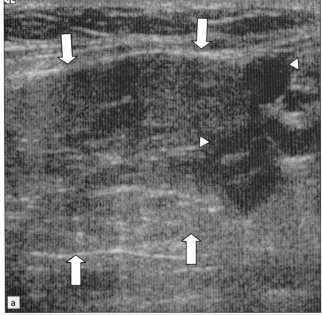

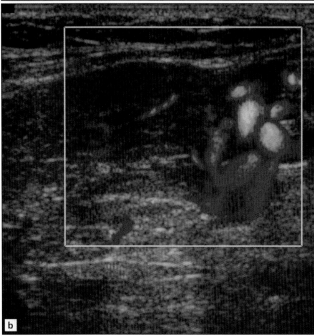

Fig. 11.32 Haemangiopericytoma. (a) The lesion (arrows) is hypoechoic and contains some prominent vascular channels (arrowheads). (b) The lesion is highly vascular with high flow seen in the vascular channels.

MYXOMA

Myxomas are uncommon benign lesions that are usually intramuscular. They have low cellularity and contain abundant myxoid ground substance, which accounts for the generally uniform appearance on imaging. On MRI myxomas are homogeneous in nature and return signal similar to that of a cyst. They may have a relatively low attenuation on CT. On ultrasound they are usually seen as hypoechoic, well-defined lesions that may contain small clefts and cysts (Fig. 11.33). Colour flow Doppler imaging is usually negative. Even if the ultrasound appearances are typical further imaging and biopsy are usually required to exclude malignancy. When multiple lesions with the typical imaging features are seen in association with fibrous dysplasia of the adjacent bone (Mazabraud's syndrome) then biopsy is not necessary (42) (Fig. 11.34).

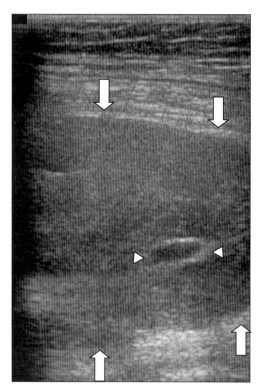

Fig. 11.33 Intramuscular myxoma. This image shows part of a well-defined uniformly hypoechic lesion (arrows) containing multiple low-level echoes. There is a typical cystic cleft (arrowheads).

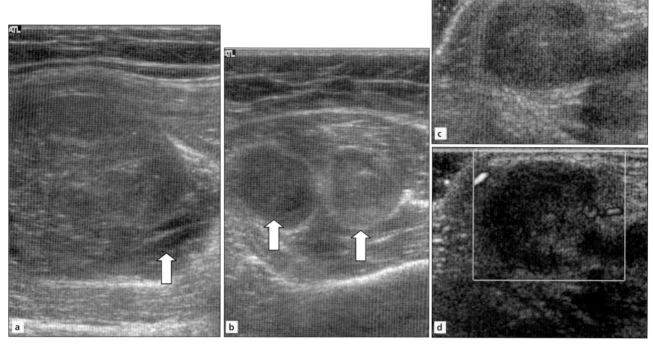

Fig. 11.34 Multiple myxomas in the thigh in Mazabaud's syndrome. (a) Typical lesion with multiple short linear echoes and cleft-like cysts (arrow). (b) Two further intramuscular lesions (arrows) are seen in a neighbouring compartment. (c) STIR MRI coronal sequence showing typical hyperintense myxoma. The abnormal heterogeneous signal in the adjacent femur represents fibrous dysplasia.

SYNOVIAL TUMOURS

Pigmented villonodular synovitis

Synovial tumours may arise from joints, tendon sheaths or bursae. They are nearly always benign. The commonest synovial lesion that may present as a mass is pigmented villonodular synovitis, a reactive or neoplastic condition of unknown aetiology. The diffuse form, which rarely occurs outside a joint, usually presents a monoarthropathy, but occasionally as a soft-tissue mass, particularly in superficial locations such as the ankle or foot. The knee is by far the commonest site. MRI is the more appropriate investigation for joint-based lesions as the intra-articular extent and bony involvement cannot be accurately assessed on ultrasound. In addition MRI is more specific as the hypertrophied synovium contains haemosiderin that returns low signal intensity on all sequences. The nodular form usually presents as a solitary mass. The commonest lesion, termed giant cell tumour of tendon sheath, is nearly always found related to the fingers or thumb. The lesion is well defined, hypoechoic or moderately hyperechoic and is usually hypervascular (43, 44) (Fig. 11.35). The nodular form may also arise from the joints, particularly the knee where Hoffa's fat pad seems to be a favoured site (Fig. 11.36). As with the diffuse form, MRI is useful in narrowing the prebiopsy diagnosis by detecting the presence of haemosiderin in the lesion.

Synovial osteochondromatosis

Synovial osteochondromatosis is a metaplastic disorder of cartilage that may occasionally present as a mass when it arises in superficial sites or in a bursa or tendon sheath. Occasionally the lesion does not appear to be related to a synovial structure. Calcification is very commonly seen and when extensive will be the prominent feature visible on ultrasound (Fig. 11.37). Intralesional vessels may be seen on Doppler. Plain films are useful in establishing the diagnosis. MRI is usually required, particularly when the lesion is arising from a joint.

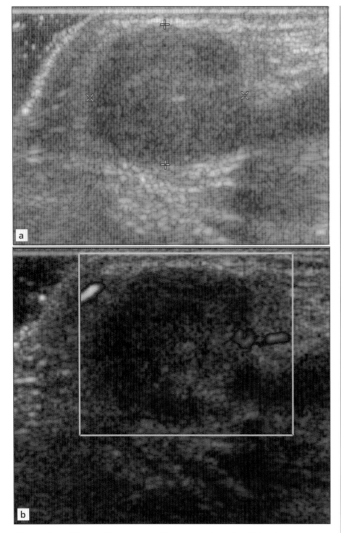

Fig. 11.35 Giant cell tumour of tendon sheath of the hand. (a) The lesion is hypoechoic and well defined and (b) shows some vascularity on power Doppler.

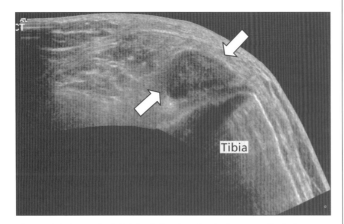

Fig. 11.36 Extended field of view sagittal ultrasound of the nodular form of pigmented villonodular synovitis. The well-defined hypoechoic lesion (arrows) is situated in Hoffa's fat pad of the knee.

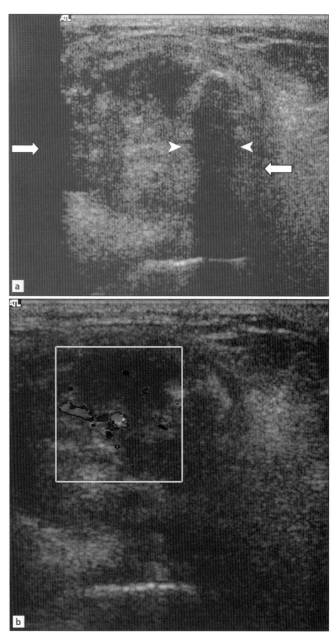

Fig. 11.37 (a) Synovial osteochondromatosis presenting as a mass on the lateral aspect of the knee (arrows). There are multiple echogenic foci representing varying degrees of mineralisation, resulting in acoustic shadowing (arrowheads). (b) The lesion is seen to be vascular on colour Doppler.

Synovial sarcomas

Synovial sarcomas are relatively common malignant tumours that usually occur in young adults. They are thought to arise from primitive mesenchymal cells, although they tend to occur around joints, particularly the knee, ankle and foot. They are usually detected early on account of their superficial location, but diagnosis may be delayed as the vast majority of periarticular masses are benign. Ultrasound appearances are nonspecific, but the diagnosis should be considered in any solid periarticular mass. Tumour calcification, which is particularly common in this lesion, will frequently be detected on ultrasound (Fig. 11.38).

CYSTS

One of the most useful features of ultrasound is the ability to differentiate cystic from solid lesions. Although ultrasound may not be able to make a specific diagnosis, a purely cyst lesion can be assumed to be benign. Cysts are usually anechoic, although they may contain some echoes that represent particulate material. In some inflammatory cysts such as an abscess or inflammatory bursitis the echoes may be so dense that the lesion may appear solid on initial inspection. By palpating the cyst with the probe these echoes can be seen to move randomly within the lesion, proving its cystic nature (45). Cysts will exhibit acoustic enhancement although this sign may also be seen with some solid lesions, particularly neuromas. The cystic nature of a cyst can be proven by using pressure to displace fluid from one part of the lesion to another although this may not be possible if the fluid is under pressure. Cysts may have solid components such as synovial hypertrophy in synovial-lined cysts or inflammatory tissue in abcesses, and when these features predominate, the lesion can mimic a neoplasm.

> **Practical tip**
>
> By palpating the cyst with the probe, echoes can be seen to move randomly within the lesion, proving its cystic nature.

> **Practical tip**
>
> The cystic nature of a cyst can also be proven by using pressure to displace fluid from one part of the lesion to another, although this may not be possible if the fluid is under pressure.

The most common nonneoplastic, nontraumatic cystic lesions are ganglions, usually arising from ligaments and tendons, synovial cysts arising from the joint and distended bursae, and meniscal or labral cysts. Cysts are therefore most commonly found around joints, particularly in the periphery where they are most readily palpable.

Ganglia

A ganglion is thought to represent mucoid degeneration of a fibrous structure, usually a tendon or ligament. Degeneneration of a synovial cyst has also been postulated as a possible mechanism as synovial lining can be detected in the neck of some lesions. However, only a minority of ganglia may be seen to communicate with the joint on arthrography. On ultrasound

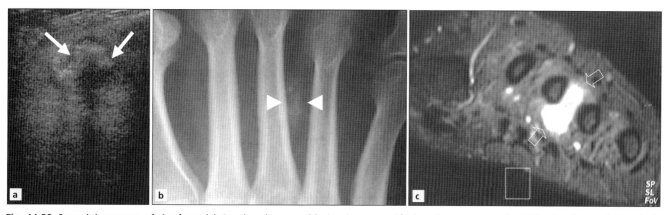

Fig. 11.38 Synovial sarcoma of the foot. (a) On the ultrasound lesion is nonspecific but the presence of calcification (arrows) is typical. (b) Plain film confirms calcification in the lesion (arrowheads). (c) STIR transverse image shows a soft-tissue mass with nonspecific features (open arrows).

lesions may be seen to communicate with a structure such as a tendon or joint capsule via a neck of varying length and width. It is important to identify the neck of the lesion at the time of imaging as at surgery this will need to be excised along with the main body of the lesion to prevent recurrence (Fig. 11.39). If the origin of the lesion is not clear or more anatomical detail is required then MRI may be helpful. The commonest symptomatic ganglion is that arising from the scapholunate ligament over the dorsum of the wrist (Fig. 11.40). An occult ganglion at this site is not palpable but may cause pain. US is a sensitive method for identifying these lesions (46, 47) and injecting with corticosteroid under ultrasound control may produce some symptomatic relief (48). In certain locations, such as the tibial tunnel, cubital tunnel or Guyon's canal ganglia may cause signs and symptoms of neural compression. When arising from a nerve root sheath the lesion may migrate within the sheath, resulting in neuropathy. The typical site for this lesion is the common peroneal nerve as it winds around the fibular head (49, 50)

(Fig. 11.41) though the more common cause of a lesion tracking along the peroneal nerve is a synovial cyst arising from the proximal tibio-fibular joint. Ganglia of the cruciates ligaments of the knee can present as a loss of knee flexion and the diagnosis is usually made on MRI. Ultrasound is useful for guiding aspiration and steroid injection (51).

Synovial cysts

Bursal swellings and distended synovial cysts can usually be diagnosed with confidence because of the typical anatomical position of the lesions (Figs 11.42 and 11.43). As with other cysts the degree of reflectivity depends on the nature of the fluid within the lesion. Synovial hypertrophy is common (Fig. 11.44) and when marked will result in a largely solid mass that can mimic a neoplasm (Fig. 11.45). Hypervascularity is often detected within the mass on colour-flow Doppler imaging, particularly in patients with an inflammatory arthropathy.

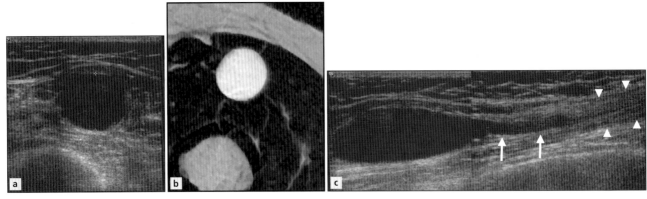

Fig. 11.39 Ganglion on the anterior aspect of the thigh. (a) Axial ultrasound section: the lesion is almost anechoic and shows acoustic enhancement. (b) Equivalent T2-weighted MR image showing homgeneous high signal intensity lesion. (c) Longitudinal section demonstrating the neck of the lesion (arrows), which can be traced down to the quadriceps tendon (arrowheads).

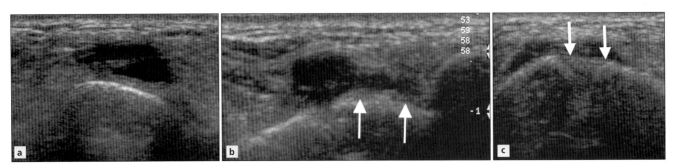

Fig. 11.40 Occult wrist ganglion. (a) Small multiloculated cyst over the dorsum of the wrist. (b) A neck (arrows) is seen extending towards the scapholunate joint. (c) The lesion is seen to originate from the scapholunate ligament (arrows).

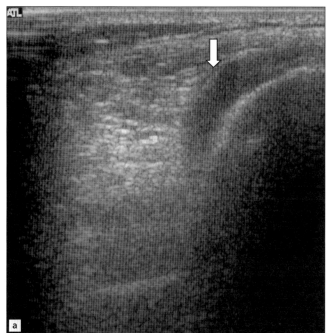

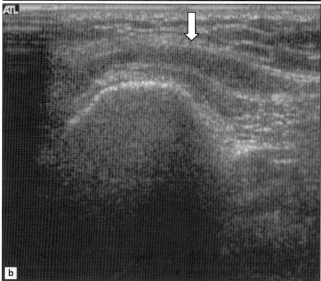

Fig. 11.41 Ganglion of the peroneal nerve in patient presenting with foot drop. The nerve is widened and hypoechoic as it winds around the neck of the fibula (arrows). At surgery, a ganglion was found dissecting along the course of the nerve.

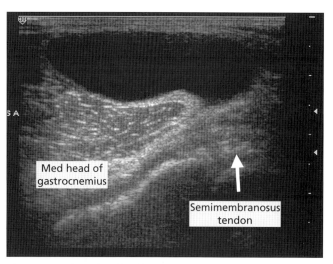

Fig. 11.42 Baker's (popliteal) cyst showing the typical configuration with the neck of the cyst situated between the medial head of gastrocnemius and semimembranosis tendon.

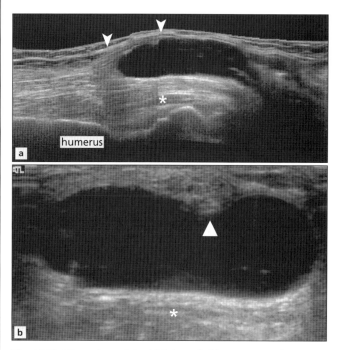

Fig. 11.43 Distention of the bicipitoradial bursa presenting as a mass in the antecubital fossa. (a) Longitudinal and (b) transverse images. A confident diagnosis can be made on account of the cystic nature of the lesion and the typical position between the brachialis (*) and biceps tendon (arrowheads).

Perimeniscal and paralabral cysts

Another cause of a periarticular cyst is a tear of the meniscus of the knee or labrum of the shoulder or hip. Meniscal cysts of the knee represent perimeniscal synovial fluid that communicates with the joint through a meniscal tear. On ultrasound cysts are usually seen as hypoechoic lesions, but may appear more echogenic (52) (Fig. 11.46). Meniscal cysts, particularly on the medial side, may migrate along the tissue planes so that the main body of

the cyst may be remote from the meniscal tear. Paralabral cysts of the shoulder and hip are not palpable but at the shoulder may be responsible for suprascapular nerve palsy in the suprascapular notch with resulting atrophy of the supraspinatus and infraspinatus muscles. If the cyst is positioned posteriorly then isolated atrophy of infraspinatus may occur (Fig. 11.47).

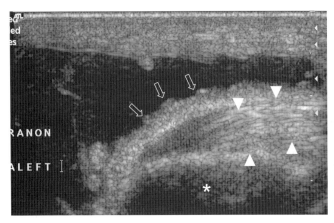

Fig. 11.44 Olecranon bursitis. The image demonstrates an anechoic fluid collection in the bursa overlying the olecranon (*) and triceps (arrowheads). The synovium is hypertrophied and its surface irregular (open arrows).

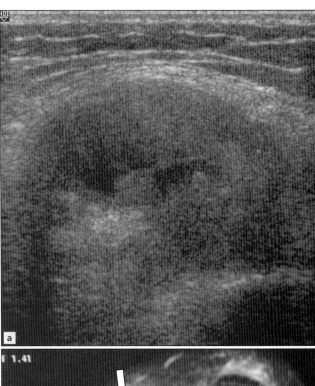

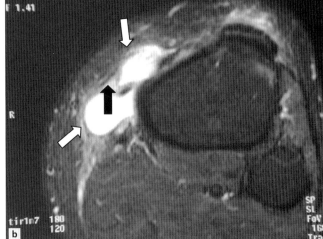

Fig. 11.45 Pes anserinus bursa. (a) The lesion appeared mainly solid on ultrasound with only a small amount of fluid in the centre of the lesion. (b) Axial STIR MR shows the lesion to be the pes anserinus bursa (arrows) closely related to the tendons of the pes anserinus on the medal side of the tibia.

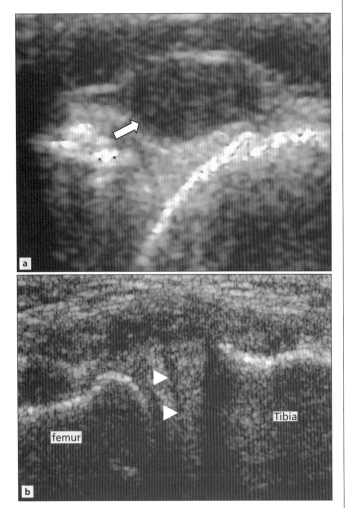

Fig. 11.46 Meniscal cyst. (a) A cyst containing echoes simulating a solid mass (arrow). (b) The lesion is seen to communicate with a tear in the medial meniscus (arrowheads).

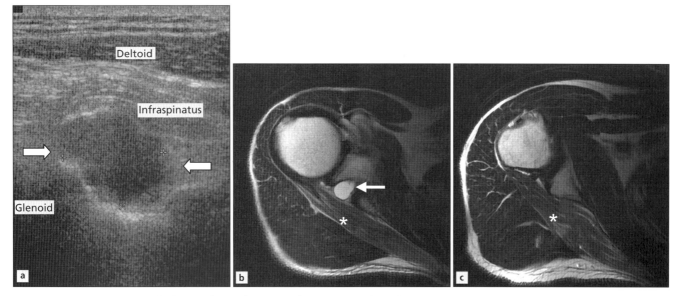

Fig. 11.47 Paraglenoid cyst. (a) The cyst (arrows) is situated in the supraglenoid notch impinging on the suprascapular nerve. Infraspinatous is echogenic, indicating atrophy. (b,c) Axial T2-weighted MRI. The cyst is seen posterior to the glenoid (arrow). There is early atrophy of the infraspinatous muscle (*).

SARCOMA

Most soft-tissue sarcomas have a similar ultrasound appearance. Typically sarcomas are large lesions in the deep tissues, particularly in the lower limbs. However, the appearances are very variable and may also present as a small superficial lesion mimicking a benign tumour (Fig. 11.48). Typically sarcomas appear as heterogeneous, but overall hypoechoic, vascular masses often with well-defined borders (Fig. 11.49). Well-differentiated liposarcomas are an exception and usually appear uniformly

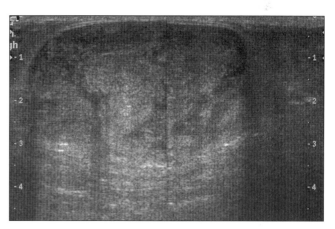

Fig. 11.49 Large undifferentiated sarcoma showing typical heterogeneous echo pattern.

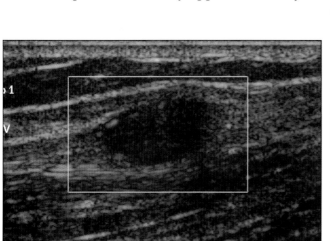

Fig. 11.48 Small well-defined lesion in the antecubital fossa with minor peripheral vascularity mimicking a benign lesion such as a neuroma. The lesion was an aggressive leiomyosarcoma.

echogenic (Fig. 11.50). Sarcomas often contain areas of necrosis and there may be tumoural mineralisation. Highly necrotic tumours may appear more uniformly hypoechoic (Fig. 11.51). Occasionally satellite lesions and enlargement of adjacent lymph nodes may be seen. Although the rare small superficial sarcomas may undergo excisional biopsy, any deep lesion will require preoperative MRI for accurate staging. MRI may also be more specific than ultrasound in providing a prebiopsy diagnosis if there are specific signal characteristics to indicate the presence of fat or fibrous tissue. Ultrasound is a convenient and easy tool for guiding percutaneous biopsy. Before any biopsy is

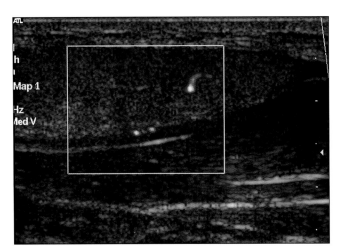

Fig. 11.50 Well-differentiated liposarcoma. The lesion is echogenic and occasional vessels are seen on power Doppler.

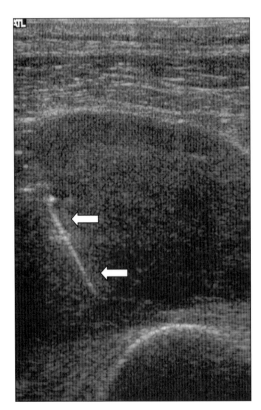

Fig. 11.51 Large highly necrotic pleomorphic sarcoma. The necrotic nature of the tumour results in a hypoechoic mass. The biopsy needle is seen within the lesion (arrows).

obtained there should be dialogue with the tumour surgeon so that the biopsy track can be excised at the time of surgery. Using ultrasound the needle can be placed with a high degree of accuracy into the viable tumour. Ultrasound can also ensure that the needle is not passed through the lesion, thus risking contamination of adjacent compartments.

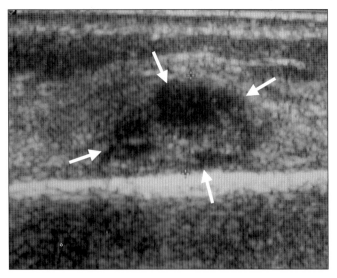

Fig. 11.52 Small deep-seated lesion (arrows) representing recurrent sarcoma.

Key point

Before any biopsy of a sarcoma is obtained there should be dialogue with the tumour surgeon so that the biopsy track can be excised at the time of surgery.

Identifying a recurrent tumour on follow-up examinations is challenging. MRI using fat suppression sequences is a sensitive method, although relatively nonspecific as differentiating a recurrent tumour from postoperative change and seroma may be difficult. Intravenous gadolinium will increased the specificity when an abnormality is seen on the unenhanced scan. Ultrasound has been shown to be an accurate method for identifying recurrence and will readily differentiate seroma from tumour (Fig. 11.52). Guided biopsy of the suspect tissue can be performed at the same time (53, 54).

OTHER MALIGNANT TUMOURS

Soft-tissue metastases are uncommon and have an appearance similar to that of other malignant tumours (Fig. 11.53). Primary soft-tissue lymphoma is also uncommon. Intramuscular lymphoma is seen as a hypoechoic ill-defined mass that may infiltrate the subcutaneous fat (55) or tissue planes (Fig. 11.54).

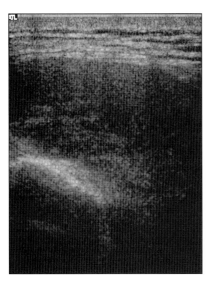

Fig. 11.53 Necrotic soft-tissue metastasis from a bladder carcinoma. There is a large nonspecific hypoechoic mass.

HAEMATOMA

Haematomas are usually not a diagnostic problem when they are temporally related to a traumatic event and have typical clinical features. However, a chronic haematoma may present as a lump with the patient having no recall of a single traumatic event. The ultrasound features are variable, ranging from an anechoic structure

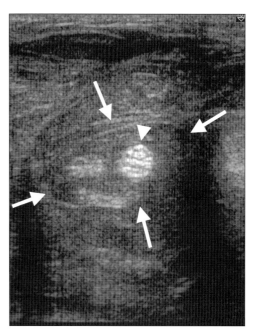

Fig. 11.54 Primary soft-tissue lymphoma. Axial scan showing extension of tumour (arrows) infiltrating along the tissue planes to surround the sciatic nerve (arrowhead).

in a completely liquidfied haematoma to an echogenic mass consisting of a solid clot (Fig. 11.55). Usually in the acute phase a mixed pattern is seen reflecting partial liquification. Chronic haematomas are usually entirely liquid and anechoic or contain low-level echoes with or

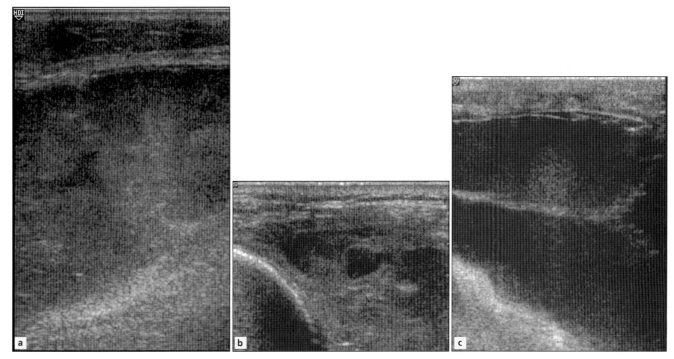

Fig. 11.55 The spectrum of findings of a haematoma. (a) Uniformly echogenic lesion in an acute haematoma. (b) Mixed echo pattern in a subacute lesion. (c) Liquefied haematoma.

without septations. Fluid/fluid levels may be seen (56). Differentiating haematoma from a necrotic sarcoma occasionally causes difficulty (57). Haematomas do not have internal Doppler signal. MRI often helps in diagnosis as blood degradation products show characteristic signal intensities. Chronic haematomas may ossify. Haematomas related to muscle tears are discussed in Chapter 12. Pseudoaneurysm is a haematoma adjacent to a defect in an artery. There is often a history of prior trauma, surgery or vascular interventional procedure. The typical appearance is of a pulsatile mass of mixed echogenicity, depending on the relative amounts of clot and fluid blood. On Doppler a jet-like swirling pulsatile blood flow is seen entering the lesion at the point of communication with the artery (Fig. 11.56). Doppler ultrasound-guided compression and ultrasound-guided injection of thrombin are useful nonsurgical techniques in aneurysms complicating arterial puncture (58, 59).

MYOSITIS OSSIFICANS

Key point

Typically an myositis ossificans is seen in the young adult or adolescent and presents as a painful, tender, ill-defined mass following an episode of trauma. However, the lesion can occur in the absence of any history of local trauma.

Myositis ossificans is a benign lesion that is usually precipitated by a single, often trivial, traumatic event. The term myositis ossificans is misleading as the lesion may occur in the subcutaneous tissues and is not usually inflammatory. Typically the lesion is seen in the young adult or adolescent and presents as a painful, tender, ill-defined mass following an episode of trauma. However, the lesion may occur in the absence of any history of local trauma. The majority of cases involve the limbs with the thigh being the commonest site. Plain films are initially unhelpful but the appearance of peripheral mineralisation after about three weeks is highly specific. Follow-up radiographs will show maturation with ossification and usually a gradual regression. CT is also nonspecific until peripheral mineralisation occurs. MRI typically shows a zonal appearance reflecting the varying

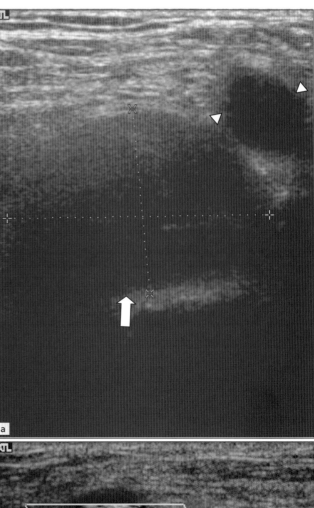

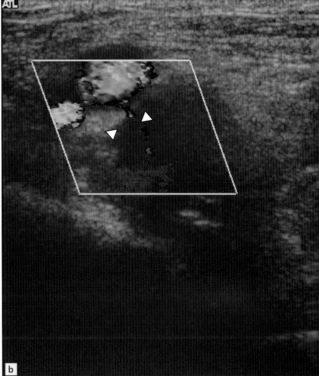

Fig. 11.56 Pseudoaneurysm. (a) There is a large mainly hypoechoic mass (arrows) in the groin lying close to the femoral artery (arrowheads). The patient had had surgery in the region a few months previously. (b) Colour flow Doppler shows a jet of blood entering the mass via a small communication to the artery (arrowheads).

layers of cellular maturation seen at histology and, after a few weeks, a low signal intensity rim representing peripheral mineralisation (60). Peripheral enhancement may be seen before mineralisation occurs (61). Extensive oedema in the adjacent muscle is typical. Ultrasound features also reflect the histology. Initially, the mass may have a nonspecific appearance, having a hypoechoic or heterogenic pattern (62) often with a highly vascular rim and vascular centre. This latter feature helps to differentiate it from abscess. Ultrasound is very sensitive in identifying early peripheral mineralisation, which will be seen as a hyperechoic zone with eventual acoustic shadowing (Fig. 11.57). As the rim matures the ultrasound beam is totally reflected and no information is obtained from the centre of the lesion (Fig. 11.58). The differential diagnosis in the early stages is a soft-tissue sarcoma and differentiation may be difficult on imaging. Although myositis ossificans tends to show a zonal pattern with peripheral vascularity and frequently central cystic areas, these features can also be seen in sarcomas. Generally, if the plain film is normal ultrasound is likely to be nonspecific. The decision to biopsy is dependent on the combined imaging and clinical features. The histology of the central portion of early lesions may look alarming with immature cells and mitotic figures and an erroneous diagnosis of malignancy may be made if sampling is inadequate.

INFECTIONS

> **Key point**
>
> On ultrasound the cystic nature of an abscess will usually be obvious. Its borders may be ill-defined and a hypoechoic rim representing oedema may be seen in surrounding lesion. Its rim is often hypervascular but no flow should be seen within the central portion of it.

The commonest infective lesion to present as a mass is an abscess. Often this arises from a known underlying lesion such as osteomyelitis but absesses may be confined to the soft tissues. On ultrasound the cystic nature of the lesion will usually be obvious. The borders of the lesion may be ill-defined and a hypoechoic rim representing

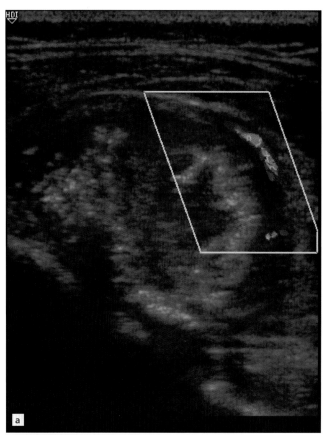

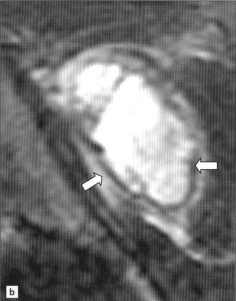

Fig. 11.57 Immature myositis ossificans. (a) The lesion has a laminar appearance with increased vasularity around the periphery. The internal structure of the lesion can still seen through the thin calcified rim. (b) Corresponding axial STIR MRI image showing a thin low-signal rim (arrows).

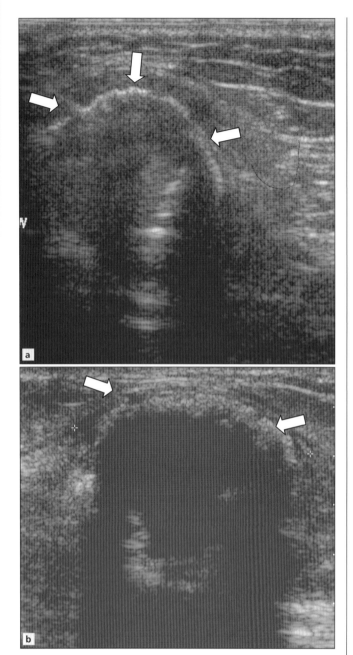

Fig. 11.58 Myositis ossificans. (a) There is an echogenic peripheral rim representing early calcification (arrows). Little detail can be seen from the centre of the lesion. (b) A more mature lesion with highly reflective rim (arrows) and acoustic shadowing.

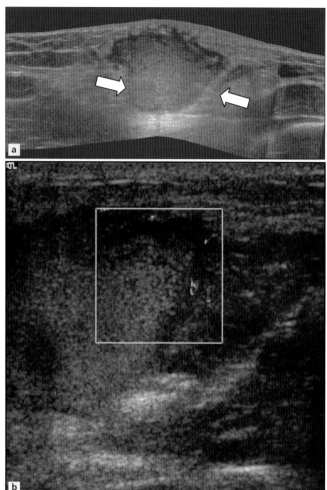

Fig. 11.59 Abscess. (a) Echogenic mass (arrows) with irregular hypoechoic inflammatory superficial margin. (b) There is marked peripheral hypervascularity.

oedema may be seen surrounding the lesion. The rim of the lesion is often hypervascular but no flow should be seen within the central portion of the abscess (63, 64) (Fig. 11.59). The echogenicity can vary. Abscesses containing thick pus and particular matter may be echogenic (Fig. 11.60). By gentle fluctuation the mass-discrete echogenic foci can be seen to circulate within the lesion, thus proving its cystic nature. It may be impossible to differatiate an abscess from a haematoma on ultrasound criteria alone. Ultrasound is an excellent tool for guiding aspiration or drain insertion (65). A relatively large bore needle may be required to successfully aspirate thick pus.

Soft-tissue fungal infections may present as a solid inflammatory mass. Fungal elements (fungal grains) may be seen as multiple discrete echogenic foci surrounded by inflammatory tissue (Fig. 11.61).

A soft-tissue abscess may be related to a foreign body. Ultrasound is an excellent technique for identifying foreign bodies, which are seen as echogenic structures that can be easily identified against the hypoechoic background of the surrounding inflammatory response (Fig. 11.62).

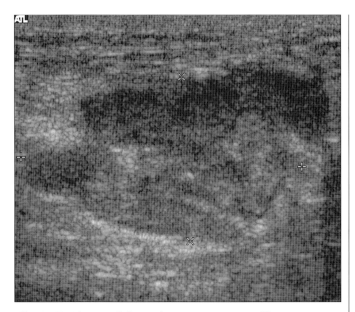

Fig. 11.60 Abscess of the groin seen as a nonspecific heterogeneous mass.

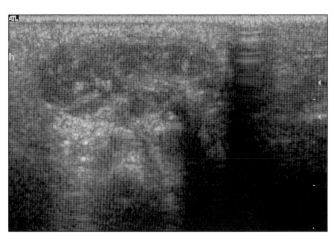

Fig. 11.61 Mycetoma of the foot. The lesion is hypoechoic but contains multiple discrete echogenic foci representing fungal grains within the inflammatory mass.

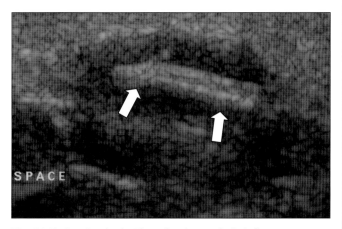

Fig. 11.62 Foreign body. There is a hypoechoic inflammatory mass surrounding an echogenic thorn (arrows).

REFERENCES

1. Salmaso GV, Taricco F. [Ultrasonographic characteristics of lipoma of the soft tissues]. Radiol Med (Torino) 1994;88(4): 373–7.
2. Ahuja AT, King AD, Kew J, King W, Metreweli C. Head and neck lipomas: Sonographic appearance. Am J Neuroradiol 1998;19(3):505–8.
3. Fornage BD, Tassin GB. Sonographic appearances of superficial soft tissue lipomas. J Clin Ultrasound 1991;19(4):215–20.
4. Matsumoto K, Hukuda S, Ishizawa M, Chano T, Okabe H. MRI findings in intramuscular lipomas. Skeletal Radiol 1999;28(3): 145–52.
5. Schultz E, Rosenblatt R, Mitsudo S, Weinberg G. Detection of a deep lipoblastoma by MRI and ultrasound. Pediatr Radiol 1993;23(5):409–10.
6. Kransdorf MJ, Moser RP Jr, Meis JM, Meyer CA. Fat-containing soft-tissue masses of the extremities. Radiographics 1991;11(1): 81–106.
7. Merton DA, Needleman L, Alexander AA, Wolfson PJ, Goldberg BB. Lipoblastoma: Diagnosis with computed tomography, ultrasonography, and color Doppler imaging. J Ultrasound Med 1992;11(10):549–52.
8. Anderson SE, Schwab C, Stauffer E, Banic A, Steinbach LS. Hibernoma: Imaging characteristics of a rare benign soft tissue tumor. Skeletal Radiol 2001;30(10):590–5.
9. Sarno A, Caliendo V, Fauciglietti P, Picciotto F, Cammarota T. [Ultrasonography, computerized tomography, and magnetic resonance in a case of hibernoma]. Radiol Med (Torino) 1995;89(5):717–9.
10. Sung MS, Kang HS, Suh JS, Lee JH, Park JM, Kim JY, Lee HG. Myxoid liposarcoma: Appearance at MR imaging with histologic correlation. Radiographics 2000;20(4):1007–19.
11. Arakawa A, Yasunaga T, Yano S, Morishita K, Nakashima K, Sato R, et al. Radiological findings of retroperitoneal leiomyoma and leiomyosarcoma: Report of two cases. Computer Med Imaging Graph 1993;17(2):125–31.
12. Freedman AM, Meland NB. Angioleiomyomas of the extremities: Report of a case and review of the Mayo Clinic experience. Plastic Reconstruct Surg 1989;83(2):328–31.
13. Hachisuga T, Hashimoto H, Enjoji M. Angioleiomyoma. A clinicopathologic reappraisal of 562 cases. Cancer 1984; 54(1):126–30.
14. McLeod AJ, Lewis E. Sonographic evaluation of pediatric rhabdomyosarcomas. J Ultrasound Med 1984;3(2):69–73.
15. Bianchi S, Abdelwahab IF, Mazzola CG, Ricci G, Damiani S. Sonographic examination of muscle herniation. J Ultrasound Med 1995;14(5):357–60.
16. Lopez Milena G, Ruiz Santiago F, Chamorro Santos C, Canadillas Barea L. Forearm soft tissue mass caused by an accessory muscle. Eur Radiol 2001;11(8):1487–9.
17. Bianchi S, Abdelwahab IF, Oliveri M, Mazzola CG, Rettagliata P. Sonographic diagnosis of accessory soleus muscle mimicking a soft tissue tumor. J Ultrasound Med 1995;14(9):707–9.
18. Rubenstein WA, Gray G, Auh YH, Honig CL, Thorbjarnarson B, Williams JJ, et al. CT of fibrous tissues and tumors with sonographic correlation. Am J Roentgenol 1986;147(5):1067–74.
19. Wang XL, De Schepper AM, Vanhoenacker F, De Raeve H, Gielen J, Aparisi F, et al. Nodular fasciitis: Correlation of MRI findings and histopathology. Skeletal Radiol 2002;31(3):155–61.
20. Frei S, de Lange EE, Fechner RE. Case report 690. Nodular fasciitis of the elbow. Skeletal Radiol 1991;20(6):468–71.
21. Meyer CA, Kransdorf MJ, Jelinek JS, Moser RP Jr. MR and CT appearance of nodular fasciitis. J Comput Assist Tomogr 1991;15(2):276–9.
22. Bianchi S, Martinoli C, Abdelwahab IF, Gandolfo N, Derchi LE, Damiani S. Elastofibroma dorsi: Sonographic findings. Am J Roentgenol 1997;169(4):1113–5.

23. Griffith JF, Wong TY, Wong SM, Wong MW, Metreweli C. Sonography of plantar fibromatosis. Am J Roentgenol 2002; 179(5):1167–72.

24. Bedi DG, Davidson DM. Plantar fibromatosis: Most common sonographic appearance and variations. J Clin Ultrasound 2001;29(9):499–505.

25. Solivetti FM, Luzi F, Bucher S, Thorel MF, Muscardin L. [Plantar fibromatosis: Ultrasonography results]. Radiol Med (Torino) 1999;97(5):341–3.

26. Eich GF, Hoeffel JC, Tschappeler H, Gassner I, Willi UV. Fibrous tumours in children: Imaging features of a heterogeneous group of disorders. Pediatr Radiol 1998;28(7):500–9.

27. Kingston CA, Owens CM, Jeanes A, Malone M. Imaging of desmoid fibromatosis in pediatric patients. Am J Roentgenol 2002;178(1):191–9.

28. Beggs, I. The ring sign: A new ultrasound sign of peripheral nerve tumours. Clinic Radiol 1998;53(11):849–50.

29. Lin J, Martel W. Cross-sectional imaging of peripheral nerve sheath tumors: characteristic signs on CT, MR imaging, and sonography. Am J Roentgenol 2001;176(1):75–82.

30. Lin J, Jacobson JA, Hayes CW. Sonographic target sign in neurofibromas. J Ultrasound Med 1999;18(7):513–7.

31. Quinn TJ, Jacobson JA, Craig JG, van Holsbeeck MT. Sonography of Morton's neuromas. Am J Roentgenol 2000;174(6):1723–8.

32. Oliver TB, Beggs I. Ultrasound in the assessment of metatarsalgia: A surgical and histological correlation. Clin Radiol 1998;53(4):287–9.

33. Derchi LE, Balconi G, De Flaviis L, Oliva A, Rosso F. Sonographic appearances of hemangiomas of skeletal muscle. J Ultrasound Med 1989;8(5):263–7.

34. Kang B, Du J, Huang J. Ultrasonographic diagnosis of hemangiomas of soft tissue. J Tongji Med Univ 1997;17(3): 168–71.

35. Yang WT, Ahuja A, Metreweli C. Sonographic features of head and neck hemangiomas and vascular malformations: review of 23 patients. J Ultrasound Med 1997;16(1):39–44.

36. Dubois J, Garel L, David M, Powell J. Vascular soft-tissue tumors in infancy: Distinguishing features on Doppler sonography. Am J Roentgenol 2002;178(6):1541–5.

37. Dubois J, Patriquin HB, Garel L, Powell J, Filiatrault D, David M, et al. Soft-tissue hemangiomas in infants and children: Diagnosis using Doppler sonography. Am J Roentgenol 1998;171(1):247–52.

38. Ogino T, Ohnishi N. Ultrasonography of a subungual glomus tumour. J Hand Surg [Br] 1993;18(6):746–7.

39. Amillo S, Arriola FJ, Munoz G. Extradigital glomus tumour causing thigh pain: A case report. J Bone Joint Surg Br 1997;79(1):104–6.

40. Lorigan JG, David CL, Evans HL, Wallace S. The clinical and radiologic manifestations of hemangiopericytoma. Am J Roentgenol 1989;153(2):345–9.

41. Juan C, Huang G, Chin S, Hsueh C, Wu C, Hsiao H, et al. Color and duplex Doppler sonography of hemangiopericytoma. J Clin Ultrasound 2001;29(1):51–5.

42. Iwasko N, Steinbach LS, Disler D, Pathria M, Hottya GA, Kattapuram S, et al. Imaging findings in Mazabraud's syndrome: Seven new cases. Skeletal Radiol 2002;31(2): 81–7.

43. Paivansalo M, Jalovaara P. Ultrasound findings of ganglions of the wrist. Eur J Radiol 1991;13(3):178–80.

44. Moschilla G, Breidahl W. Sonography of the finger. Am J Roentgenol 2002;178(6):1451–7.

45. Loyer EM, Kaur H, David CL, DuBrow R, Eftekhari FM. Importance of dynamic assessment of the soft tissues in the sonographic diagnosis of echogenic superficial abscesses. J Ultrasound Med 1995;14(9):669–71.

46. Blam O, Bindra R, Middleton W, Gelberman R. The occult dorsal carpal ganglion: Usefulness of magnetic resonance imaging and ultrasound in diagnosis. Am J Orthop 1998;27(2):107–10.

47. Cardinal E, Buckwalter KA, Braunstein EM, Mih AD. Occult dorsal carpal ganglion: Comparison of US and MR imaging. Radiology 1994;193(1):259–62.

48. Breidahl WH, Adler RS. Ultrasound-guided injection of ganglia with coricosteroids. Skeletal Radiol 1996;25(7):635–8.

49. Leijten FS, Arts WF, Puylaert JB. Ultrasound diagnosis of an intraneural ganglion cyst of the peroneal nerve. Case report. J Neurosurg 1992;76(3):538–40.

50. Pedrazzini M, Pogliacomi F, Cusmano F, Armaroli S, Rinaldi E, Pavone P. Bilateral ganglion cyst of the common peroneal nerve. Eur Radiol 2002;12(11):2803–6.

51. DeFriend DE, Schranz PJ, Silver DA. Ultrasound-guided aspiration of posterior cruciate ligament ganglion cysts. Skeletal Radiol 2001;30(7):411–4.

52. Seymour R, Lloyd DC. Sonographic appearances of meniscal cysts. J Clin Ultrasound 1998;26(1):15–20.

53. Choi H, Varma DG, Fornage BD, Kim EE, Johnston DA. Soft-tissue sarcoma: MR imaging vs sonography for detection of local recurrence after surgery. Am J Roentgenol 1991;157(2): 353–8.

54. Pino G, Conzi GF, Murolo C, Schenone F, Magliani L, Imperiale A, et al. Sonographic evaluation of local recurrences of soft tissue sarcomas. J Ultrasound Med 1993;12(1):23–6.

55. Beggs I. Primary muscle lymphoma. Clin Radiol 1997;52(3): 203–12.

56. Giovagnorio F, Andreoli C, De Cicco M. [The echographic and computed tomographic assessment of "spontaneous" hematomas of the abdominal wall]. 1997;94(5):481–5.

57. Doyle AJ, Miller MV, French JG. Ultrasound of soft-tissue masses: Pitfalls in interpretation. Australas Radiol 2000;44(3): 275–80.

58. Friedman SG, Pellerito JS, Scher L, Faust G, Burke B, Safa T. Ultrasound-guided thrombin injection is the treatment of choice for femoral pseudoaneurysms. Arch Surg 2002;137(4): 462–4.

59. Steinkamp HJ, Werk M, Felix R. Treatment of postinterventional pseudoaneurysms by ultrasound-guided compression. Invest Radiol 2000;35(3):186–92.

60. De Smet AA, Norris MA, Fisher DR. Magnetic resonance imaging of myositis ossificans: Analysis of seven cases. Skeletal Radiol 1992;21(8):503–7.

61. Cvitanic O, Sedlak J. Acute myositis ossificans. Skeletal Radiol 1995;24(2):139–41.

62. Fornage BD, Eftekhari F. Sonographic diagnosis of myositis ossificans. J Ultrasound Med 1989;8(8):463–6.

63. Arslan H, Sakarya ME, Bozkurt M, Unal O, Dilek ON, Harman M. The role of power Doppler sonography in the evaluation of superficial soft tissue abscesses. Eur J Ultrasound 1998;8(2): 101–6.

64. Breidahl WH, Newman JS, Taljanovic MS, Adler RS. Power Doppler sonography in the assessment of musculoskeletal fluid collections. Am J Roentgenol 1996;166(6):1443–6.

65. Cardinal E, Bureau NJ, Aubin B, Chhem RK. Role of ultrasound in musculoskeletal infections. Radiol Clin North Am 2001;39(2):191–201.

Ultrasound of muscle injury

12

Philip Robinson

INTRODUCTION

> **Key point**
>
> Although the evaluation of muscle injuries by MR imaging has been extensively described, ultrasound has a number of distinct advantages over this technique, including dynamic muscle assessment, speed of examination, relative cost and the ability to perform real-time intervention.

Although for the investigation of pathology in any body system there are a number of complimentary imaging techniques, musculoskeletal ultrasound has become established as a pivotal investigation in the assessment of muscle injury (1–3). Prior to the advent of MR imaging ultrasound was increasingly used in the assessment of muscle injury but subsequently went into relative decline when MR imaging became more widely available (2). However, in the past decade the development of new transducer technology has allowed the demonstration of muscular architecture at a resolution higher than can currently be obtained on MR imaging (1–3). Although the evaluation of muscle injuries by MR imaging has been extensively described (4–6), ultrasound now has a number of distinct advantages over this technique (1–3, 7). These advantages include dynamic muscle assessment, speed of examination, relative cost and the ability to perform real-time intervention. Additionally ultrasound can demonstrate the muscle structure surrounding a lesion that can often be obscured by oedema on MR imaging (1–3).

Specialists and primary care physicians are increasingly requesting imaging evaluation of muscle injury. Muscle tears and strains form a significant proportion of injuries in professional sports (30%) where accurate assessment of muscle injury can be important in planning rehabilitation (8). Although initial research and development has concentrated on providing diagnostic and prognostic information in professional athletes (4–6), as the public and referrers' expectations have risen these imaging techniques are now being applied to recreational athletes and for the assessment and rehabilitation of patients after polytrauma. This chapter will discuss the role of ultrasound in assessing acute muscle injury and its subsequent complications.

EXAMINATION TECHNIQUE

Initial assessment of muscle injury commences with a brief clinical history and pertinent physical examination of the patient. This allows the subsequent ultrasound examination to be targeted towards the most relevant areas (2).

The majority of skeletal muscles lie superficially within the body and therefore are optimally assessed by linear transducers, which allow increased near resolution and a larger near field of view compared to curved array transducers (1, 2, 9). Modern multifrequency transducers (centre frequency greater than 10 MHz) allow visualisation of most muscle groups. However, lower-frequency linear (8.5 MHz) or curved array transducers (5 MHz) may have to be used in obese or very muscular patients especially in the gluteal region and proximal thigh. The choice of the optimal transducer is always tailored to the individual muscle region and may have to be altered several times during the examination. In the majority of muscle examinations the use of thick coupling gel is adequate for assessment; however, a stand-off may be necessary for the investigation of muscle hernias as even light skin pressure can maintain the hernia in reduction (10).

> **Practical tip**
>
> In the majority of muscle examinations the use of thick coupling gel is adequate for assessment; however, a stand-off may be necessary for the investigation of muscle hernias as even light skin pressure can maintain the hernia in reduction.

Although linear transducers do allow an increased near field of view compared to curved transducers this is still relatively small. A dual-screen facility allows real-time comparison of two different areas (usually the asymptomatic opposite side) but it can also be used in a single area to double the transducer's field of view (Fig. 12.1) (1). However, modern software now

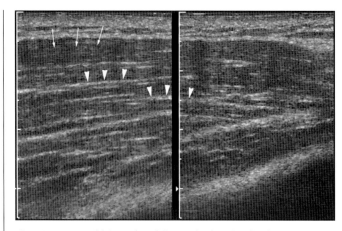

Fig. 12.1 Normal biceps brachii muscle, longitudinal sonogram. Dual-screen facility has been used to extend the transducer field of view. Note the echogenic linear perimysium (arrowheads) with intervening hypoechoic fascicles (small arrows).

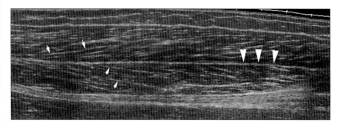

Fig. 12.2 Normal biceps femoris muscle, extended field of view (Siescape), longitudinal sonogram. Note the bipennate structure with parallel echogenic perimysium (small arrowheads) converging obliquely on the main myotendinous area (large arrowheads).

allows composite image formation, which can extend the transducer's field of view to 60 cm (11, 12). These panoramic images are collated by image registration during probe motion over an anatomical area (11, 12). The composite image can be constructed in any plane with maintenance of resolution and measurement accuracy (Fig. 12.2) (11–13). This feature can be most useful for measuring muscle lesions larger than the transducer's normal field of view and also for demonstrating pathology and surrounding anatomy to nonimaging clinicians. Otherwise, this feature does not seem to significantly add to the user's primary diagnostic ability (14).

After obtaining the optimal transducer setting, examination begins with longitudinal and transverse scanning of the symptomatic area. Fortunately in the majority of muscle injuries, the symptomatic area accurately locates the muscle lesion and is usually focal, rarely affecting the

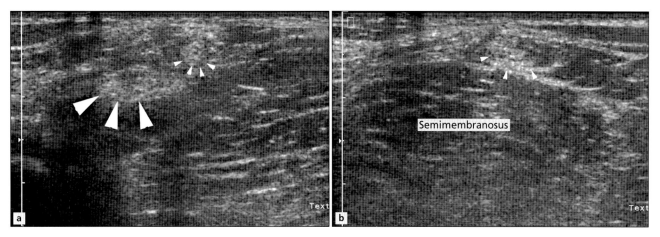

Fig. 12.3 Normal posterior muscles and tendons at the level of the knee joint, transverse sonograms. (a) The relationship of the semimembranosus (large arrowheads) and semitendinosus tendons (small arrowheads) can be determined. (b) At a level superior to (a) the semimembranosus muscle is predominant with more superficial semitendinosus tendon (arrowheads).

whole limb or even muscle group (4, 6, 8, 15). Once the abnormality is located, the examiner must be confident of the anatomy being examined and the exact position of the pathology. This can be achieved by moving to the nearest anatomical area where the underlying muscular and tendinous anatomy can be defined and then scanning back to the area of abnormality, following the muscles and tendons in a continuous manner. This is usually best achieved in the transverse plane. For example, in the case of a hamstring injury define the anatomy of the individual muscles and tendons at the posterior aspect of the knee (Fig. 12.3) and then scan transversally in a continuous fashion to the area of pathology, identifying which muscle (or muscles) is affected (Fig. 12.4).

Practical tip

Confidence in the anatomy being examined and the exact position of the pathology can be achieved by moving the transducer to the nearest anatomical area where the underlying muscular and tendinous anatomy can be defined and then scanning back to the area of abnormality, following the muscles and tendons in a continuous manner.

Key point

After assessing the appearance of any pathology at rest, the abnormal area and surrounding tissues should be assessed dynamically with active and/or passive contraction.

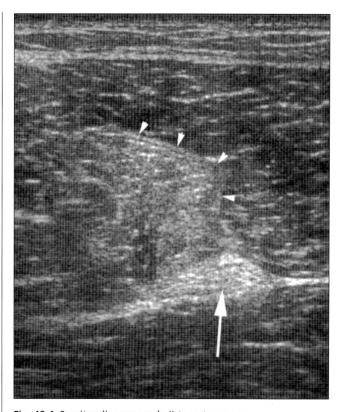

Fig. 12.4 Semitendinosus grade II tear, transverse sonogram. After scanning transversely from the level of Fig. 12.3b, the area of abnormality can be identified within semitendinosus extending to the intervening fascia between biceps femoris and semitendinosus (arrowheads). Note proximity to the sciatic nerve (large arrow).

After assessing the appearance of any pathology at rest, the abnormal area and surrounding tissues should be assessed dynamically with active and/or passive contraction (1, 2, 7). This allows the consistency of the abnormality (e.g. solid or cystic), alteration in muscle function and any movement of disrupted fibres (helping differentiate grades of tears) to become more apparent (Fig. 12.5) (1, 2, 7). Additional manoeuvres, especially in the case of muscle hernias, may be required as the hernia may only become apparent when the patient is standing (see the section Muscle hernia) (10).

Doppler interpretation is rarely necessary in assessing muscle injury except where there is clinical doubt regarding other underlying pathology (e.g. soft-tissue sarcoma, inflammatory lesion or vascular abnormality) (1, 2). At present 3D imaging has little practical application although it has potential as a research tool. One application may include the more accurate assessment of muscle volume involved by injury, which may subsequently offer a more accurate prognosis for individual injuries (16, 17).

MUSCLE PHYSIOLOGY AND ANATOMY; NORMAL ULTRASOUND APPEARANCES

Key point

In athletes and young adults the main area of weakness in the muscle–tendon–bone unit is the myotendinous junction, where the transformation zone between the muscle fibrils and tendon is relatively inelastic. Conversely in the immature skeleton the weakest area is the bone–tendon interface (leading to avulsion fracture), while in the older population, it is usually the degenerate tendon that tears.

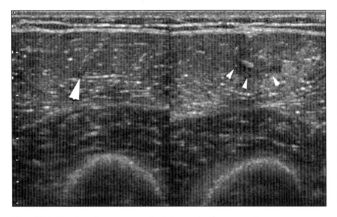

Fig. 12.5 Rectus femoris grade I tear, dual-screen view, transverse sonograms. Left-hand image shows minor hypoechoic area (large arrowhead) within the muscle. The right-hand image has been taken during active contraction and demonstrates more marked distraction of the tear at the myotendinous junction with hypoechoic fluid (small arrowheads).

The function of muscle is to generate force through active contraction of the muscle fibrils within the muscle belly. This active force is transmitted to bone via the relatively inactive muscle tendons (4). In athletes and young adults the main area of weakness in this muscle–tendon–bone unit is the myotendinous junction where the transformation zone between the muscle fibrils and tendon is relatively inelastic (5, 8, 18). Conversely in the immature skeleton the weakest area is the bone–tendon interface (leading to avulsion fracture), while in the older population, it is usually the degenerate tendon that tears (3). This explains why indirect muscle injuries are relatively uncommon in these latter two population groups.

Physiologically muscles are relatively inhomogeneous, consisting of two groups of muscle fibrils: T1 (slow twitch) and T2 fibres (fast twitch) (5, 18, 19). Postural muscles consist mainly of T1 fibres, which are mitochondrial rich and therefore can perform sustained low-energy contractions (5, 18, 19). T2 fibres depend on the glycolytic pathway and muscles rich in this fibre type produce much more forceful and rapid contractions (4, 18, 19). The arrangement of muscle fibres also determines muscle physiology, with purely linear arrangements optimal for distance movement (postural muscles), whereas pennate (featherlike) arrangements are better for producing maximal force (Fig. 12.2) (2, 4). Thus muscles that have a predominance of T2 fibres, have a pennate arrangement and span more than two joints are subject to the greatest intrinsic forces and are therefore more susceptible to indirect muscle injury (see the section Indirect muscle injury) (6, 8, 18).

Key point

Muscles that have a predominance of T2 fibres, have a pennate arrangement and span more than two joints are subject to the greatest intrinsic forces and are therefore more susceptible to indirect muscle injury.

The forces present within a muscle are also dependent on the way the muscle contracts. Isotonic contraction occurs when a constant load is applied to a muscle and its length changes. In concentric contractions, the muscle shortens, whereas in eccentric contraction the muscle lengthens. Eccentric contractions have been shown to produce greater intrinsic forces than concentric contractions (4, 8, 20–22).

Microscopically muscle bellies consist of individual muscle fibres that form groups or fascicles enveloped by connective tissue known as endomysium (23, 24). The muscle fibres and fascicles are predominantly of low echogenicity on ultrasound compared to adjacent fascia and nervous tissue (Fig. 12.1) (1, 9, 25). Fascicles are grouped and enclosed by fibroadipose septa or perimysium, which is a relatively thicker connective tissue, again rich in blood vessels, nervous tissue and adipose tissue (3, 23). Because of its thickness the perimysium appears relatively echogenic on ultrasound and in pennate muscle is seen on longitudinal scanning as multiple parallel lines forming oblique angles (separated by the hypoechoic fascicles) with the echogenic myotendinous junction (Fig. 12.2) (1, 2). Finally another thick layer of echogenic fascia called the epimysium surrounds the entire muscle (Fig. 12.6). Because of their linear configuration these septa are also susceptible to anisotropy (see Chapter 1). In the transverse plane the fibres are hypoechoic with the intervening septa seen as echogenic dots (Fig. 12.6) (1, 2).

During exercise, blood flow through the muscle and connective tissues can increase 20-fold with resultant muscle swelling and displacement of the overlying fascial planes (a volume increase of 10–15%) (1, 26, 27). Oedema has been identified on MR imaging in normal subjects after exercise but no significant change in echotexture has been described on ultrasound (28–33).

MUSCLE INJURY

Accessory muscles

There are a number of accessory muscles throughout the body that have the potential to be misdiagnosed both clinically and radiologically as a soft-tissue mass. The problem is compounded as these muscles can occasionally be symptomatic (34–36).

> **Key point**
>
> As an accessory muscle, the accessory soleus has the potential to be misdiagnosed both clinically and radiologically as a soft-tissue mass. It lies deep to soleus and the Achilles tendon, inserting into the upper calcaneus anteromedial to the Achilles tendon.

The accessory soleus is a prime example of this and lies deep to soleus and the Achilles tendon, inserting into the upper calcaneus anteromedial to the Achilles tendon (Fig. 12.7) (34–36). There is a minimal distal tendon and therefore the muscle belly extends to the superior margin of the calcaneus. Symptoms can occur after exercise when it can also be felt as a palpable mass behind the ankle (34–36). This is probably a type of compartment syndrome due to increased blood flow and swelling in the limited pre-Achilles space (see Chronic complications) (34–36).

On ultrasound the muscle appears as a soft-tissue mass deep to the Achilles tendon but

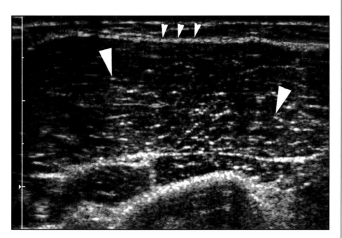

Fig. 12.6 Normal biceps brachii muscle, transverse sonogram. In this plane the perimysium are seen as multiple echogenic dots (large arrowheads). The thick echogenic epimysium surrounds the entire muscle (small arrowheads).

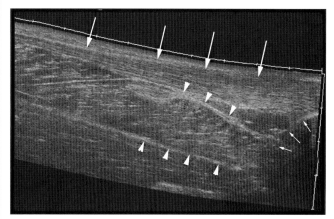

Fig. 12.7 Accessory soleus muscle, longitudinal sonogram. A thickened Achilles tendon is present (large arrows) passing distally to insert onto the calcaneus (small arrows). A soft-tissue mass with typical muscle echo texture (arrowheads) occupies the pre-Achilles space anterior to the Achilles tendon extending distally to insert into the calcaneus (small arrows).

with normal muscle architecture filling the pre-Achilles space (Fig. 12.7).

Other accessory muscles include the accessory flexor digitorum longus, which passes through the tarsal tunnel adjacent to the flexor hallucis longus. Below the medial malleolus the tendon merges with the flexor digitorum longus but the muscle can occasionally cause local mass effect and tarsal tunnel syndrome (35).

Treatment of symptomatic accessory muscles includes fasciotomy or surgical release.

Acute muscle injury

This is a common clinical occurrence both in the general population and in professional sports where it can account for over one-third of all acute injuries (8). Injuries can be classified as direct (e.g. contusion, laceration) or indirect (e.g. delayed onset muscle soreness, strain or tear) (4, 8, 15).

Direct muscle injury

Muscle contusion. Muscle contusion occurs secondary to direct trauma, causing muscle fibre disruption and haematoma by compression of muscle against bone (8). Pathologically the dominant process is haematoma, which begins to organise within two to three days. Healing occurs with muscle regeneration and/or fibrosis proportional to the extent of the injury (4, 37).

Muscle contusion is commonly seen in contact sports ("dead leg") or as part of polytrauma usually in the lower limb. This is a clinical diagnosis obtained from patient history but on examination muscle function is relatively normal given the degree of pain (38–41). Clinically the patient can be graded according to the restriction of joint movement nearest the site of impact. The grading system is divided into mild, moderate or severe, with mild being joint movement greater than two-thirds of full range, moderate a third to two-thirds of full range and severe less than a third of full range (41).

> **Key point**
>
> The clinical grading system for muscle contusion is divided into mild, moderate or severe, with mild being joint movement greater than two-thirds of full range, moderate a third to two-thirds of full range and severe less than a third of full range.

> **Practical tip**
>
> On ultrasound an acute contusion (0–48 hr) appears ill defined with irregular margins and marked echogenic swelling of the fascicles and entire muscle.

On ultrasound an acute contusion (0–48 hr) appears ill defined with irregular margins and marked echogenic swelling of the fascicles and entire muscle (Fig. 12.8) (42). In severe clinical

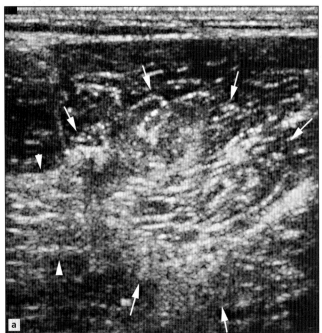

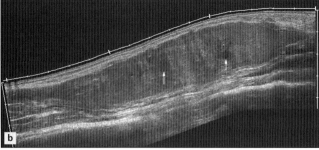

Fig. 12.8 Acute haematoma. (a) Semitendinosus contusion, transverse sonogram. Professional soccer player who received a direct blow during a tackle. Ill-defined echogenic swelling affecting the deep aspect of semitendinosus (arrows) and extending across the intervening septum into semimembranosus (small arrowheads). (b) Biceps haemorrhage, longitudinal sonogram. Thirteen-year-old boy with leukaemia and platelet count of 12. Muscle became acutely swollen after blood pressure measurement. Entire muscle is swollen with diffuse ill-defined increase in echotexture and some focal hypoechoic areas appearing (arrows).

cases dynamic imaging confirms that a complete tear is not present and documents the extent of muscle damage (Fig. 12.9). At 48 to 72 hr ultrasound appearances become better defined with a clearer echogenic margin and the main area of the haematoma appearing hypoechoic (Figs 12.9 and 12.10) (1). Subsequently as the

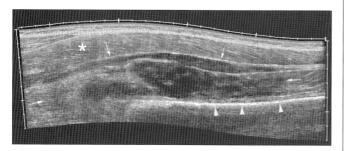

Fig. 12.9 Muscle contusion anterior thigh, longitudinal sonogram (Siescape). Soccer player struck on thigh during tackle 10 days earlier presenting with increasing thigh pain. Vastus intermedius and the deep aspect of rectus femoris are largely replaced by an extensive loculated hypoechoic haematoma (arrows). The haematoma abuts the femur (arrowheads) and is displacing the long head of rectus femoris (*). The haematoma required surgical evacuation due to incipient compartment syndrome.

haematoma begins to organise, the echogenic periphery gradually fills in towards the centre (Fig. 12.10) (42, 43). In the following weeks the contusion can be monitored for regeneration of muscle, scar tissue or more rarely myositis ossificans (see Chronic complications) (38, 44). However, in sporting injuries, the majority of contusions heal with normal muscle regeneration and chronic complications are relatively rare (8).

> **Key point**
>
> In sporting injuries, the majority of contusions heal with normal muscle regeneration and chronic complications are relatively rare.

Muscle laceration. Muscle laceration is a direct penetrating injury that incises through the skin, subcutaneous tissues and underlying muscle. Usually the superficial injury heals well; however, the underlying muscle injury has a high incidence of linear scar formation (Fig. 12.11)

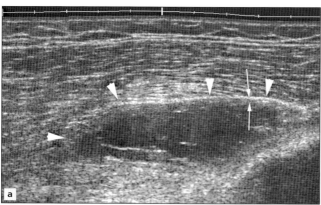

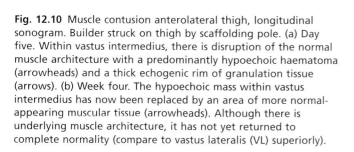

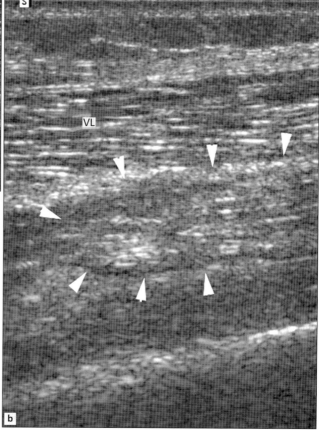

Fig. 12.10 Muscle contusion anterolateral thigh, longitudinal sonogram. Builder struck on thigh by scaffolding pole. (a) Day five. Within vastus intermedius, there is disruption of the normal muscle architecture with a predominantly hypoechoic haematoma (arrowheads) and a thick echogenic rim of granulation tissue (arrows). (b) Week four. The hypoechoic mass within vastus intermedius has now been replaced by an area of more normal-appearing muscular tissue (arrowheads). Although there is underlying muscle architecture, it has not yet returned to complete normality (compare to vastus lateralis (VL) superiorly).

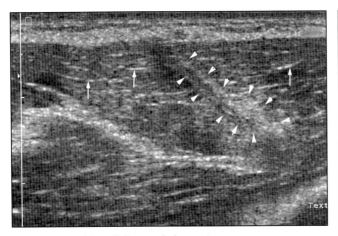

Fig. 12.11 Brachioradialis muscle laceration, transverse sonogram. Previous laceration due to assault with screwdriver. Thick irregular echogenic structure (arrowheads) disrupting the normal muscle architecture. The scar extends through the muscle, crossing the normal anatomical boundaries with echogenic perimysium seen on either side (arrows).

(4). Scar formation within the muscle decreases its ability to shorten and therefore also decreases its ability to generate tension on contraction (21, 44).

Lacerations are most commonly seen in trauma cases but can be associated with particular sports, for example ice hockey. Although in most cases, this decrease in function is not clinically relevant, if the muscles are required for a specific task or sporting activity, the limitations in developing maximal range of movement or power are more significant.

Ultrasound demonstrates the scar as a linear echogenic structure with relatively normal surrounding muscle architecture (Fig. 12.11). The scar does not follow any normal anatomical plane and is thicker, longer and more irregular than normal septa (Fig. 12.11). Studies are currently evaluating the use of antifibrotic agents to inhibit this process in trauma patients (45).

Indirect muscle injury

Indirect muscle injury is one of the commonest mechanisms of injury occurring at all levels of sporting activity (8). In professional athletes the incidence and muscle groups affected vary according to the sport. Certainly in soccer the incidence has been estimated at 30–38% of all injuries (8, 46) and in common with many other sports (47–51) the lower limb is most commonly affected (8, 46, 52).

Delayed onset muscle soreness. Delayed onset muscle soreness (DOMS) occurs when specific muscle groups undergo unaccustomed strenuous exercise (39, 51, 53). This usually occurs in recreational athletes who sporadically participate in sports. However, this can also occur in professional athletes with exercise of muscle groups not normally used in their own sport or when training is intensified after a previous injury. Pathologically the underlying mechanism is not clearly understood (39). At a microscopic level there is thought to be disruption of muscle fibrils, particularly at the myotendinous junction where there are also large concentrations of pain receptors (39). Some studies have shown muscle enzymes to be elevated after 24 hr and whether this results from direct fibril damage or from secondary lysosomal release is not known (8, 54, 55).

Key point

DOMS presents as a diffuse muscle pain develops 12 to 24 hours after activity, affecting multiple limbs and exacerbated by eccentric contraction.

Clinically diffuse muscle pain develops 12 to 24 hr after activity, affecting multiple limbs and exacerbated by eccentric contraction (15, 51, 53). This helps to clinically differentiate DOMS from a muscle tear or strain, which usually causes immediate focal pain and is exacerbated by concentric contraction. Additionally DOMS usually resolves within 7 days without any specific treatment (4, 8).

Key point

Delayed onset muscle soreness usually resolves within 7 days without any specific treatment.

Because this is a clinical diagnosis imaging is rarely necessary in the majority of cases (2). However, in athletes when it can occur if training is intensified after injury, imaging can be useful in excluding other causes of severe pain if the clinical history is not clear. MR imaging can show oedema in multiple muscles, but this is not a specific or sensitive finding with the abnormality persisting up to 82 days after clinical resolution (19, 37). Ultrasound is usually normal but its role lies in excluding a significant muscle strain or tear, which allows appropriate rehabilitation to continue.

Muscle tear or strain. Muscle strain or tear is an indirect injury caused by excessive force applied across the muscle rather than direct trauma (6, 8). Muscles with increased T2 fibrils, which span two joints and perform forceful eccentric contractions, are more susceptible to this form of injury as they experience the greatest intrinsic forces (as previously mentioned) (6, 8). Specific muscles, especially rectus femoris and biceps femoris, are more commonly affected than others within a synergistic group (47–51, 56). Hamstring injury is particularly common in a number of sports because this group of muscles spans the hip and knee joints and undergoes forceful eccentric contraction when resisting knee extension during sprinting (4, 20, 22, 55).

Key point

Muscles with increased T2 fibrils, which span two joints and perform forceful eccentric contractions, are more susceptible to muscle tear or strain as they experience the greatest intrinsic forces. Specific muscles, especially rectus femoris and biceps femoris, are more commonly affected than others within a synergistic group.

As has already been mentioned the myotendinous portion of the muscle is the commonest area to be injured in athletes but the junction of the muscle fibres and epimysium is also susceptible to injury (see the next section) (57). It should be remembered that the myotendinous junction is histologically much more extensive than is apparent on imaging and can extend throughout 60% of the total muscle length (58, 59). On exceeding the elastic limit of the muscle the fibrils and fascicles are disrupted with haemorrhage from the torn vascular fascia predominating in the first 24 hr (6, 8). Subsequently there is marked muscle oedema with an inflammatory infiltrate (6, 8). After 48 hr organisation begins to occur along with early

muscle regeneration (1). Subsequent muscle healing can take from 3 to 16 weeks, depending on the extent of injury. The ability of myocytes to regenerate by cell recruitment from the adjacent endomysium is good (60). However, if the injury is extensive there is always a potential for fibrous scar tissue to form (see Chronic complications) (55).

Key point

Clinical grading system of muscle strain:

  I. muscle strain less than 5% loss of function with mild evidence of haematoma or oedema.

  II. more severe than grade I but with some function preserved.

  III. complete muscle tear with no objective function and occasionally a palpable gap in the muscle belly.

Clinically, muscle strain or tear is characterised by immediate focal pain and decreased function, which can be due to muscle disruption or associated reactive spasm in adjoining muscles (6, 8, 15, 55). Occasionally a subcutaneous ecchymosis can occur but this usually develops 12 to 24 hr later (8). There is a well-established clinical grading system that has three components (61). Grade I injury is less than 5% loss of function with mild evidence of haematoma or oedema (61). If there is little clinical history these findings can overlap with the clinical features of muscle contusion (8). Grade II injury is more severe but with some function preserved. Clinical grade III strains are complete muscle tears with no objective function and occasionally a palpable gap in the muscle belly. It is well recognised that differentiation of these clinical grades can be difficult and thus ultrasound has a potentially important role in these situations (1, 2, 5, 15, 19, 62, 63).

In imaging terms various grading systems that have tried to correlate findings with the clinical grading system have been described. On ultrasound examination, grade I muscle injuries can show normal appearances or a small area of focal disruption (less than 5% of the muscle volume) with haematoma and perifascial fluid relatively common (Figs 12.5 and 12.12) (8, 15, 62).

Grade II injuries correspond to a partial tear with muscle fibre disruption seen (over 5%) but not affecting the whole muscle belly (2, 7). Initially the haematoma is echogenic but after 24 hr with oedema and the influx of inflammatory cells it becomes relatively echo-poor (Fig. 12.13). Subsequent organisation is seen with peripheral echogenic granulation tissue (Fig. 12.13). Again tearing of the blood vessel-rich muscle fascia is common and perifascial fluid tracking along the muscle boundaries can be identified (6). This form of intermuscular haematoma is relatively common in hamstring injuries but is less significant than a true intramuscular haematoma that implies a much more severe injury (5, 63). The oedema and haematoma associated with these injuries can obscure underlying muscle detail on MRI examination, leading to potential overgrading. Dynamic ultrasound assessment of the muscle can identify disrupted portions of the muscle with separation of the frayed ends on contraction or with transducer pressure, termed the "bell-clapper" sign. This sign is specific for muscle fibre disruption but can occur in a partial or complete tear (Fig. 12.14a) (25).

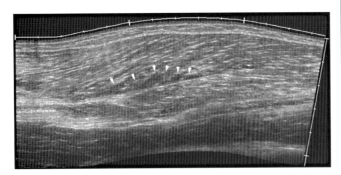

Fig. 12.12 Grade I muscle tear biceps femoris, longitudinal sonogram. Professional soccer player 4 days after injury. There is disruption of the proximal myotendinous junction of biceps femoris with loss of normal muscle architecture replaced by hypoechoic haematoma (arrowheads).

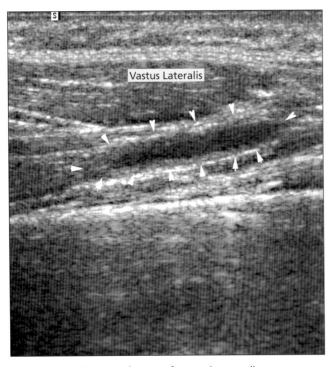

Fig. 12.13 Grade II muscle tear of vastus intermedius, longitudinal sonogram. Professional soccer player 6 days after injury. Distal myotendinous tear with hypoechoic haematoma (arrowheads), which has developed an echogenic rim of granulation tissue.

Key point

Ultrasound grade of muscle injuries:

I. normal appearance or a small area of focal disruption (less than 5% of the muscle volume) with haematoma and perifascial fluid relatively common.

II. partial tear with muscle fibre disruption seen (over 5%) but not affecting the whole muscle belly.

III. complete muscle tear with frayed margins and bunching of the muscle on dynamic stressing.

Grade III injuries are complete muscle tears with frayed margins and bunching of the muscle on dynamic stressing (Fig. 12.14) (7). Again fluid can decompress through tears in the muscle fascia and extend along the epimysium and neurovascular bundles (Fig. 12.15) (6). This can cause clinical confusion because pressure on adjacent nerves causes referred symptoms in any grade of injury. Ultrasound imaging can identify this complication, especially in the lower limb where the sciatic nerve can be irritated by haematoma from adjacent hamstring tears (Figs 12.15 and 12.16). The sciatic nerve is easily

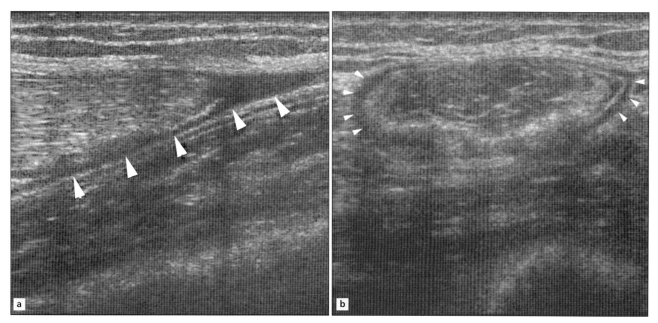

Fig. 12.14 Grade III muscle tear rectus femoris. (a) Longitudinal sonogram shows disruption of distal myotendinous junction of rectus femoris with bunching of the proximal muscle belly and distal hypoechoic fluid extending along the fascia (arrowheads), giving the bell-clapper sign. (b) Transverse sonogram at the level of the retracted muscle shows swollen muscle with disrupted architecture and perifascial fluid (arrowheads).

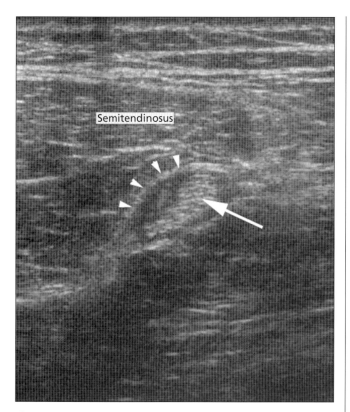

Fig. 12.15 Sciatic nerve irritation, transverse sonogram. Grade II muscle tear of biceps femoris associated with perifascial fluid tracking. The sciatic nerve is easily visualised (large arrow) with surrounding fluid in its investing fascia (arrowheads). The patient complained of pain extending down the entire leg consistent with sciatic nerve irritation.

identified on ultrasound and not obscured by oedema as can often occur with MR imaging.

Ultrasound has been shown to be a useful tool in assessing the sequential stages of muscle repair and therefore aiding rehabilitation planning (1, 7). As already mentioned in high-grade injuries, the hypoechoic haematoma begins to organise with an echogenic rim, which gradually fills in over a number of weeks (Fig. 12.17). Studies have shown that if the athlete resumes activities at this point, there is an increased risk of re-tear (58). If the haematoma is large and causing marked local mass effect aspiration may provide temporary symptomatic relief (under ultrasound guidance if necessary). However, routine evacuation of smaller haematomas does not seem to be of significant clinical benefit with rapid recurrence and no acceleration of healing (57).

Subsequent follow-up ultrasound imaging can show the appearance of more normal-appearing muscle architecture over the following weeks (Fig. 12.17). Once this is the predominant finding, it is suggested that more rigorous rehabilitation can occur (1). Conversely if the healing process demonstrates predominant scar formation management can be appropriately altered (please

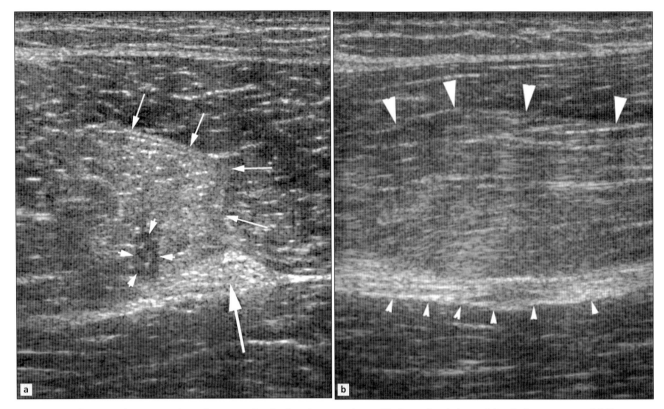

Fig. 12.16 Grade II muscle tear semimembranosus. Professional soccer player 10 days after injury with sciatic symptoms. (a) Transverse sonogram shows the muscle tear with a predominance of echogenic granulation tissue (small arrows) and a small hypoechoic area remaining inferiorly (arrowheads). The muscle injury abuts the sciatic nerve (large arrow), explaining the patient's referred symptoms. (b) Longitudinal sonogram in the same patient shows the muscle injury (large arrowheads) causing marked swelling of the muscle and displacing the sciatic nerve (small arrowheads) inferiorly.

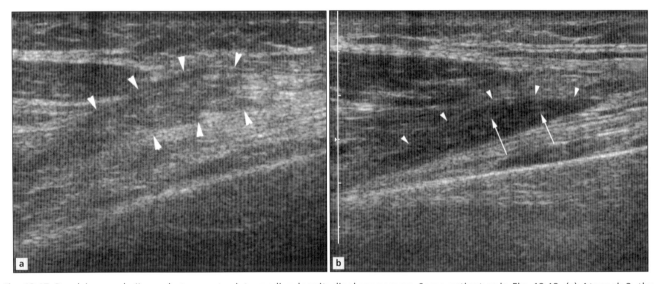

Fig. 12.17 Resolving grade II muscle tear vastus intermedius, longitudinal sonograms. Same patient as in Fig. 12.13. (a) At week 3, the previous hypoechoic haematoma has now filled in with echogenic material (arrowheads). Normal muscle architecture is not evident at present. (b) Two weeks later (week 5), more normal-appearing hypoechoic muscle echo texture is appearing (arrowheads) with linear echogenic perimysium (arrows).

see later). The MR imaging features of healing muscle tears have not been shown to be as clinically helpful with marked signal abnormality persisting throughout the different stages of healing (33, 64).

Key point

Aponeurosis distraction is a specific type of grade II muscle injury that occurs at the aponeurotic margin of two synergistic muscles. When it occurs in the medial head of gastrocnemius, it is known as "tennis leg".

Aponeurosis distraction. Aponeurosis distraction is a specific type of grade II muscle injury that occurs at the aponeurotic margin of two synergistic muscles. The muscles most frequently involved include the medial gastrocnemius and soleus, soleus and flexor hallucis longus or semimembranosus and semitendinosus (Fig. 12.16) (57). When this occurs in the medial head of gastrocnemius it is known as "tennis leg"

(Fig. 12.18) (4, 57). Again this muscle is at risk of injury because it spans two joints, consists of T2 fibres and undergoes eccentric loading during forced knee extension and ankle dorsiflexion (4, 57). The aponeurosis between the two muscles is a particularly weak area as the soleus consists mainly of T1 fibres and is relatively inelastic compared to the gastrocnemius (4). The Achilles tendon itself is usually not injured.

Ultrasound demonstrates a grade II injury with muscle fibre disruption adjacent to the aponeurosis and the presence of perifascial fluid and haematoma (Fig. 12.18). These injuries respond well to conservative treatment, although scarring can occur in the region of the aponeurosis (Fig. 12.19) (57).

Rhabdomyolysis. This condition rarely occurs secondary to trauma or in otherwise fit and healthy individuals. Muscle necrosis can occur for a variety of reasons including infection, inflammatory disease, infarction or prolonged pressure in an unconscious patient (e.g. drug overdose) (1). The clinical history should help differentiate these conditions from other types of muscle injury.

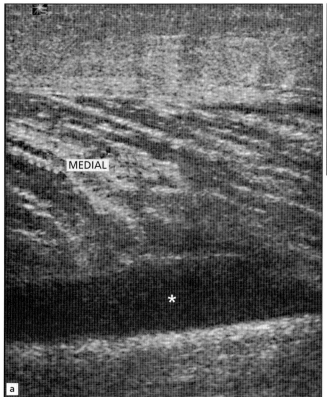

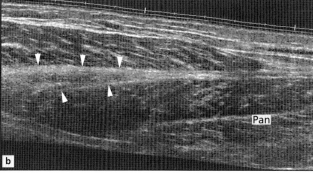

Fig. 12.18 "Tennis leg". (a) Acute injury one day prior to ultrasound examination. Grade II tear of the medial head of gastrocnemius from the aponeurosis with haematoma (*). (b) Subacute injury 15 days earlier (different patient to that in a). Echogenic granulation tissue (arrowheads) extends along the border of the medial gastrocnemius and soleus.

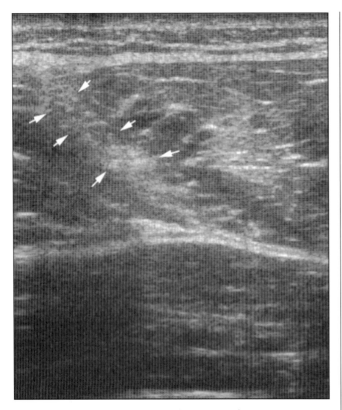

Fig. 12.19 Aponeurotic scarring of the rectus femoris, transverse sonogram. Professional soccer player with previous grade II muscle tear. One year later, there is thick irregular echogenic tissue (small arrows) at the margin of the rectus femoris and vastus lateralis consistent with scarring. This area was nontender and showed full movement on dynamic testing with no tethering evident.

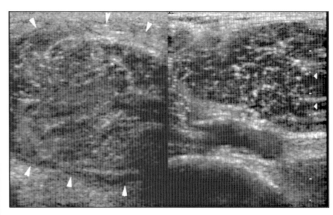

Fig. 12.20 Pyomyositis of biceps femoris, dual-screen facility, transverse sonograms. Intravenous drug abuser with increased fluctuant swelling of the thigh. The left-hand image shows a markedly swollen biceps femoris (arrowheads) compared to the right-hand image of the asymptomatic side. Throughout the muscle the normally hypoechoic fasicles have a more echogenic appearance with reduced echogenicity of the intervening septa.

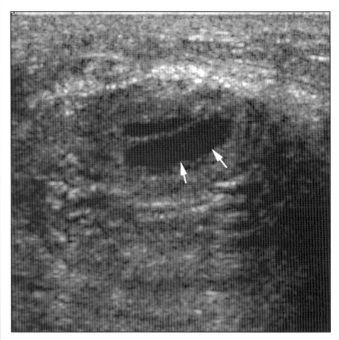

Fig. 12.21 Pyomyositis of biceps femoris with abscess, transverse sonogram. Same patient as in Figure 12.19, 4 days later. There is now an irregular hypoechoic fluid collection (arrows) consistent with an abscess.

The ultrasound features are nonspecific and include muscle swelling with relatively hyperechoic fibres and hypoechoic septa due to oedema (Fig. 12.20) (1, 65). This is usually best appreciated by comparison to normal musculature in the same or opposite limb. As necrosis continues hyperechoic foci appear, which can progress to full necrosis or abscess (Fig. 12.21) (1, 65, 66). If necessary, free hand aspiration or drainage can be performed under ultrasound guidance.

CHRONIC COMPLICATIONS

Fibrous scarring

As has previously been mentioned, muscle cells have a good ability to regenerate and the tendency for muscle injury to heal by fibrosis depends on the extent and type of injury (8, 55). Muscle lacerations have a high incidence of repair by scarring but in other types of injury this usually occurs only when they are more severe (4). Scar tissue can start to form as soon as 2 weeks post-injury and usually occurs adjacent to the epimysium (Fig. 12.19) (2).

Clinically the presence of scar tissue can restrict muscle function and the ability of an athlete to return to the previous level of activity (8). The contractile strength of the muscle is

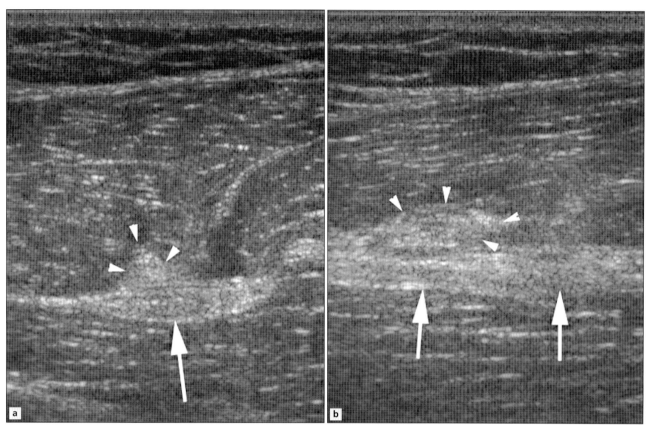

Fig. 12.22 Muscle scar involving the sciatic nerve. Professional soccer player with previous semitendinosus muscle tear presenting with tightness and referred leg pain on sprinting. (a) Transverse sonogram shows the sciatic nerve (large arrow) and adjacent nodular area of echogenic scar tissue (arrowheads). (b) Longitudinal sonogram of the same area clearly demonstrates the sciatic nerve (large arrows) with the nodular scar tissue impinging on its superior aspect (arrowheads).

reduced and makes it more susceptible to re-injury (6, 58). Scar tissue can also involve adjacent nervous tissue and cause referred symptoms (Fig. 12.22).

Ultrasound detects fibrotic scarring as an echogenic focus, which usually takes a well-defined linear pattern in distraction injuries (e.g. laceration or muscle strain/tear) (Figs 12.22 and 12.23) or a stellate pattern with compression injuries (e.g. contusion) (8, 55). Dynamic stressing on ultrasound can assess the relative inelasticity of this tissue and any adherence to adjacent structures (Fig. 12.23).

Myositis ossificans

Myositis ossificans is a rare complication of muscle injury and usually develops after injuries associated with a large haematoma or contusion. However, it has been reported that in up to 40% of cases the patient has no recollection of any significant trauma (1).

Pathologically this process represents heterotropic nonneoplastic bone formation. This is laid down in a lamellar fashion and is thought to develop within the layers of blood products formed within the original haematoma (67). Peripheral calcification appears at 6 to 8 weeks with mature ossification present by 6 months (68–70). Again in the majority of cases this tends to resolve without treatment (18, 68).

Clinically the development of myositis ossificans should be suspected when the degree of pain and soft-tissue swelling persists and is out of proportion to the original injury (8). Classically as a simple contusion should be resolving, pain does not only persist, but actually increases in severity (8, 55). The commonest muscle group involved by this condition are the quadriceps as they are most commonly affected by muscle contusion.

Prior to the development of calcification or ossification ultrasound appearances are similar to an organising haematoma. However, an

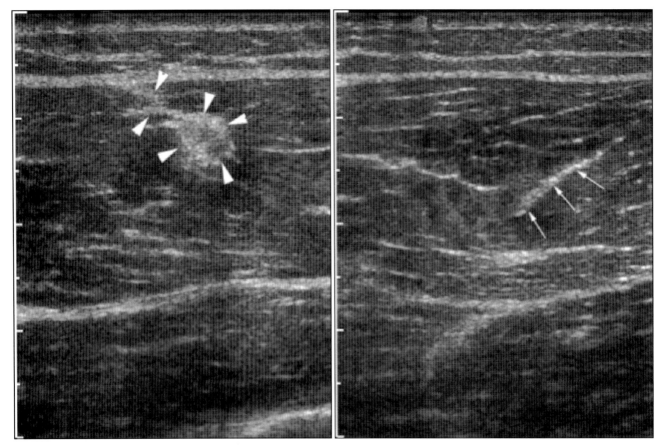

Fig. 12.23 Rectus femoris myotendinous scar. Soccer player with previous right rectus femoris grade II muscle tear. Left-hand image shows the myotendinous junction, which is nodular and irregular with echogenic scar tissue (arrowheads). The right-hand image shows the opposite limb with a more normal linear echogenic myotendinous junction (arrows).

advantage of ultrasound is that it can demonstrate the relatively well-defined peripheral margins and borders with adjacent soft tissues (68, 69). This is especially important if clinicians suspect other pathology such as an underlying neoplastic process. Performing MR imaging at this stage can show an extremely heterogenous appearance with surrounding oedema that can easily be misinterpreted as malignant (67, 71).

Ultrasound also demonstrates the peripheral calcification and ossification before it is clearly evident on plain film or MR imaging (68, 69). The main differential for this appearance is a parosteal neoplasm; however, ultrasound can demonstrate the preserved soft-tissue planes around the well defined calcification/ossification (Fig. 12.24), indicating a nonaggressive process. The density of the ossification can sometimes limit the ability to demonstrate the intact underlying periosteum of the adjacent bone (Fig. 12.24), which is also important for excluding a neoplastic process. However, if necessary,

CT scanning can be used to better define this relationship (Fig. 12.24c) (1, 2).

Other rarer causes of muscle calcification and ossification include previous inflammatory myositis, severe burns and neurological injury (1).

Muscle atrophy/hypertrophy

Atrophy of an injured muscle can commence as soon as 5 to 10 days after injury (72, 73). If this persists, it will become irreversible after approximately 4 months (Fig. 12.25) (72, 73). Obviously with the majority of injuries this rarely occurs, but if atrophy is detected despite a relatively minor muscle injury then damage to the supplying nerves or containing fascia should be suspected (1, 2).

Muscle hypertrophy can occur in synergistic muscles adjacent to an injured muscle as they are recruited to maintain overall function. Pseudo-hypertrophy of injured muscle can occur with fat deposition in the atrophic muscle, causing apparent muscle swelling (1, 72).

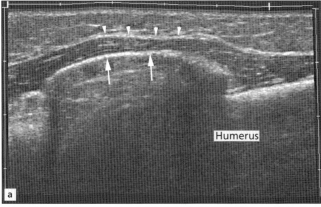

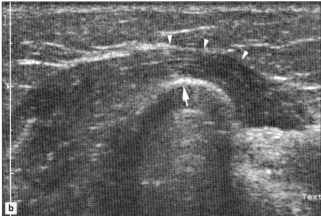

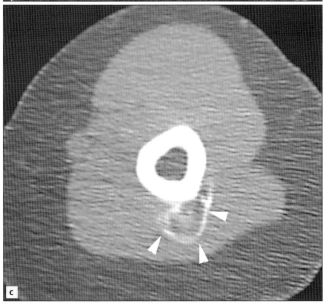

Fig. 12.24 Myositis ossificans left arm. Twenty-nine-year-old woman who presented with increasing pain and swelling 8 months after a fall. (a) Longitudinal sonogram shows a linear area of dense ossification within the triceps muscle. It lies superior to the humerus, displacing the triceps muscle and fascia superiorly (arrowheads). The interface with the surrounding soft tissues is smooth and homogeneous. (b) Transverse sonogram shows echogenic ossification (arrow) within triceps (arrowheads). However, the underlying relationship with the humerus cannot be determined due to acoustic shadowing. (c) Axial CT image shows predominant peripheral ossification separate from the underlying humerus.

Muscle hernia

A muscle hernia is defined as protrusion of muscular tissue through a defect in the containing epimysium (fascia) (74). This commonly occurs in the anterior and lateral muscle groups of the lower leg (especially tibialis anterior) (Fig. 12.26) but is also recognised with rectus femoris and the hamstrings (Fig. 12.27) (10). It is thought that the fascia overlying tibialis anterior has an area of potential weakness due to penetrating branches of the peroneal nerve and associated vasculature (55).

Clinically there may be a history of previous trauma or surgery but this is not universal. The hernia usually presents as a mass that may only appear after exercise or on standing (10). The hernia may be painful on exertion; however, quite frequently the main problem is cosmetic and it must be remembered that surgical treatment is not without complication (75). The clinical differential diagnosis includes an incompetent perforating vein.

This is one of the few occasions where a stand-off may be necessary so that transducer pressure does not maintain the hernia in reduction. Ultrasound can accurately identify the thick echogenic muscle fascia and any defect is seen as a hypoechoic gap (Fig. 12.26) (10). Dynamic manoeuvres can be performed to reproduce the muscle hernia if it is currently reduced (Figs 12.26 and 12.27). On acute herniation the muscle may appear hyperechoic due to compression of the fascial planes within it.

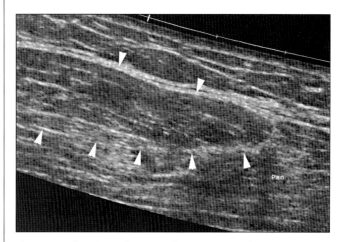

Fig. 12.25 Chronic grade III muscle tear semitendinosus, longitudinal sonogram. The retracted proximal component (arrowheads) has lost much of its normal echo texture and is atrophic.

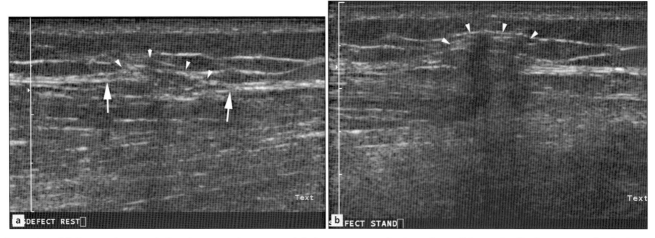

Fig. 12.26 Tibialis anterior muscle hernia presenting as a nodule in an amateur hockey player. (a) Longitudinal sonogram (with the patient lying down) shows a defect in the muscle fascia (large arrows) and protrusion of muscle through the gap (arrowheads). (b) On standing, the prolapsing muscle becomes more prominent (arrowheads).

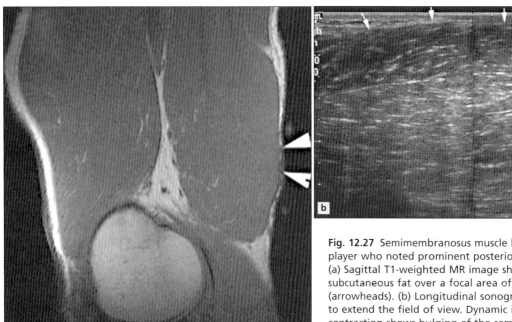

Fig. 12.27 Semimembranosus muscle hernia. Professional soccer player who noted prominent posterior thigh bulge on exercising. (a) Sagittal T1-weighted MR image shows possible reduction of subcutaneous fat over a focal area of semimembranosus (arrowheads). (b) Longitudinal sonogram using dual-screen facility to extend the field of view. Dynamic image obtained on muscle contraction shows bulging of the semimembranosus into the subcutaneous fat with no evidence of an echogenic fascia (small arrows).

However, if chronic it may appear hypoechoic due to a degree of oedema or necrosis (10). Because of its small size and its variable presentation on dynamic manoeuvres, MR imaging can be relatively ineffective in demonstrating these lesions (10, 19).

Compartment syndrome

Compartment syndrome is caused by an acute increase in intramuscular pressure that cannot disseminate due to the restricting muscle fascia (8, 55). Normal pressures within a muscle compartment are between 0–4 mmHg; however, if this pressure exceeds 15 mmHg blood flow can be compromised and muscle necrosis occur (53).

This can develop after indirect muscle tears but is more commonly associated with direct trauma and intramuscular haematomas (Fig. 12.9) caused by skeletal fractures (especially of the tibia) (76, 77). In this situation, diagnosis is nearly always clinical as this is a medical emergency and urgent surgical decompression is necessary.

In terms of sporting activity, exertional compartment syndrome can occur acutely with the increase in blood flow on exercise, causing muscle swelling and an acute rise in intracompartmental pressure. Again this is most common in the leg, affecting the anterior and deep posterior musculature (8, 53, 77–79). The patient usually presents with pain and paraesthesia after exercise (55, 79). Appearances on imaging are nonspecific and not reliable in making the diagnosis (Fig. 12.9). On ultrasound the muscle can appear echogenic with relative sparing of periseptal areas still receiving sufficient blood flow from the adjacent fascia (1). Studies evaluating a muscle cross-sectional area on ultrasound both before and after exercise describe two different patterns in symptomatic patients. In one group the muscle compartment cannot expand with a relatively rigid fascia compared to normal subjects where muscle volume can increase by 10 to 15%. In the other symptomatic group, although the muscle compartment does expand during exercise, there is a slow reduction in volume post-exercise compared to normal subjects (1).

Practical tip

On ultrasound a muscle with compartment syndrome can appear echogenic with relative sparing of periseptal areas still receiving sufficient blood flow from the adjacent fascia, however, generally imaging appearances can be non-specific and are not reliable.

The treatment of exertional compartment syndromes consists of fasciotomy but significant morbidity can result due to subsequent muscle dysfunction, herniation or scarring (1).

CONCLUSION

Modern transducer development has pushed musculoskeletal ultrasound to the forefront as an investigative tool for a number of muscle pathologies. Its exquisite demonstration of muscle architecture, surrounding fascia and neurovascular structures, along with its real-time dynamic capability should always make it the initial imaging technique for muscle injury. Its importance lies not only in refining the initial clinical diagnosis but also in providing an accurate assessment of muscle repair and complications after injury.

REFERENCES

1. Van Holsbeeck M, Introcasco J. Musculoskeletal ultrasound, 2nd ed. St Louis: Mosby; 2001.
2. Fornage BD. The case for ultrasound of muscles and tendons. Semin Musculoskelet Radiol 2000;4(4):375–91.
3. Graf P, Schuler P. Sonographie am Stutz und Bewegungsapparat bei Erwachsenen und Kindern. Weinheim: Editions Medizin VCH;1988.
4. Mink JH. Muscle injuries. In: Deutsch A, Mink JH, Kerr R, editors. MRI of the foot and ankle. New York: Raven Press; 1992:281–312.
5. Fleckenstein JL, Shellock FG. Exertional muscle injuries: magnetic resonance imaging evaluation. Top Magn Reson Imaging 1991;3(4):50–70.
6. Speer KP, Lohnes J, Garrett WE, Jr. Radiographic imaging of muscle strain injury. Am J Sports Med 1993;21(1):89–95; discussion 96.
7. Takebayashi S, Takasawa H, Banzai Y, Miki H, Sasaki R, Itoh Y, et al. Sonographic findings in muscle strain injury: clinical and MR imaging correlation. J Ultrasound Med 1995;14(12):899–905.
8. Peterson L, Renstrom P. Sports injuries. Chicago: Year Book Medical; 1986.
9. Fornage BD. Ultrasonography of muscles and tendons. In: Examination technique and atlas of normal anatomy of the extremities. New York: Springer-Verlag; 1989.
10. Bianchi S, Abdelwahab IF, Mazzola CG, Ricci G, Damiani S. Sonographic examination of muscle herniation. J Ultrasound Med 1995;14(5):357–60.
11. Weng L, Tirumalai AP, Lowery CM, Nock LF, Gustafson DE, Von Behren PL, et al. US extended-field-of-view imaging technology. Radiology 1997;203(3):877–80.
12. Fornage BD, Atkinson EN, Nock LF, Jones PH. US with extended field of view: Phantom-tested accuracy of distance measurements. Radiology 2000;214(2):579–84.
13. Barberie JE, Wong AD, Cooperberg PL, Carson BW. Extended field-of-view sonography in musculoskeletal disorders. Am J Roentgenol 1998;171(3):751–7.
14. Lin EC, Middleton WD, Teefey SA. Extended field of view sonography in musculoskeletal imaging. J Ultrasound Med 1999;18(2):147–52.
15. Noonan TJ, Garrett WE, Jr. Muscle strain injury: Diagnosis and treatment. J Am Acad Orthop Surg 1999;7(4):262–9.
16. Slavotinek JP, Varrell G, Fon GT. Hamstring injuries in footballers: The prevalance and prognostic value of MRI findings. Radiology 2000;217(P):191.
17. Pomeranz SJ, Heidt RS, Jr. MR imaging in the prognostication of hamstring injury. Work in progress. Radiology 1993;189(3):897–900.
18. Noonan TJ, Garrett WE, Jr. Injuries at the myotendinous junction. Clin Sports Med 1992;11(4):783–806.
19. Steinbach L, Fleckenstein J, Mink J. MR imaging of muscle injuries. Semin Musculoskeletal Radiol 1998;1:128–41.
20. Shellock FG, Fukunaga T, Mink JH, Edgerton VR. Exertional muscle injury: Evaluation of concentric versus eccentric actions with serial MR imaging. Radiology 1991;179(3):659–64.
21. Garrett WE, Jr, Safran MR, Seaber AV, Glisson RR, Ribbeck BM. Biomechanical comparison of stimulated and nonstimulated skeletal muscle pulled to failure. Am J Sports Med 1987;15(5):448–54.
22. Markee J, Logue J, Williams M. Two-joint muscles of the thigh. J Bone Joint Surg Am 1955;38:125–142.
23. Clemente C. Gray's anatomy. Philadelphia: Lea & Febiger; 1985.
24. Agur A. Grant's atlas of anatomy, 9th ed. Baltimore, MD: Williams and Wilkins; 1991.
25. Fornage BD, Touche DH, Segal P, Rifkin MD. Ultrasonography in the evaluation of muscular trauma. J Ultrasound Med 1983;2(12):549–54.

26. Matin P. Basic principles of nuclear medicine techniques for detection and evaluation of trauma and sports medicine injuries. Semin Nucl Med 1988;18(2):90–112.

27. Sjogaard G, Adams RP, Saltin B. Water and ion shifts in skeletal muscle of humans with intense dynamic knee extension. Am J Physiol 1985;248(2 Pt 2):R190–6.

28. Fleckenstein JL, Canby RC, Parkey RW, Peshock RM. Acute effects of exercise on MR imaging of skeletal muscle in normal volunteers. AJR Am J Roentgenol 1988;151(2):231–7.

29. Archer BT, Fleckenstein JL, Bertocci LA, Haller RG, Barker B, Parkey RW, et al. Effect of perfusion on exercised muscle: MR imaging evaluation. J Magn Reson Imaging 1992;2(4):407–13.

30. Fisher MJ, Meyer RA, Adams GR, Foley JM, Potchen EJ. Direct relationship between proton T2 and exercise intensity in skeletal muscle MR images. Invest Radiol 1990;25(5):480–5.

31. Fleckenstein JL, Bertocci LA, Nunnally RL, Parkey RW, Peshock RM. 1989 ARRS Executive Council Award. Exercise-enhanced MR imaging of variations in forearm muscle anatomy and use: importance in MR spectroscopy. AJR Am J Roentgenol 1989;153(4):693–8.

32. Fleckenstein JL, Haller RG, Bertocci LA, Parkey RW, Peshock RM. Glycogenolysis, not perfusion, is the critical mediator of exercise-induced muscle modifications on MR images. Radiology 1992;183(1):25–6; discussion 26–7.

33. Shellock FG, Fukunaga T, Mink JH, Edgerton VR. Acute effects of exercise on MR imaging of skeletal muscle: concentric vs eccentric actions. AJR Am J Roentgenol 1991;156(4):765–8.

34. Romanus B, Lindahl S, Stener B. Accessory soleus muscle. A clinical and radiographic presentation of eleven cases. J Bone Joint Surg Am 1986;68(5):731–4.

35. Burks JB, DeHeer PA. Tarsal tunnel syndrome secondary to an accessory muscle: A case report. J Foot Ankle Surg 2001; 40(6):401–3.

36. Bianchi S, Abdelwahab IF, Oliveri M, Mazzola CG, Rettagliata P. Sonographic diagnosis of accessory soleus muscle mimicking a soft tissue tumor. J Ultrasound Med 1995;14(9): 707–9.

37. Marcantonio DR, Cho GJ. Focus on muscle in orthopedic MRI. Semin Musculoskelet Radiol 2000;4(4):421–34.

38. Zarins B, Ciullo JV. Acute muscle and tendon injuries in athletes. Clin Sports Med 1983;2(1):167–82.

39. Armstrong RB. Mechanisms of exercise-induced delayed onset muscular soreness: A brief review. Med Sci Sports Exerc 1984;16(6):529–38.

40. Stauber W. Eccentric action of muscles: Physiology, injury, and adaption. In: Stauber W, editor. Exercise and Sports Sciences Reviews. Philadelphia: Franklin Institute; 1988:158–85.

41. Jackson DW, Feagin JA. Quadriceps contusions in young athletes. Relation of severity of injury to treatment and prognosis. J Bone Joint Surg Am 1973;55(1):95–105.

42. Aspelin P, Ekberg O, Thorsson O, Wilhelmsson M, Westlin N. Ultrasound examination of soft tissue injury of the lower limb in athletes. Am J Sports Med 1992;20(5):601–3.

43. Lehto M, Alanen A. Healing of a muscle trauma. Correlation of sonographical and histological findings in an experimental study in rats. J Ultrasound Med 1987;6(8):425–9.

44. Garrett WE, Jr. Injuries to the muscle-tendon unit. Instr Course Lect 1988;37:275–82.

45. Fukushima K, Badlani N, Usas A, Riano F, Fu F, Huard J. The use of an antifibrosis agent to improve muscle recovery after laceration. Am J Sports Med 2001;29(4):394–402.

46. Hawkins RD, Hulse MA, Wilkinson C, Hodson A, Gibson M. The association football medical research programme: an audit of injuries in professional football. Br J Sports Med 2001;35(1): 43–7.

47. Berson BL, Rolnick AM, Ramos CG, Thornton J. An epidemiologic study of squash injuries. Am J Sports Med 1981;9(2):103–6.

48. Burkett LN. Causative factors in hamstring strains. Med Sci Sports 1970;2(1):39–42.

49. Canale ST, Cantler ED, Jr, Sisk TD, Freeman BL, 3rd. A chronicle of injuries of an American intercollegiate football team. Am J Sports Med 1981;9(6):384–9.

50. Krejci V, Koch P. Muscle and tendon injuries in athletes. Chicago: Year Book Medical Publishers; 1980.

51. Newham DJ, Mills KR, Quigley BM, Edwards RH. Pain and fatigue after concentric and eccentric muscle contractions. Clin Sci (Lond) 1983;64(1):55–62.

52. McMaster WC, Walter M. Injuries in soccer. Am J Sports Med 1978;6(6):354–7.

53. Zabetakis P. Muscle soreness and rhabdomyolysis. In: Nicholas J, Hershman E, editors. The lower extremity and spine in sports medicine. St Louis: Mosby; 1986:59–81.

54. Schwane JA, Johnson SR, Vandenakker CB, Armstrong RB. Delayed-onset muscular soreness and plasma CPK and LDH activities after downhill running. Med Sci Sports Exerc 1983;15(1):51–6.

55. Nicholas J, Hershman E. The lower extremity and spine in sports medicine. St Louis: Mosby; 1986.

56. Southmayd W, Hoffman M. Sports health: The complete book of athletic injuries. New York: Quick Fox; 1981.

57. Bianchi S, Martinoli C, Abdelwahab IF, Derchi LE, Damiani S. Sonographic evaluation of tears of the gastrocnemius medial head ("tennis leg"). J Ultrasound Med 1998;17(3): 157–62.

58. Taylor DC, Dalton JD, Jr, Seaber AV, Garrett WE, Jr. Experimental muscle strain injury. Early functional and structural deficits and the increased risk for reinjury. Am J Sports Med 1993;21(2):190–4.

59. Garrett WE, Jr, Califf JC, Bassett FH, 3rd. Histochemical correlates of hamstring injuries. Am J Sports Med 1984;12(2): 98–103.

60. Bullough P, Vigorita V. Atlas of orthopaedic pathology. New York: Gower Medical; 1984.

61. O'Donoghue D. Principles in the management of specific injuries. In: O'Donoghue D, editor. In treatment of injuries to athletes, 4th ed. Philadelphia: Saunders; 1984:39–91.

62. Garrett WE, Jr. Muscle strain injuries: clinical and basic aspects. Med Sci Sports Exerc 1990;22(4):436–43.

63. Baker BE. Current concepts in the diagnosis and treatment of musculotendinous injuries. Med Sci Sports Exerc 1984; 16(4):323–7.

64. Fleckenstein JL, Weatherall PT, Parkey RW, Payne JA, Peshock RM. Sports-related muscle injuries: Evaluation with MR imaging. Radiology 1989;172(3):793–8.

65. Weinberg WG, Dembert ML. Tropical pyomyositis: Delineation by gray scale ultrasound. Am J Trop Med Hyg 1984;33(5): 930–2.

66. Yagupsky P, Shahak E, Barki Y. Non-invasive diagnosis of pyomyositis. Clin Pediatr (Phila) 1988;27(6):299–301.

67. De Smet AA, Norris MA, Fisher DR. Magnetic resonance imaging of myositis ossificans: Analysis of seven cases. Skeletal Radiol 1992;21(8):503–7.

68. Bodley R, Jamous A, Short D. Ultrasound in the early diagnosis of heterotopic ossification in patients with spinal injuries. Paraplegia 1993;31(8):500–6.

69. Peck RJ, Metreweli C. Early myositis ossificans: a new echographic sign. Clin Radiol 1988;39(6):586–8.

70. Booth DW, Westers BM. The management of athletes with myositis ossificans traumatica. Can J Sport Sci 1989;14(1): 10–6.

71. Shirkhoda A, Armin AR, Bis KG, Makris J, Irwin RB, Shetty AN. MR imaging of myositis ossificans: variable patterns at different stages. J Magn Reson Imaging 1995;5(3):287–92.

72. Petersilge CA, Pathria MN, Gentili A, Recht MP, Resnick D. Denervation hypertrophy of muscle: MR features. J Comput Assist Tomogr 1995;19(4):596–600.

73. Booth FW. Physiologic and biochemical effects of immobilization on muscle. Clin Orthop 1987(219):15–20.

74. Miniaci A, Rorabeck CH. Tibialis anterior muscle hernia: A rationale for treatment. Can J Surg 1987;30(2):79–80.

75. Miniaci A, Rorabeck CH. Compartment syndrome as a complication of repair of a hernia of the tibialis anterior. A case report. J Bone Joint Surg Am 1986;68(9):1444–5.

76. Ehman RL, Berquist TH. Magnetic resonance imaging of musculoskeletal trauma. Radiol Clin North Am 1986;24(2):291–319.

77. Mubarak SJ, Hargens AR. Acute compartment syndromes. Surg Clin North Am 1983;63(3):539–65.

78. Balduini FC, Shenton DW, O'Connor KH, Heppenstall RB. Chronic exertional compartment syndrome: Correlation of compartment pressure and muscle ischemia utilizing ^{31}P-NMR spectroscopy. Clin Sports Med 1993;12(1):151–65.

79. Martens MA, Backaert M, Vermaut G, Mulier JC. Chronic leg pain in athletes due to a recurrent compartment syndrome. Am J Sports Med 1984;12(2):148–51.

Ultrasound imaging of joint disease

13

Philip J O'Connor and Andrew J Grainger

Increasingly in both the literature and clinical practice modalities such as MRI and ultrasound are quoted as having a potential role in the assessment of articular disease (1–5). This chapter focuses on the role of ultrasound in patients with joint pain and covers both articular and periarticular disorders. The technical aspects of joint ultrasound examination, the imaging findings, developing roles and the current evidence base for diagnostic/therapeutic impact will be discussed.

Ultrasound is an extension of the clinical examination with improvements in image quality and user interface fuelling clinical interest in ultrasound.

TECHNICAL ASPECTS OF ULTRASOUND

Musculoskeletal ultrasound requires high-frequency probes in order to achieve the necessary resolution for accurate diagnosis. Fortunately the majority of joints are relatively superficial and can be imaged effectively using probe frequencies of approximately 7.5 MHz or higher. These probes should be linear array, with curvilinear probes rarely required for musculoskeletal imaging especially with electronic curvilinear conversion of linear transducers increasingly available. The development of extended field of view and three-dimensional techniques are of debatable value in diagnostic terms but are extremely useful when demonstrating an abnormality to clinicians or colleagues (Fig. 13.1).

To achieve high diagnostic yield the examiner should use the highest possible probe frequency to visualise the tissue of interest. The image should be focused on the area of interest, utilising the lowest frame rate possible to allow dynamic assessment of the tissue. Artefacts are common in musculoskeletal ultrasound; of these, tissue anisotropy and beam edge artefacts are important and require further discussion. Linear array probes are sensitive in the detection of tendon anisotropy, which can be diagnostically useful in itself.

Anisotropy results from tissues that contain multiple parallel linear sound interfaces such as tendons or muscles that cause

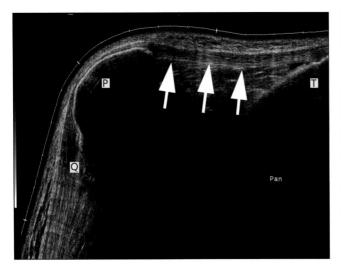

Fig. 13.1 Extended field-of-view image of the extensor mechanism of the knee, showing the advantage of being able to demonstrate large anatomical structures in a single image. Here the tibia (T), patella (P) and quadriceps tendon (Q) are shown along with the patellar tendon (arrows).

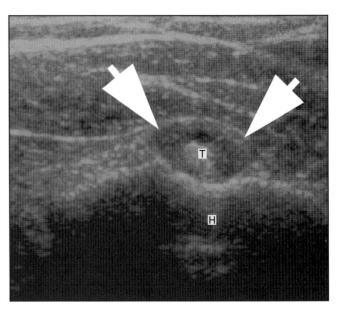

Fig. 13.2 Effect of anisotropy demonstrated in the long head of biceps tendon. (a) With the transducer face positioned parallel to the tendon the tendon appears brightly echogenic (T) against the surrounding synovial thickening (arrows) in this patient with long head of biceps tenosynovitis. (b) Moving the probe so the beam is no longer perpendicular to the tendon causes the tendon to loose its echogenic appearance and become difficult to distinguish from the surrounding synovium. H = humerus.

preferential reflection of the beam in one direction. If these structures are not visualised with the transducer array perpendicular to the long axis of the linear interfaces there is reflection of the beam away from the transducer, causing a dramatic reduction in echogenicity (ultrasound brightness) of the tissue. This mimics disease of these structures and represents a pitfall in the assessment of tendons and muscles. It can, however, also be of value, allowing the identification of tendons as a result of their changing echogenicity, especially when there is surrounding tenosynovitis present (Fig. 13.2). Multibeam compound imaging is a relatively recent technical innovation that reduces anisotropic effects.

Beam edge artefact is most evident around the margins of large tendons. It results in a very characteristic appearance at the edge of these tendons with loss of signal and distal acoustic shadowing that can mimic or obscure fluid or inflammation in the paratenon. Joint ultrasound should be methodical and cover all areas of the joint in the longitudinal and transverse planes. For small joints the transducer should have a small surface area or "footprint" to allow good skin contact, giving maximal acoustic access to the joint and reducing the risk of misinterpretation as a result of artefact. The use of a stand-off can be awkward and is rarely required with modern ultrasound equipment.

Near-field resolution is normally of high enough quality to allow diagnosis. Joint motion is particularly important in the demonstration of small joint effusions. Even limited active motion increases intra-articular pressure, squeezing out fluid into ultrasonically visible areas. In the hand, asking the patient to make a fist or splay the fingers increases the "acoustic window" for the transducer and can be helpful when detecting erosions.

APPLICATION OF ULTRASOUND IN RHEUMATOLOGY

Diagnostic ultrasound has the ability to image the body's soft tissues, cartilage and bone surface at high resolution. It can distinguish fluid from solid tissue, either in terms of appearance alone or by guiding accurate aspiration. Combining this with its real-time dynamic imaging capability and inherent close clinical correlation (you must be with the patient to perform an ultrasound) gives us a symptom-based, anatomical and functional assessment, ideal for the evaluation of articular and periarticular disorders.

The uses of ultrasound in joint disease fall into three main groups: diagnosis, assessment of treatment response or disease activity, and ultrasound-guided therapy. The first two groups represent the differing impact of imaging findings in diagnostic and therapeutic terms and will be discussed together for each imaging abnormality. Ultrasound-guided therapy refers to local injection treatment with needle placement guided by ultrasound and will be discussed separately. Diagnosis can also result from ultrasound-guided needling from either synovial biopsy or fluid aspiration for analysis.

INTRA-ARTICULAR ABNORMALITIES

Joint Effusion

Practical tip

Active or passive joint movement while scanning causes redistribution of any fluid present and can push fluid into ultrasonically visible areas.

Key point

The presence of effusion is a sensitive predictor of joint disease, but is unfortunately completely nonspecific.

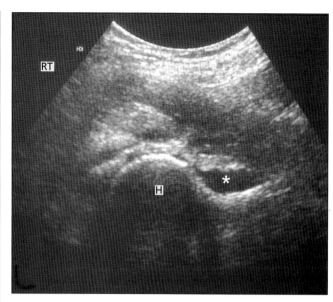

Fig. 13.3 Hip joint effusion. Here the typical anechoic appearance of simple fluid (*) is seen within this hip joint. H = femoral head.

Ultrasound is extremely sensitive in the detection of even small amounts of joint fluid. Active or passive joint movement while scanning causes redistribution of any fluid present and can push fluid into ultrasonically visible areas. Simple fluid is anechoic with no internal echoes (Fig. 13.3). The fluid is compressible and can be moved with probe pressure and demonstrates distal acoustic enhancement with no demonstrable vascularity (Fig. 13.4). Occasionally it can be difficult to differentiate simple fluid from underlying cartilage, which is also anechoic, but in the majority of cases a thin bright interface is seen between cartilage and fluid. More

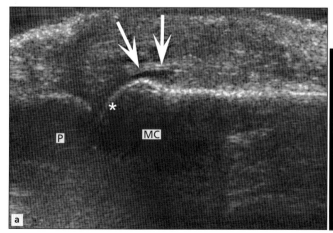
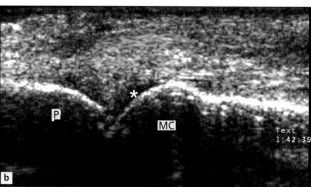

Fig. 13.4 Joint effusion in metacarpophalangeal (MCP) joint. (a) Fluid (arrows) is seen within the capsule of this MCP joint. It is indistinguishable from the anechoic hyaline cartilage overlying the metacarpal head (*). (b) With compression the fluid is no longer seen, although the noncompressible cartilage remains clearly visible. MC = metacarpal, P = proximal phalanx.

complex fluid contains internal structure as a result of proteinaceous fluid, fibrinous exudates, crystal deposition or cellular debris. Good acoustic access to the joint normally does not cause diagnostic difficulty, while compression of complex fluid normally shows random free movement of the internal echoes in the fluid; this would not be the case with solid tissue. With the increasing sensitivity of modern colour flow and power Doppler imaging, a lack of Doppler flow is becoming increasingly reliable in differentiating between complex fluid and synovitis (Fig. 13.5). The presence of effusion is a sensitive predictor of joint disease, but is unfortunately completely nonspecific. The main therapeutic impact is in the exclusion of intra-articular fluid, making articular disease much less likely. This is especially important in the setting of infection where the absence of joint effusion effectively excludes septic arthritis.

It must be remembered that in the immature skeleton infection frequently affects the metaphyseal region, and this area must also be examined to exclude periosteal reaction or subperiosteal abscess formation.

In some cases, ultrasound may still not allow a confident diagnosis. Ultrasound has a role in this setting allowing guided aspiration or washout of the joint to be performed to help differentiate between synovitis, complex fluid and infection.

Synovitis

> **Key point**
>
> Because synovitis varies in its activity and extracellular fluid content, it has a spectrum of appearances from hyperechoic to virtually anechoic.

> **Practical tip**
>
> Differentiating synovitis from effusion fluid can be difficult; compression using the probe can be helpful, with fluid displaced rather than deformed by the probe.

Synovium is not seen at ultrasound unless it is thickened, in which case it appears as hypoechoic intra-articular tissue (Fig. 13.6a). However, exact appearances vary according to the amount of extracellular fluid in the synovial tissue. Fluid whether free, intra- or extra-cellular is an excellent transmitter of sound, being of low acoustic impedance and containing little or no

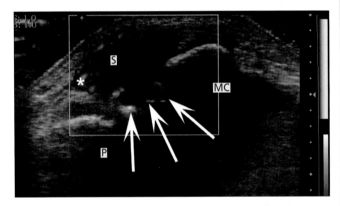

Fig. 13.5 Synovitis and bone erosion in MCP joint of patient with rheumatoid arthritis. Power Doppler signal (*) is demonstrated in the thickened low reflective synovium (S) on the dorsal aspect of this MCP joint. The synovium extends into an erosion (arrows) seen as a break in the cortex on the metacarpal head. MC = metacarpal, P = proximal phalanx.

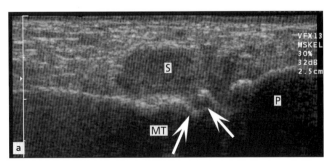
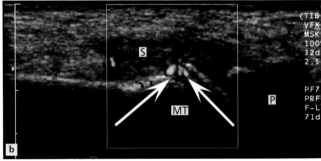

Fig. 13.6 Synovitis and bone erosion in metatarsophalangeal joint of patient with rheumatoid arthritis. (a) Low reflective synovium (S) is seen distending the capsule of this second metatarsophalangeal joint. An erosion in the metatarsal head is shown (arrows). (b) With power Doppler the enhanced vascularity of the synovium is seen. Note how the vascular synovium extends into the erosion. MT = metatarsal, P = proximal phalanx.

acoustic interfaces. The higher the extracellular fluid content, the lower the echogenicity. Because synovitis varies in its activity and extracellular fluid content, it thus has a spectrum of appearances from hyperechoic to virtually anechoic. Synovitis in inflammatory disease tends to occur at characteristic sites such as the radial or ulnar aspects of the metacarpophalangeal (MCP) joints (6) or the suprapatellar pouch of the knee. Differentiating synovitis from effusion fluid can be difficult; compression using the probe can be helpful with fluid displaced rather than deformed (Fig. 13.4).

Authors have attempted to use synovial vascularity as demonstrated by colour or power Doppler as a diagnostic tool, although these data are preliminary and sometimes conflicting (7–9) (Fig. 13.6b). When performing small joint scanning the usual rule of comparing with the opposite site does not always help, as the most common small joint arthropathies can be symmetrical.

There is now increasing evidence that clinical examination is insensitive when compared with ultrasound and MRI (10–12). Ostergaard et al. (13) compared ultrasound with MRI for the detection of knee pathology in patients with rheumatoid arthritis (RA). Using MRI as gold standard they concluded that ultrasound was 100% sensitive for the detection of synovial fluid and Baker's cysts but less sensitive (although specific) for detecting synovial hypertrophy. Rubaltelli et al. compared ultrasound synovial thickness with arthroscopic findings in 13 RA and 14 psoriatic arthritis knees and found good correlations for the suprapatellar and medial recess compartments (14).

Power Doppler ultrasound detects significantly more synovitis, as measured by increased synovial blood flow, than clinical assessment (6). Studies have also showed that most synovitis occurred on the radial aspect of the joint, which may correlate with the greater number of erosions seen at this site (15). Published data suggest that there is a substantial incidence of subclinical synovial disease in patients with both inflammatory and mechanical arthritis (16). There are currently differing views in the rheumatological literature regarding the primacy of synovitis in the pathogenesis of inflammatory arthropathy. Opinion is split between authors who claim a direct link between synovitis and joint damage and those who suggest these are uncoupled processes. The authors believe the former is the case and that the demonstration of synovitis will be the most important measure of therapeutic response and thus outcome in patients with inflammatory arthropathy. In terms of outcome measures, ultrasound would be a more sensitive, less specific outcome measure than erosion but would have the huge advantage of imaging the therapeutically targeted abnormality. This combined with advantages over MR of cost savings, multisite assessment and patient compliance make a compelling argument for the use of ultrasound in the assessment of inflammatory arthritis.

The introduction of power Doppler ultrasound (PDUS) has provided a new technique for the imaging of arthritis that has been looked at in a number of studies. PDUS has demonstrated hyperaemia around effusions due to inflammatory joint disease compared to effusions without inflammatory origin (17). In the authors' experience this is particularly true of effusions with an infective aetiology (Fig. 13.7). PDUS has been shown to perform well when compared with clinical disease activity assessment and traditional greyscale US (6), with histopathology correlation studies in the knee in RA and osteoarthritis (OA) (18, 19) and MRI correlation in small joints in RA (9). Studies indicate that PDUS has potential applications in disease activity assessment in RA (6, 20, 21) and in the monitoring of therapeutic response (7, 22, 23).

Currently the application of PDUS to rheumatological imaging is handicapped by a lack of consensus with regard to standard examination technique or technical parameters. A wide variation in methodology exists in the published literature. Reproducibility is a major problem and it is critical that studies to assess both inter- and intraobserver reliability are performed. Variables such as operator experience, training influence and choice of US machine are all important. Movement of the transducer or patient (enhancing the Doppler effect) can result in "flash" artefact, which can compromise interpretation (24). Increasing the pulse repetition frequency, reducing gain and altering the persistence help to minimise flash artefact. Bone cortex can also produce artefact deep to the tissue–bone interface (25). Excess pressure from the transducer can result in vessel occlusion and hence a reduction in blood flow and decreased power Doppler signal. This can be reduced by using a stand-off gel pad or water bath

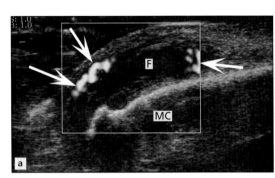
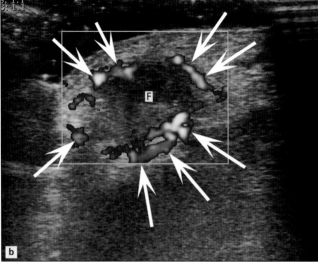

Fig. 13.7 Septic arthritis in MCP joint. A large joint effusion is seen (F). Due to the complex nature of the fluid it appears of low reflectivity, rather than the anechoic appearance of simple fluid (compare with Fig. 13.3). There is intense peripheral enhancement with power Doppler (arrows) in the surrounding synovium seen here in both longitudinal (a) and transverse (b) sections. MC = metacarpal.

technique. Similarly using a large quantity of acoustic jelly is a more practical but effective way of minimising pressure effect. All these factors need to be taken into account when performing PDUS examinations.

Joint space and cartilage abnormality

> **Key point**
>
> Bone erosions are cortical breaks that are the cornerstone of the diagnosis of inflammatory arthropathy, and are the most important imaging prognostic indicator.

Bone erosions are cortical breaks that are the cornerstone of the diagnosis of inflammatory arthropathy, and are the most important imaging prognostic indicator (Fig. 13.8). Ultrasound can identify erosions (26, 27) but few studies are validated (10, 15). In comparison to plain radiographs, ultrasound's multiplanar, real-time, high-resolution imaging of the bone surface has been shown to detect 6.5 times as many erosions in 7.5 times as many patients in early RA and 3.4 times as many erosions in 2.7 times as many patients in late RA (15).

Larger joints have also been studied in inflammatory arthropathy. Alasaarela *et al.* (28) compared ultrasound with conventional

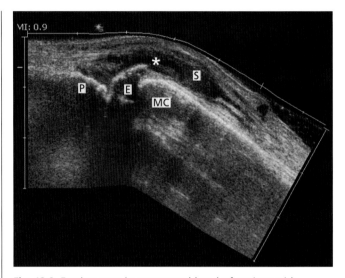

Fig. 13.8 Erosion seen in metacarpal head of patient with rheumatoid arthritis. The erosion is seen as a break in the cortex of the metacarpal head (E) on this extended field-of-view longitudinal image. Note also the associated synovitis (S) and joint effusion (*). MC = metacarpal, P = proximal phalanx.

radiography, CT and MRI in the detection of humeral head erosions, again in long-standing RA. They found MRI, CT and ultrasound were all more sensitive than radiography, with MRI and ultrasound superior to CT in detecting small erosions.

The morphology or site of erosion has no diagnostic implication with no difference documented in the literature as to lesion appearances in RA, seronegative and crystal disease. However, no studies have specifically addressed this issue.

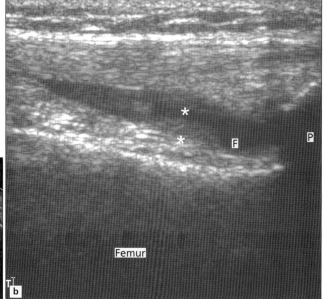

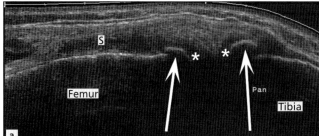

Fig. 13.9 Osteoarthritis of the knee. (a) Extended field-of-view longitudinal section over the medial aspect of the knee shows osteophytes (arrows) arising from the femur and tibia at the joint margin. The osteophytes arise at the edge of the articular cartilage (*). Associated synovial thickening is seen (S), indicating the inflammatory component of the disease. (b) Longitudinal section through the suprapatellar pouch demonstrates further synovitis (*) and a joint effusion (F). P = patella.

Ultrasound can demonstrate a number of features of OA and has a limited role in the assessment of mechanical arthritis. These include loss of joint space and cartilage (29, 30), meniscal abnormalities (31), osteophytes, Baker's cysts (32) and synovitis. Ultrasound may have a role in determining which patients with mechanical arthritis have an inflammatory element more suited to treatment with intra-articular steroids. In addition it can clarify diagnosis; knee joint line pain is common and ultrasound can usefully demonstrate meniscal degeneration and perimeniscal inflammatory change suitable for local steroid therapy in patients with or without established OA (33) (Figs 13.9a, 13.9b).

In patients with chondrocalcinosis (pseudo-gout), ultrasound can demonstrate crystal deposition on cartilage, which is seen as a dense white line running parallel with the articular margin (34, 35) (Fig. 13.10). This should not be confused with a cartilage–fluid interface line, which is an artefact seen in synovitic joints or lines occurring when there is gas entrapment within microfissures of degenerative cartilage. Gouty crystals cannot usually be seen unless complexes have calcified (Fig. 13.11), although a speckled appearance is seen within diseased joints.

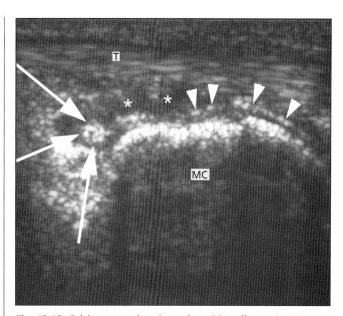

Fig. 13.10 Calcium pyrophosphate deposition disease in MCP joint. Synovitis is shown in this MCP joint (*), but in addition the normally anechoic hyaline cartilage shows foci of intense reflectivity (arrowheads) due to crystal deposition (chondrocalcinosis). An area of crystal deposition is demonstrated separately within the joint (arrows). T = extensor tendon, MC = metacarpal.

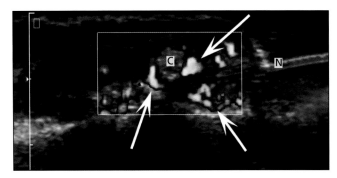

Fig. 13.11 Gouty tophus adjacent to distal interphalangeal joint. A urate crystal (C) is seen surrounded by hypervascular inflammatory tissue (arrows). The nail bed (N) is visible on the right of the image.

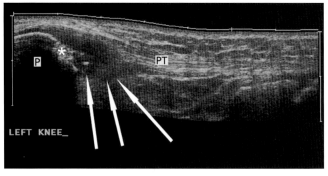

Fig. 13.12 Proximal patellar tendon enthesitis in a patient with ankylosing spondylitis. At the enthesis the patellar tendon is thickened and has lost its normal striation and echogenicity (arrows). The lower pole of the patella shows bony erosion with some new bone proliferation (*). P = patella, PT = patellar tendon.

Apart from identifying and guiding aspiration of effusions, the clinical impact of imaging in crystal disease is as yet unproven.

Entheseal abnormalities

An enthesis is a point of union between a tendon, ligament or capsule and bone (36, 37). Inflammation of this site, known as enthesitis, is a characteristic feature of a group of rheumatic conditions known as the spondyloarthropathies (SpA) but can be seen in other conditions such as gout or secondary to mechanical stresses. The outcome of SpA is generally better than RA, with early diagnosis conferring useful prognostic information.

The literature mainly refers to detection of enthesitis in larger structures such as the plantar fascia (38, 39) and Achilles (40) and patellar (41) tendons.

Key point

Typical early ultrasound findings of enthesitis can occur either in the tendon or in the adjacent bone.

Typical early ultrasound findings of enthesitis can occur either in the tendon or in the adjacent bone. The tendon changes seen are those of tendinopathy. This is a noninflammatory process associated with disruption of the tendon fibrils. Increasing amounts of glycoprotein matrix produce an increase in the water content of the tendon, fibroblast and tenocyte proliferation and neovascularisation. In ultrasound terms this manifests itself as loss of the normal organised tendon structure with increased tendon thickness.

The tendon becomes more hypoechoic (increased fluid content) with vascular in growth from the paratenon. These changes are essentially an adaptive response to stress and are thus amplified in areas of biomechanical stress.

An inflammatory infiltrate is seen in areas of tendon disease. This occurs when there is macrotrauma (partial or full thickness tearing) or as direct extension of inflammatory change from the paratenon into the tendon.

Key point

Differentiation between an osteophyte and enthesophyte is not difficult, as an osteophyte forms close to the joint line and generally lies in an intra-articular position, whereas enthesophytes form some distance away from the joint line at the site of the tendon, ligament or capsular junction with bone.

Changes are also seen at the bone surface of the enthesis and are a combination of erosion and proliferative new bone formation (Fig. 13.12). Differentiation between an osteophyte and enthesophyte is, in practice, not difficult. An osteophyte forms close to the joint line and generally lies in an intra-articular position. The bone is well formed with little in the way of surrounding inflammatory change, and joint space loss is usually present. Enthesophytes form some distance away from the joint line at the site of the tendon, ligament or capsular junction with bone. There is frequently surrounding inflammatory change, characterised by low reflectivity and hypervascularity of the surrounding soft tissues, and erosion of the bone

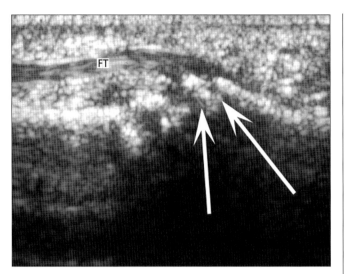

Fig. 13.13 Early flexor tendon enthesitis in a patient with psoriatic arthritis. Longitudinal section along volar aspect of DIP joint shows some thickening of the flexor tendon (FT) at its insertion. There is bony irregularity and proliferation at the enthesis site on the distal phalanx (arrows).

cortex. Entheseal erosion occurs more at sites of compression such as the deep aspect of the plantar fascia, or Achilles or patellar tendons. The earliest change seen in enthesitis is that of irregularity of the bone surface where there is fine periosteal new bone formation (Fig. 13.13). This is the ultrasound equivalent of the periostitis seen on conventional radiography.

Ultrasound has been shown to demonstrate periosteal change earlier than radiography in the setting of infection and tumours and it would be reasonable to assume the same would be the case for developing enthesitis. Another common association with SpA is the presence of bursal disease, e.g. infrapatellar or retrocalcaneal bursitis.

Assessment of enthesitis in the hand is difficult, with seronegative patients frequently presenting with dactylitis or sausage finger. Most authors agree that the universal finding on ultrasound is a flexor tenosynovitis with nonspecific subcutaneous oedema (42–44).

Key point

With seronegative patients frequently presenting with dactylitis or sausage finger, most authors agree that the universal finding on ultrasound of enthesitis in the hand is a flexor tenosynovitis with nonspecific subcutaneous oedema.

PERIARTICULAR ABNORMALITIES

Periarticular masses

When faced with a periarticular mass, one of the first and most useful roles of ultrasound is to distinguish a solid mass from a cystic structure.

Establishing a mass as cystic substantially reduces the differential diagnosis and, in many cases, allows a diagnosis to be made.

Cysts

As with joint effusions discussed above, simple encysted fluid is anechoic and there is acoustic enhancement of the tissues deep to the fluid.

Unless the cystic structure communicates with a joint or tendon sheath into which it can be decompressed, cysts are not normally compressible.

Bursae

One of the most common causes of a periarticular cystic structure is fluid seen within a bursa. Bursae are pouches of fluid that facilitate movement between adjacent structures by reducing friction. Two types of bursae are recognised: synovial-lined bursae, which tend to occur in well-recognised positions and may communicate with the adjacent joint, and adventitial bursae. The latter have no synovial lining and are acquired as a result of friction between two structures, leading to the collection of fluid within the tissues separating them. They are much more variable in location and may develop at specific sites relating to a patient's occupation or a sporting activity. Bursae normally contain only a trace of fluid. However, if a bursa becomes inflamed as a result of repetitive trauma, such as may occur with exercise, it will become more distended with fluid and appear as a cystic structure. Associated with the fluid distension there may be thickening of the bursal synovial lining that can often be appreciated at ultrasound. Thickened bursal synovium shows a range of ultrasound appearances similar to those seen in joint synovitis (Fig. 13.14).

Although the fluid will often appear anechoic, the presence of haemorrhage or infection will lead to fluid with a more complex and echogenic appearance. Bursae around individual joints can be very variable. However, the distribution of synovial bursae around some joints is more predictable, including the subacromial bursa of the shoulder, the retrocalcaneal bursa of the ankle and a number of bursae about the knee. Bursae may communicate with the adjacent joint, as with the gastrocnemius–semimembranosus bursa of

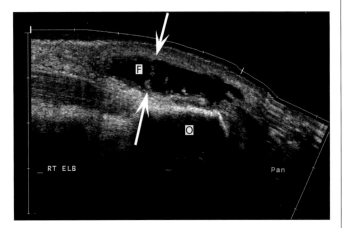

Fig. 13.14 Olecranon bursitis. Fluid is seen within the olecranon bursa (F) on this longitudinal section. There is associated synovial thickening (arrows). O = olecranon.

the knee. When distended this is familiar as popliteal or Baker's cyst and has a characteristic appearance that should be sought before diagnosis is made (Fig. 13.15). In other cases joint communication is variable, as with the iliopsoas bursa, which may or may not communicate with the hip.

However, the majority of bursae show no communication and represent isolated pockets of fluid. In these cases a pathological communication with the adjacent joint may still occur.

This occurs between the glenohumeral joint and subacromial bursa in cases of full thickness rotator cuff tear where fluid can communicate between the two structures through the tear. The possibility of communication with a joint should be considered when a distended bursa is identified because, in these cases, bursal distension may be the result of a primary joint abnormality resulting in a joint effusion that then tracks into and distends the bursa. Bursae known to communicate with a joint can thus indicate pathology in the joint; for instance, the popliteal

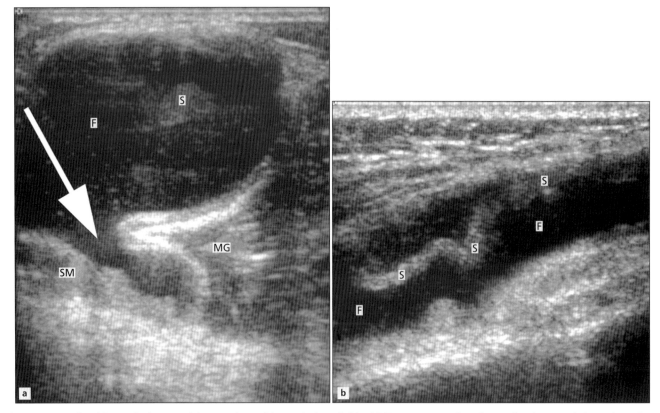

Fig. 13.15 Popliteal bursa (Baker's cyst) in a patient with psoriatic arthritis. (a) Transverse section shows the characteristic neck to the Baker's cyst (arrow) as the cyst arises between the medial head of gastrocnemius (MG) and the semimembranosus (SM). Frond-like thickened synovium (S) is seen surrounded by the bursal fluid (F). (b) Longitudinal section of the same patient with fluid (F) and a thickened synovitic septum (S) demonstrated within the cyst.

cyst in adults is often seen secondary to a primary knee abnormality (45–47). Around the knee, bursitis is particularly commonly seen anteriorly in the prepatellar bursa (Fig. 13.16) or superficial infrapatellar bursa, and medially associated with the tendons of the pes anserinus at their tibial insertion (the pes anserine bursa). Bursae are not confined to adults and a Baker's cyst is a relatively common cause of a popliteal fossa mass in children. Bursae may leak or rupture. Rupture of a popliteal cyst is a well-recognised cause of calf swelling and pain (Fig. 13.6b).

Synovial cysts and recesses

Occasionally, out-pouches from joints are seen on ultrasound as fluid-filled structures adjacent to a joint. No confusion exists if a communication is readily demonstrated with the joint. However, in some cases the communication is less readily demonstrated. Knowledge of the potential sites where these may be seen can help in making the diagnosis. Such synovial recesses are particularly common around the knee and the anterior aspect of the shoulder. There is some overlap between bursae and synovial recesses; the distinction in the case of the popliteal cyst is clearly blurred and some authors would think of it as a synovial recess of the joint (48).

Cysts associated with fibrocartilage lesions

In addition to the hyaline cartilage seen overlying the articular surfaces of synovial joints, many joints also contain fibrocartilaginous structures.

Examples include the menisci of the knee and the labrum of the hip and shoulder. In contrast to the anechoic appearance of hyaline cartilage, fibrocartilage appears highly reflective on ultrasound (Fig. 13.17). Para-articular cysts may be seen associated with tears of these fibrocartilaginous structures. Most commonly these are seen about the knee in association with meniscal tears. Diagnosis can often be made on ultrasound without recourse to other imaging as the cyst can be seen to communicate with a tear in the meniscus (Fig. 13.18). They are thought to occur when synovial fluid is forced through the tears, forming a cystic structure at the articular surface of the meniscus (47, 49). Meniscal cysts have, in the past, been thought to be more commonly associated with tears of the lateral meniscus.

However, more recent literature using MRI has indicated that medial and lateral meniscal cysts occur with more equal frequency than previously thought and the earlier discrepancy may reflect the increased difficulty of detecting medial

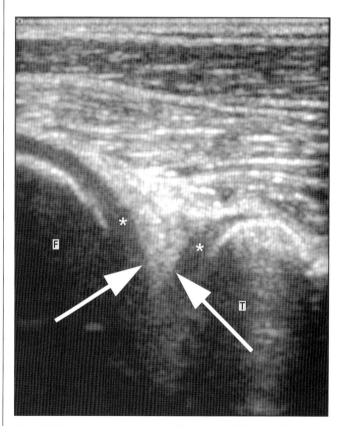

Fig. 13.17 Normal appearances of hyaline and fibrocartilage at the knee. Longitudinal section over the medial aspect of the knee shows the brightly reflective fibrocartilaginous medial meniscus (arrows) and the low-reflective articular hyaline cartilage (*) overlying the femur (F) and tibia (T).

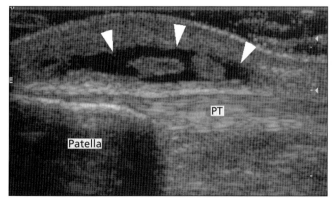

Fig. 13.16 Pre-patellar bursitis. Longitudinal section over the anterior aspect of the knee shows the fluid-filled bursa (arrowheads) lying anterior to the patella and patellar tendon (PT).

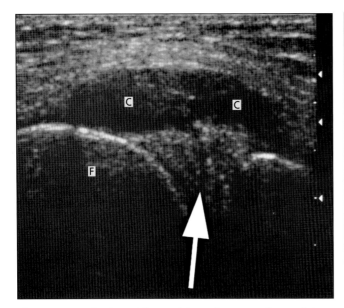

Fig. 13.18 Meniscal cyst (C) seen lying adjacent to the medial meniscus on this longitudinal section. A cleft representing the meniscal tear is seen extending through the meniscus (arrow). F = femur

meniscal cysts clinically (50). Difficulty stems from the medial meniscal cyst being confined deep to the medial collateral ligament and so presenting much later as a palpable mass. The presence of structures confining the cyst means that some meniscal cysts can track some distance from the meniscus before becoming clinically palpable. Ultrasound usually still shows the narrow, often complex track connecting the main cyst to the meniscal tear. As indicated above, cysts may be seen in association with fibrocartilaginous structures in other joints. In particular these are seen as paralabral cysts in association with tears of the glenoid labrum (51, 52) and acetabular labrum (53). Parts of the glenoid labrum are amenable to ultrasound examination and reports exist of the effective use of ultrasound in the diagnosis of glenoid labral pathology (54, 55). However, the anterior labrum (most commonly affected in cases of instability) remains difficult to visualise and the superior labrum and biceps anchor are not shown with ultrasound. As a result, MR arthrography remains the imaging modality of choice for glenoid labral lesions but, where present, a related cyst can often be readily identified and the possibility of a labral tear inferred. Little has been published on the direct visualisation of acetabular labral tears on ultrasound.

Again parts of the labrum are well shown, but MR arthrography remains the imaging modality of choice when labral pathology is suspected.

However, as with the glenoid labrum a tear can be inferred when a paralabral cyst is seen on ultrasound.

Occasionally symptoms arise from paralabral cysts as a result of pressure on adjacent nerves (51, 56). The ultrasound appearance of such nerve entrapments and percutaneous ultrasound-guided aspiration of the cyst has been described (57).

Ganglion cysts

Ganglion cysts are often seen adjacent to joints and are particularly common around the wrist and ankle. They are mucin-filled cystic structures and are often septated. On ultrasound they appear as well-defined anechoic lesions and may have a demonstrable communication with the joint or an adjacent tendon sheath. As with other masses they may compress adjacent neurovascular structures and this may be the patient's primary presentation.

Other periarticular cystic structures

Benign and malignant masses may appear cystic owing to foci of necrosis or degeneration.

This is particularly common in the case of schwannomas, a benign nerve sheath tumour. These arise from nerves and have a fusiform appearance. Knowledge of the location of the major nerves about the joint helps in making the diagnosis. In addition, the tumour will often have a "rat tail" appearance at the point where the nerve enters and leaves the lesion. In the majority of cases of malignant tumours that have cystic components owing to necrosis, the lesion will still show more solid elements, allowing the distinction from more benign cysts to be made, or at least raising the suspicions of the examiner sufficiently to prompt further investigation. Ultrasound may be particularly useful in guiding biopsy of cystic tumours since a more solid component of the mass, more likely to yield diagnostic tissue, can be targeted.

Abscess collections can occur around joints and again will appear as cystic masses. Often the fluid in an abscess is echogenic and, where this is the case, pressure with the probe can set the fluid moving within the cavity, confirming the fluid nature of the contents. The fluid centre of the abscess cavity will appear avascular with Doppler imaging.

However, the wall of the abscess, which may be thick and irregular, may appear hypervascular, owing to increased perfusion about the collection.

Again, ultrasound will be useful in guiding aspiration and drainage of abscess collections.

Solid masses

If ultrasound demonstrates a solid mass close to a joint, the differential diagnosis is somewhat larger. It is important to exclude normal structures such as accessory muscles as a cause of the mass. Apart from using knowledge of the usual sites for accessory muscles, which are particularly common in the calf and around the ankle, consideration of the echo pattern of the structure under investigation also helps: does it look like muscle? Having confirmed that the solid mass is genuine, further clues as to the nature of the mass can be gained from its relationship to other normal structures. Nerve sheath tumours will arise from nerves and show the rat-tail appearance previously mentioned. They may also characteristically show a "ring" sign consisting of an echogenic ring seen within the tumour on ultrasound (58). However, distinction between different masses on the basis of echo pattern is often not possible. Even when a particular underlying cause is suspected, further imaging and usually biopsy, often under ultrasound guidance, are required to confirm the findings.

In the context of periarticular soft-tissue disease, two synovial-based masses warrant special consideration.

Pigmented villonodular synovitis (PVNS) and synovial chondromatosis arise from joint synovium. PVNS is seen on ultrasound as a focal or diffuse mass or thickening of joint, tendon or bursal synovium. There may be associated bone erosion. There are no specific features relating to the echo characteristics of the mass and, when suspected, MRI is often a more helpful imaging modality because the signal characteristics of the lesion can be distinguishing. Synovial chondromatosis is a benign metaplastic proliferation of cartilaginous nodules within synovium. Again it can arise within the synovium of joints, bursae or tendon sheaths. Although ultrasound appearances may be nonspecific, cartilage nodules may undergo ossification (synovial osteochondromatosis), in which case the synovial mass will be seen to be associated with multiple calcific bodies with a typical ultrasound appearance of bright surface reflectivity and posterior acoustic shadowing.

Ligaments

Many ligaments are amenable to ultrasound examination and disruption of these structures can be demonstrated at ultrasound. Large ligaments, such as the medial collateral ligament of the knee, are readily seen and have an ultrasound appearance similar to that of tendons, comprising parallel echogenic fibrils arranged longitudinally along the length of the ligament. As with tendons, ligaments are subject to anisotropic artefact and a scrupulous technique must be adopted to ensure the ligament is imaged parallel to the face of the ultrasound transducer (2).

Ultrasound readily identifies the medial collateral ligament (MCL) of the knee running between the medial femoral condyle and medial tibial metaphysis. It is seen as a trilaminar structure comprising deep and superficial components of the ligament separated by a low reflective layer of fibroadipose tissue. Disruption of the ligament may involve its avulsion with a piece of bone from its origin or insertion, or a partial or full thickness tear of the ligament itself.

Although partial thickness tears can involve either the deep or superficial component of the MCL, the deep component is far more commonly torn (59). A ligamentous strain is seen as low reflective change and thickening of the ligament, while a tear will be seen as a low reflective fissure traversing the ligament, usually in a zigzag fashion (Fig. 13.19).

As with examination of tendons, dynamic stressing of the ligament under investigation is an important part of the examination (60). When viewing the MCL of the knee, a tear can often be better appreciated with the application of varus stress to the joint.

> **Practical tip**
>
> When viewing the medial collateral ligament of the knee, a tear can often be better appreciated with the application of varus stress to the joint.

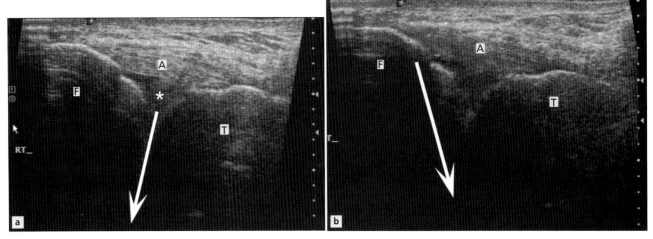

Fig. 13.19 Normal anterior talofibular ligament (ATFL). Here the beam-steering function on the ultrasound machine is used to utilise the inherent anisotropy of the ligament (A) and better define its boundaries. (a) The beam has been directed perpendicular to the ligament, which is seen as a brightly reflective fascicular structure. Its superficial border is difficult to distinguish from the adjacent subcutaneous fat although its deep border is seen contrasting with the joint fluid (*). (b) The beam has now been directed obliquely relative to the ligament, which now appears dark and its superficial border becomes obvious. Arrow indicates direction of ultrasound beam. F = fibula, T = talus.

Other ligaments readily demonstrated at ultrasound include collateral ligaments of the elbow (61, 62), the ulnar collateral ligament of the first metacarpophalangeal joint (63–66) and lateral collateral ligaments of the ankle (67, 68) (Fig. 13.19).

Although reports concerning the value of ultrasound in diagnosis of cruciate ligament disruption in the knee do exist (60, 69–71), the authors have found ultrasound of virtually no use in this situation. In cases of suspected cruciate ligament disruption MRI remains the imaging modality of choice at the authors' institution.

Tendons

Examination of the tendons around a joint forms an important part of joint examination. Swelling suspected as arising from a joint may in fact represent synovial thickening of a tendon sheath in a patient with tenosynovitis. Tendinopathic change and tears should also be looked for in the periarticular tendons.

Particular mention should be made of the examination of tendons about the hip in the context of snapping hip syndrome. This condition manifests as an audible or palpable snapping at the hip during movement. Although these symptoms may result from intra-articular pathology, such as a loose body or labral tear, extra-articular causes include the snapping of tendons over bony prominences about the hip. Two tendons are commonly involved. The iliopsoas tendon may snap over the iliopectineal eminence of the pelvis, or the iliotibial band (ITB) may snap over the greater trochanter. In both cases dynamic demonstration of the snapping tendon can be achieved with ultrasound. The tendon is seen to jerk abnormally over the bony prominence at the same time as the snap is felt or heard (72).

In the popliteal fossa, patients may experience a snapping sensation as the result of an abnormal, jerky movement between the semitendinosus and semimembranosus tendons as the knee is moved between flexion and extension. Again, jerky movement can be demonstrated and shown to correspond with the snapping sensation using dynamic scanning. A bursa may be seen between the two tendons.

The ITB may be associated with symptoms at its distal end as it passes over the lateral femoral condyle at the knee. Here the condition of ITB friction syndrome may be seen. This condition is commonly seen in athletes and is sometimes known as runner's knee. Symptoms result from inflammation in the ITB and surrounding soft tissues as a result of friction between it and the prominent lateral femoral condyle. Changes are best seen on ultrasound soon after exercise. The ITB may be seen to be thickened with low reflective change and an associated bursa lying between the ITB and the lateral femoral condyle may be distended (73, 74).

ULTRASOUND-GUIDED MUSCULOSKELETAL INTERVENTION

Diagnostic and therapeutic injections are of value in the assessment and treatment of both joint disease and soft-tissue lesions. Diagnostic injections are those performed into or around a structure where local anaesthetic is instilled to determine whether patient symptoms arise from that area. When steroid is injected alone or in addition to local anaesthetic, the injection is considered therapeutic. These injections have often been performed with little validation of either results or the pathology being injected. Surveys of rheumatological practice have shown little consensus between clinicians in virtually all aspects of these treatments (75). The conditions being treated, site of injection, frequency of injection and injection technique all varied widely. Injections can be into joints or aimed at treating a variety of extra-articular conditions. Examples include subacromial subdeltoid bursal injections in patients with shoulder impingement syndrome or rotator cuff disease, greater trochanteric bursitis, tenosynovitis, calcification associated with inflammatory change, plantar fasciitis and carpal tunnel syndrome.

Two published studies showed extremely poor accuracy of joint injections without imaging guidance, reporting an accuracy of 42–51% for large joint injection and only 29% for subacromial bursal injections (76, 77). For these injections to be of reliable diagnostic and therapeutic value, the exact site of injection must be known. Ultrasound can and should help clarify this situation by both delineating the abnormality present and recording the site of injection. Ultrasound allows the operator to dynamically image needle placement and distribution of any injection performed.

Needle placement technique is similar in all applications regardless of the type of needle being positioned or whether the intention is to aspirate, biopsy or inject. Needle visualisation in musculoskeletal ultrasound is generally excellent because of the high-resolution (7.5–17 MHz) transducers typically employed and also the comparatively superficial situation of the structures of interest.

Needle placements around deeper structures, such as the deep greater trochanteric bursa or hip joints, are more difficult but even in these cases the use of transducer guides is rarely needed.

There are a variety of techniques available for optimising needle visualisation. Choosing a needle path as parallel as possible to the face of the transducer improves needle conspicuity by providing a single, strong sound interface that should render the needle visible regardless of the acoustic properties of the surrounding tissues. The real-time nature of ultrasound also helps in that a moving interface is much easier to localise. This is done using small regular backwards and forwards movement of the needle and is especially useful when injecting relatively deep structures. If the structure of interest is, as is often the case in pathological states, hypoechoic relative to surrounding tissues, the needle tip becomes more visible on entering the lesion simply as a result of increased acoustic contrast. Occasionally there is still diagnostic doubt as to the site of the needle tip. In these cases injection of sterile saline, which is almost invariably accompanied by a small amount of gas, is advised. This will be ultrasonically visible and will localise the injection site regardless of whether the needle tip can be demonstrated.

Applications

Joint Aspiration

Ultrasound-guided joint aspirations are frequently performed. Aspiration helps diagnose the nature of an arthropathy with the usual objective being to confirm or exclude the presence of infection or crystal disease. The majority of joints can be aspirated under direct needle visualisation.

The hip is the most common joint requiring ultrasound-guided aspiration. On occasions this can be difficult in the adult as lower-frequency transducers are required to achieve the beam penetration necessary to visualise the hip. These transducers inherently have a lower spatial resolution; this combined with an oblique needle approach makes visualisation of the needle more difficult. From a diagnostic viewpoint this also makes differentiation between complex fluid and synovial or capsular thickening problematic with aspiration often the only diagnostic option. For more superficial joints if synovial or periarticular hyperaemia is present there is an increased risk of infection, which serves as a useful guide as to which joints require aspiration.

For superficial joints a 21-G needle or less usually suffices. For the hip, however, an 18- or 20-G needle should be used; if no effusion fluid is initially aspirated, there are possible manoeuvres to increase diagnostic yield. Injecting a small amount (2–3 ml) of nonbactericidal saline into the joint with reaspiration of the fluid for microbacteriological assessment can be performed. If there is difficulty with reaspirating this fluid from the joint then asking the patient to take the weight of the leg on the affected side increases the intra-articular pressure in the hip, allowing easier reaspiration.

This manoeuvre can also be of value during initial aspiration as effusions pool posterior, with increased intra-articular pressure redistributing any joint fluid present. Samples can then be sent for routine microbacteriological analysis either in dry sample pots or in blood culture medium.

Diagnostic and therapeutic injections

Ultrasound-guided intervention offers an extension to the diagnostic capabilities of musculoskeletal ultrasound. This is under-utilised at present and, if applied more widely either by clinicians or radiologists, would help develop a more measured objective approach to therapy. A diagnostic injection is one targeted at a specific anatomical site with or without ultrasound abnormality. The purpose of the injection is to determine whether the patient's symptoms arise from this area by the assessment of response to local anaesthetic. Therapeutic injections are similar to diagnostic injections but also contain glucocorticosteroid to give an anti-inflammatory effect. Certain steroids also inhibit fibroblasts (78) and have an action to decrease aberrant neuronal discharges (79, 80), which could be of specific value in entheseal disorders such as plantar fasciitis. In general it is best to think of long-acting corticosteroids as a form of long-acting analgesia that reduces patient symptoms though probably has little effect on outcome. The use of steroid injections basically translates to "inject conditions that would get better on their own but hurt while they do". An example of this is shoulder impingement, where it is difficult to rehabilitate patients in the acute

setting without adequate pain relief to allow effective physiotherapy.

In this type of case, injection of the subacromial bursa can be of value and it would be advisable to accompany the corticosteroid with a substantial volume of local anaesthetic to give a "washout" effect to the injection (Fig. 13.20). Injections around large weight-bearing tendons, such as the Achilles tendon or patellar tendon, should be avoided and only performed after extensive discussion of the risks and benefits with both the patient and the clinical team.

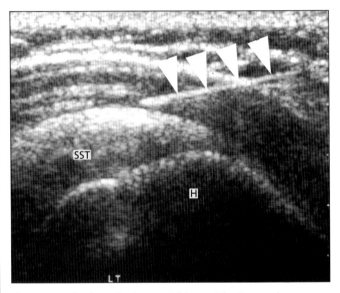

Fig. 13.20 Injection of subacromial bursa. The image shows a needle (arrowheads) being positioned in the subacromial bursa prior to injection. SST = supraspinatus tendon, H = humeral head.

VALIDATION, COMPETENCY AND TRAINING

Despite its many benefits, problem areas in the use of musculoskeletal ultrasound in rheumatology remain.

Validation studies, especially in terms of reproducibility, are required. However, the most contentious issue that remains between radiologists and rheumatologists is who performs ultrasound. In the authors' institution radiologists and rheumatologists practice musculoskeletal ultrasound together without any perceived conflict of interest. In our view, the main issue is one of training and assuring that the staff performing these examinations are competent and can be demonstrated to have undertaken appropriate training. In developing areas in the assessment of inflammatory arthropathies, such as ultrasound, it is quite reasonable for rheumatologists to develop and validate training schemes. Where techniques are already well established, for example more general musculoskeletal ultrasound of soft-tissue masses or shoulder disease, the practitioner should undertake training that conforms to the requirements of, or is agreed as appropriate by, the professional body of the sonologists already performing these studies.

REFERENCES

1. Wakefield RJ, Gibbon WW, Emery P. The current status of ultrasonography in rheumatology. Rheumatology (Oxford) 1999;38(3):195–8.
2. Wang SC, Chhem RK, Cardinal E, Cho KH. Joint sonography. Radiol Clin North Am 1999;37(4):653–68.
3. Lin J, Fessell DP, Jacobson JA, Weadock WJ, Hayes CW. An illustrated tutorial of musculoskeletal sonography: Part I, introduction and general principles. Am J Roentgenol 2000;175(3):637–45.
4. Manger B, Kalden JR. Joint and connective tissue ultrasonography—A rheumatologic bedside procedure? A German experience. Arthritis Rheum 1995;38(6):736–42.
5. Grassi W, Cervini C. Ultrasonography in rheumatology: An evolving technique. Ann Rheum Dis 1998;57(5):268–71.
6. Hau M, Schultz H, Tony HP, Keberle M, Jahns R, Haerten R, et al. Evaluation of pannus and vascularization of the metacarpophalangeal and proximal interphalangeal joints in rheumatoid arthritis by high-resolution ultrasound (multidimensional linear array). Arthritis Rheum 1999; 42(11):2303–8.
7. Newman JS, Laing TJ, McCarthy CJ, Adler RS. Power Doppler sonography of synovitis: assessment of therapeutic response— Preliminary observations. Radiology 1996;198(2):582–4.
8. Rubin JM. Musculoskeletal power Doppler. Eur Radiol 1999; 9(Suppl 3):S403–6.
9. Szkudlarek M, Court-Payen M, Strandberg C, Klarlund M, Klausen T, Ostergaard M. Power Doppler ultrasonography for assessment of synovitis in the metacarpophalangeal joints of patients with rheumatoid arthritis: A comparison with dynamic magnetic resonance imaging. Arthritis Rheum 2001;44(9):2018–23.
10. Backhaus M, Kamradt T, Sandrock D, Loreck D, Fritz J, Wolf KJ, et al. Arthritis of the finger joints: A comprehensive approach comparing conventional radiography, scintigraphy, ultrasound, and contrast-enhanced magnetic resonance imaging. Arthritis Rheum 1999;42(6):1232–45.
11. Koski JM, Anttila P, Hamalainen M, Isomaki H. Hip joint ultrasonography: Correlation with intra-articular effusion and synovitis. Br J Rheumatol 1990;29(3):189–92.
12. Conaghan PG, Wakefield R, O'Connor P, Gibbon W, Brown C, Emery P. The metacarpophalangeal joints in early arthritis: A comparison of clinical, radiographic, MRI and ultrasonographic findings. Ann Rheum Dis 1999;28(Suppl).
13. Ostergaard M, Court-Payen M, Gideon P, Wieslander S, Cortsen M, Lorenzen I, et al. Ultrasonography in arthritis of the knee. A comparison with MR imaging. Acta Radiol 1995;36(1): 19–26.
14. Rubaltelli L, Fiocco U, Cozzi L, Baldovin M, Rigon C, Bortoletto P, et al. Prospective sonographic and arthroscopic evaluation of proliferative knee joint synovitis. J Ultrasound Med 1994;13(11):855–62.
15. Wakefield RJ, Gibbon WW, Conaghan PG, O'Connor P, McGonagle D, Pease C, et al. The value of sonography in the detection of bone erosions in patients with rheumatoid arthritis: A comparison with conventional radiography. Arthritis Rheum 2000;43(12):2762–70.
16. Wakefield R, Gibbon W, O'Connor P, et al. High resolution ultrasound demonstrates synovitis in the majority of patients with knee osteoarthritis. Arthritis Rheum 1998;41(Suppl):S146.
17. Breidahl WH, Newman JS, Taljanovic MS, Adler RS. Power Doppler sonography in the assessment of musculoskeletal fluid collections. Am J Roentgenol 1996;166(6):1443–6.
18. Walther M, Harms H, Krenn V, Radke S, Faehndrich TP, Gohlke F. Correlation of power Doppler sonography with vascularity of the synovial tissue of the knee joint in patients with osteoarthritis and rheumatoid arthritis. Arthritis Rheum 2001;44(2):331–8.
19. Schmidt WA, Volker L, Zacher J, Schlafke M, Ruhnke M, Gromnica-Ihle E. Colour Doppler ultrasonography to detect pannus in knee joint synovitis. Clin Exp Rheumatol 2000; 18(4):439–44.
20. Qvistgaard E, Rogind H, Torp-Pedersen S, Terslev L, Danneskiold-Samsoe B, Bliddal H. Quantitative ultrasonography in rheumatoid arthritis: Evaluation of inflammation by Doppler technique. Ann Rheum Dis 2001; 60(7):690–3.
21. Carotti M, Salaffi F, Manganelli P, Salera D, Simonetti B, Grassi W. Power Doppler sonography in the assessment of synovial tissue of the knee joint in rheumatoid arthritis: A preliminary experience. Ann Rheum Dis 2002;61(10):877–82.
22. Stone M, Bergin D, Whelan B, Maher M, Murray J, McCarthy C. Power Doppler ultrasound assessment of rheumatoid hand synovitis. J Rheumatol 2001;28(9):1979–82.
23. Hau M, Kneitz C, Tony HP, Keberle M, Jahns R, Jenett M. High resolution ultrasound detects a decrease in pannus vascularisation of small finger joints in patients with rheumatoid arthritis receiving treatment with soluble tumour necrosis factor alpha receptor (etanercept). Ann Rheum Dis 2002;61(1):55–8.
24. Bude RO, Rubin JM. Power Doppler sonography. Radiology 1996;200(1):21–3.
25. Cardinal E, Lafortune M, Burns P. Power Doppler US in synovitis: Reality or artifact? Radiology 1996;200(3):868–9.
26. Grassi W, Filippucci E, Farina A, Salaffi F, Cervini C. Ultrasonography in the evaluation of bone erosions. Ann Rheum Dis 2001;60(2):98–103.
27. McGonagle D, Gibbon W, O'Connor P, Blythe D, Wakefield R, Green M, et al. A preliminary study of ultrasound aspiration of bone erosion in early rheumatoid arthritis. Rheumatology (Oxford) 1999;38(4):329–31.
28. Alasaarela E, Suramo I, Tervonen O, Lahde S, Takalo R, Hakala M. Evaluation of humeral head erosions in rheumatoid arthritis: A comparison of ultrasonography, magnetic resonance imaging, computed tomography and plain radiography. Br J Rheumatol 1998;37(11):1152–6.
29. Grassi W, Lamanna G, Farina A, Cervini C. Sonographic imaging of normal and osteoarthritic cartilage. Semin Arthritis Rheum 1999;28(6):398–403.
30. Iagnocco A, Coari G, Zoppini A. Sonographic evaluation of femoral condylar cartilage in osteoarthritis and rheumatoid arthritis. Scand J Rheumatol 1992;21(4):201–3.
31. Rutten MJ, Collins JM, van Kampen A, Jager GJ. Meniscal cysts: Detection with high-resolution sonography. Am J Roentgenol 1998;171(2):491–6.
32. Helbich TH, Breitenseher M, Trattnig S, Nehrer S, Erlacher L, Kainberger F. Sonomorphologic variants of popliteal cysts. J Clin Ultrasound 1998;26(3):171–6.
33. Bergin D, Keogh C, O'Connell M, Rowe D, Shah B, Zoga A, et al. Atraumatic medial collateral ligament oedema in medial compartment knee osteoarthritis. Skeletal Radiol 2002;31(1):14–8.

34. Coari G, Iagnocco A, Zoppini A. Chondrocalcinosis: Sonographic study of the knee. Clin Rheumatol 1995;14(5): 511–4.

35. Kellner H, Zoller W, Herzer P. Ultrasound findings in chondrocalcinosis. Z Rheumatol 1990;49(3):147–50.

36. Benjamin M, McGonagle D. The anatomical basis for disease localisation in seronegative spondyloarthropathy at entheses and related sites. J Anat 2001;199(Pt 5): 503–26.

37. Nipple GA, Sitaj S. Enthesopathy. Clin Rheum Dis 1979; 5:957–87.

38. Cardinal E, Chhem RK, Beauregard CG, Aubin B, Pelletier M. Plantar fasciitis: Sonographic evaluation. Radiology 1996;201(1): 257–9.

39. Gibbon WW, Long G. Ultrasound of the plantar aponeurosis (fascia). Skeletal Radiol 1999;28(1):21–6.

40. Fornage BD. Achilles tendon: US examination. Radiology 1986;159(3):759–64.

41. Davies SG, Baudouin CJ, King JB, Perry JD. Ultrasound, computed tomography and magnetic resonance imaging in patellar tendinitis. Clin Radiol 1991;43(1):52–6.

42. Olivieri I, Barozzi L, Favaro L, Pierro A, de Matteis M, Borghi C, et al. Dactylitis in patients with seronegative spondylarthropathy. Assessment by ultrasonography and magnetic resonance imaging. Arthritis Rheum 1996;39(9): 1524–8.

43. Kane D, Greaney T, Bresnihan B, Gibney R, FitzGerald O. Ultrasonography in the diagnosis and management of psoriatic dactylitis. J Rheumatol 1999;26(8):1746–51.

44. Wakefield RJ, Emery P, Veale D. Ultrasonography and psoriatic arthritis. J Rheumatol 2000;27(6):1564–5.

45. Fielding JR, Franklin PD, Kustan J. Popliteal cysts: A reassessment using magnetic resonance imaging. Skeletal Radiol 1991;20(6):433–5.

46. Janzen DL, Peterfy CG, Forbes JR, Tirman PF, Genant HK. Cystic lesions around the knee joint: MR imaging findings. Am J Roentgenol 1994;163(1):155–61.

47. Murphey MD, Gross TM, Rosenthal HG, Neff JR. Magnetic resonance imaging of soft tissue and cystic masses about the knee. Top Magn Reson Imaging 1993;5(4):263–82.

48. Morrison JL, Kaplan PA. Water on the knee: Cysts, bursae, and recesses. Magn Reson Imaging Clin N Am 2000;8(2): 349–70.

49. Burk DL, Jr, Dalinka MK, Kanal E, Schiebler ML, Cohen EK, Prorok RJ, et al. Meniscal and ganglion cysts of the knee: MR evaluation. Am J Roentgenol 1988;150(2):331–6.

50. Tasker AD, Ostlere SJ. Relative incidence and morphology of lateral and medial meniscal cysts detected by magnetic resonance imaging. Clin Radiol 1995;50(11):778–81.

51. Tirman PF, Feller JF, Janzen DL, Peterfy CG, Bergman AG. Association of glenoid labral cysts with labral tears and glenohumeral instability: Radiologic findings and clinical significance. Radiology 1994;190(3):653–8.

52. Tung GA, Entzian D, Stern JB, Green A. MR imaging and MR arthrography of paraglenoid labral cysts. Am J Roentgenol 2000;174(6):1707–15.

53. Schnarkowski P, Steinbach LS, Tirman PF, Peterfy CG, Genant HK. Magnetic resonance imaging of labral cysts of the hip. Skeletal Radiol 1996;25(8):733–7.

54. Taljanovic MS, Carlson KL, Kuhn JE, Jacobson JA, Delaney-Sathy LO, Adler RS. Sonography of the glenoid labrum: A cadaveric study with arthroscopic correlation. Am J Roentgenol 2000;174(6):1717–22.

55. Hammar MV, Wintzell GB, Astrom KG, Larsson S, Elvin A. Role of us in the preoperative evaluation of patients with anterior shoulder instability. Radiology 2001;219(1):29–34.

56. Robinson P, White LM, Lax M, Salonen D, Bell RS. Quadrilateral space syndrome caused by glenoid labral cyst. Am J Roentgenol 2000;175(4):1103–5.

57. Hashimoto BE, Hayes AS, Ager JD. Sonographic diagnosis and treatment of ganglion cysts causing suprascapular nerve entrapment. J Ultrasound Med 1994;13(9):671–4.

58. Beggs I. The ring sign: A new ultrasound sign of peripheral nerve tumours. Clin Radiol 1998;53(11):849–50.

59. Bouffard JA, Dhanju J. Ultrasonography of the knee. Semin Musculoskelet Radiol 1998;2(3):245–70.

60. Friedl W, Glaser F. Dynamic sonography in the diagnosis of ligament and meniscal injuries of the knee. Arch Orthop Trauma Surg 1991;110(3):132–8.

61. Martinoli C, Bianchi S, Giovagnorio F, Pugliese F. Ultrasound of the elbow. Skeletal Radiol 2001;30(11):605–14.

62. Sasaki J, Takahara M, Ogino T, Kashiwa H, Ishigaki D, Kanauchi Y. Ultrasonographic assessment of the ulnar collateral ligament and medial elbow laxity in college baseball players. J Bone Joint Surg Am 2002;84-A(4):525–31.

63. Hergan K, Mittler C. Sonography of the injured ulnar collateral ligament of the thumb. J Bone Joint Surg Br 1995;77(1):77–83.

64. Hoglund M, Tordai P, Muren C. Diagnosis by ultrasound of dislocated ulnar collateral ligament of the thumb. Acta Radiol 1995;36(6):620–5.

65. Jones MH, England SJ, Muwanga CL, Hildreth T. The use of ultrasound in the diagnosis of injuries of the ulnar collateral ligament of the thumb. J Hand Surg [Br] 2000;25(1):29–32.

66. Schnur DP, DeLone FX, McClellan RM, Bonavita J, Witham RS. Ultrasound: A powerful tool in the diagnosis of ulnar collateral ligament injuries of the thumb. Ann Plast Surg 2002;49(1): 19–22.

67. Fessell DP, van Holsbeeck M. Ultrasound of the foot and ankle. Semin Musculoskelet Radiol 1998;2(3):271–82.

68. Milz P, Milz S, Putz R, Reiser M. 13 MHz high-frequency sonography of the lateral ankle joint ligaments and the tibiofibular syndesmosis in anatomic specimens. J Ultrasound Med 1996;15(4):277–84.

69. Ptasznik R, Feller J, Bartlett J, Fitt G, Mitchell A, Hennessy O. The value of sonography in the diagnosis of traumatic rupture of the anterior cruciate ligament of the knee. Am J Roentgenol 1995;164(6):1461–3.

70. Skovgaard Larsen LP, Rasmussen OS. Diagnosis of acute rupture of the anterior cruciate ligament of the knee by sonography. Eur J Ultrasound 2000;12(2):163–7.

71. Miller TT. Sonography of injury of the posterior cruciate ligament of the knee. Skeletal Radiol 2002;31(3):149–54.

72. Pelsser V, Cardinal E, Hobden R, Aubin B, Lafortune M. Extraarticular snapping hip: Sonographic findings. Am J Roentgenol 2001;176(1):67–73.

73. Ptasznik R. Ultrasound in acute and chronic knee injury. Radiol Clin North Am 1999;37(4):797–830, x.

74. Bonaldi VM, Chhem RK, Drolet R, Garcia P, Gallix B, Sarazin L. Iliotibial band friction syndrome: Sonographic findings. J Ultrasound Med 1998;17(4):257–60.

75. Haslock I, MacFarlane D, Speed C. Intra-articular and soft tissue injections: A survey of current practice. Br J Rheumatol 1995;34(5):449–52.

76. Jones A, Regan M, Ledingham J, Pattrick M, Manhire A, Doherty M. Importance of placement of intra-articular steroid injections. BMJ 1993;307(6915):1329–30.

77. Eustace JA, Brophy DP, Gibney RP, Bresnihan B, FitzGerald O. Comparison of the accuracy of steroid placement with clinical outcome in patients with shoulder symptoms. Ann Rheum Dis 1997;56(1):59–63.

78. Aronow L. Effects of glucocorticoids on fibroblasts. Monogr Endocrinol 1979;12:327–40.

79. Devor M, Govrin-Lippmann R, Raber P. Corticosteroids suppress ectopic neural discharge originating in experimental neuromas. Pain 1985;22(2):127–37.

80. Pataky PE, Graham WP, 3rd, Munger BL. Terminal neuromas treated with triamcinolone acetonide. J Surg Res 1973;14(1): 36–45.

Doppler imaging in the musculoskeletal system

14

James L Teh

INTRODUCTION

> **Key point**
>
> Important roles of Doppler US in the musculoskeletal system are to differentiate between a solid lesion and a cyst, monitoring inflammatory disease progression and assess response to therapy and possibly help differentiate between benign and malignant soft-tissue masses.

Many pathological conditions affecting the musculoskeletal system result in alteration of regional blood flow. In these circumstances, Doppler ultrasound plays a crucial role in supporting and confirming the diagnosis. There are many diverse applications for Doppler ultrasound. The demonstration of blood flow within a low-echogenicity mass allows differentiation of a solid lesion from a cyst. Inflammatory and infective conditions are often associated with increased blood flow, and detection of these changes gives very useful additional information to the greyscale findings. More recently, the ability to detect small changes in blood flow has led to the use of Doppler imaging for monitoring disease progression and assessing response to therapy. There is also growing evidence that Doppler imaging may help differentiate benign from malignant soft-tissue masses. The field is rapidly evolving with the increasing availability of new techniques such as echo-contrast agents, blood flow quantification and harmonic imaging.

BASIC PHYSICS

The Doppler principle, first described in 1842 by the Austrian physicist Christian Doppler, is a wave theory that forms the basis of blood flow detection on ultrasound. There is a shift of frequency in a wave when a source moves relative to the receiver, which is commonly recognised as a drop in the pitch of a siren as an emergency vehicle approaches and passes by.

The relative change in the transmitted and received ultrasound frequency is called *Doppler shift* and is proportional to the velocity of the moving source,

$$\text{Doppler shift} = 2fv \cos \theta / c,$$

where f is the ultrasound frequency, v is the velocity of the blood, θ is the angle between beam and direction of blood flow and c is the velocity of ultrasound in tissue. The values for f and c are known and thus the velocity of the blood v can be calculated when the angle of insonation θ is taken into account.

Colour Doppler vs power Doppler

Colour Doppler provides information on blood flow across the entire real-time image by encoding the mean Doppler shift at a particular position in colour, and superimposing this upon the greyscale image. Power Doppler on the other hand displays the total integrated power in the Doppler signal in colour. There are three main problems that may arise from using colour Doppler for imaging the musculoskeletal system that are not encountered with power Doppler, these being background noise, aliasing and angle dependency (1).

Random noise

> **Key point**
>
> The most significant drawback of using colour Doppler is that random noise may appear as flow in any direction.

The most significant drawback of using colour Doppler is that random noise may appear as flow in any direction. This arises because noise has a random frequency shift, which the system interprets as flow. As the Doppler gain is turned up, noise increases, which results in filling up of the image background with random flow artefact. Ultimately, the detection of true flow becomes impossible (Fig. 14.1a). On power Doppler sonography, noise always has a uniformly low power. Therefore, when the Doppler gain is increased, the result is a uniformly coloured background rather than a random distribution of colours. Any real flow will therefore manifest as a much stronger signal than the background noise, and remain detectable (Fig. 14.1b). This allows a much greater sensitivity to flow compared to colour Doppler, increasing the dynamic range.

> **Key point**
>
> Power Doppler sonography allows a much greater sensitivity to flow compared to colour Doppler, increasing the dynamic range.

Aliasing

Aliasing is a phenomenon that occurs when an analogue signal is sampled at a frequency lower than half of its maximum frequency. When this occurs, all the frequencies above the half of the sampling frequency (the Nyquist frequency) are back-folded in the low-frequency region. In

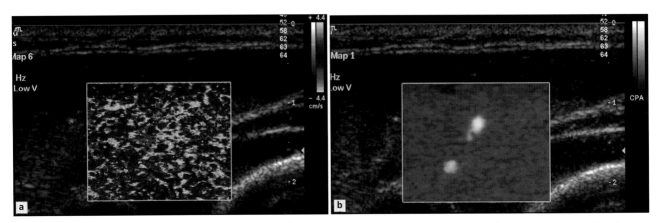

Fig. 14.1 Noise. (a) Transverse scan of the forearm demonstrating the effect of backgound noise on detection of flow with colour Doppler. (b) With power Doppler the background noise does not obscure true flow.

colour Doppler mode, aliasing may cause vessels to appear discontinuous. In addition, aliasing may distort direction and speed information. Power Doppler is free from aliasing, as the signal is calculated from the integral of the Doppler power spectrum. As a consequence, however, power Doppler does not display any information on direction and velocity.

Key point

Power Doppler is free from aliasing, as the signal is calculated from the integral of the Doppler power spectrum. As a consequence, however, power Doppler does not display any information on direction and velocity.

Angle dependency

Colour Doppler imaging is, by nature, angle-dependent. If the direction of flow is perpendicular to the angle of insonation, there is loss of Doppler signal. This may be partly counteracted by steering the beam to detect this flow, but because the beam cannot be continuously steered in all directions, regions of undetected flow invariably occur. Colour Doppler may therefore miss vessels if they course perpendicular to the ultrasound beam, resulting in an underestimation of vascularity. Furthermore, the colour Doppler signal alters according to the direction of flow, and if a vessel changes direction across the ultrasound field, it will change colour, which may result in difficulty tracking vessels. Unlike colour Doppler, power Doppler is relatively angle-independent. This is because power in a Doppler signal is related to the number of moving scatterers in a field, i.e. flowing red blood cells. If the angle of insonation is altered, their mean Doppler shift will change, but their power remains unaltered.

Power Doppler also allows better boundary detection and definition, and more accurate three-dimensional depiction of vascular anatomy. Compared to colour Doppler, the main disadvantage of power Doppler is its extreme sensitivity to motion. However, the development of motion suppression techniques, such as weighted temporal averaging, has largely

overcome this shortfall. With this technique, there is increased persistence of the displayed Doppler signal, which may lead to a slow response in the image or image lag (2).

Key point

Compared to colour Doppler, the main disadvantage of power Doppler is its extreme sensitivity to motion.

To summarise, colour Doppler, although well suited to evaluating high-velocity flow, is less effective in depicting low-velocity microvascular flow, and power Doppler, therefore, is the preferred method of Doppler evaluation of blood flow in most musculoskeletal conditions. Although information on the direction of flow is not provided, the increased sensitivity of power Doppler means that smaller vessels and slower flow can be demonstrated, allowing a more complete depiction of the vasculature.

Ultrasound contrast agents

The potential applications of ultrasound contrast agents in the musculoskeletal system are diverse, but at present, their use is not widespread. Currently, the best available ultrasound contrast agents are encapsulated microbubbles, which are bubbles measuring less than 7μm in diameter, that have been stabilised by an outer shell (3, 4). The small size of these bubbles allows unimpeded passage across the pulmonary circulation. Flowing within the bloodstream, microbubbles behave as active reflectors, oscillating within the ultrasound beam. They possess a natural resonant frequency at which they can absorb and scatter ultrasound very efficiently. When microbubbles are insonated at their resonant frequency, the oscillations produced become distorted, generating a "harmonic frequency". Combined with harmonic imaging, ultrasound contrast agents allow visualisation of blood flow, hitherto undetectable on standard Doppler sonography (4). With harmonic imaging, the ultrasound probe emits at the fundamental frequency and receives at the second harmonic frequency, which is twice the value of the fundamental frequency. As soft tissue produces only a negligible harmonic effect, the predominant signal produced is by the flowing contrast agent—leading to substantial enhancement of flow signal.

> **Practical tip**
>
> Combined with harmonic imaging, ultrasound contrast agents allow visualisation of blood flow, hitherto undetectable on standard Doppler sonography.

DOPPLER ULTRASOUND SETTINGS

All modern ultrasound machines have preset profiles that optimise imaging parameters, according to the region being scanned. It is important, however, to understand how the various settings may alter the image, as the parameters may need to be customised.

Doppler gain

With musculoskeletal imaging, the Doppler gain threshold should be set such that there is no signal seen within bone (5). This is because the bone surface is a strong specular reflector and spurious Doppler signal may occur at the cortical–soft-tissue interface. This is different from other anatomical areas where the gain is usually set to just above the noise floor level.

> **Practical tip**
>
> Doppler gain threshold should be set such that there is no signal seen within bone.

Doppler filter level

The Doppler filter reduces the amount of background noise, allowing a cleaner signal to be obtained. If the filter is set too high, then slow flow in a vessel may be missed. In practice, filtration should initially be set at the lowest possible level and then increased gradually to obtain the optimal image.

> **Practical tip**
>
> Doppler filtration should initially be set at the lowest possible level and then increased gradually to obtain the optimal image.

Colour persistence

Persistence refers to the amount of frame-averaging that occurs in obtaining an image. A high level of persistence results in the summation of several frames, leading to a high signal-to-noise ratio, at the expense of an impaired response rate, with less information obtained on pulsatile flow. Conversely, a low persistence results in a rapid response rate, but a poor signal-to-noise ratio.

Velocity scale setting

In colour Doppler imaging, the velocity scale setting is directly related to the pulse repetition frequency, or sampling frequency. If the scale is set too low this will result in aliasing. If the scale is set too high, the result will be poor colour sensitivity at slower velocity flow.

Sample volume

The sample box size determines the volume of tissue from which information is obtained. A large sample volume will result in a decrease in the pulse repetition frequency, which in turn increases motion sensitivity. Although it may be useful to include adjacent areas of normal tissue to demonstrate the differences in blood flow, as a rule, the sample box size should be kept as small as possible.

> **Practical tip**
>
> The sample box size with power Doppler imaging should be kept as small as possible.

DOPPLER ULTRASOUND TECHNIQUE AND PRACTICAL TIPS

An ultrasound examination of a musculoskeletal organ should ideally include Doppler interrogation. This will allow regional blood flow to be evaluated, which may help to confirm or refute a suspected diagnosis. In addition, the routine use of Doppler allows familiarisation with normality, which is crucial to recognising abnormal findings. A linear array transducer, operating at a minimum of 7MHz, is essential to obtain optimal scan quality.

Transducer pressure

As most musculoskeletal structures are superficial, it is crucial to only exert a minimum amount of transducer pressure when examining patients. If the soft tissues are compressed, the vascular structures will become compromised, leading to an underestimation of blood flow. A jelly stand-off is a simple and effective method for ensuring that only minimum transducer pressure is applied (Fig. 14.2).

> **Practical tip**
>
> As most musculoskeletal structures are superficial, it is crucial to only exert a minimum amount of transducer pressure when examining patients with Doppler ultrasound.

Examine structures in a relaxed state

If a tendon or muscle is examined in a state of contraction or tension, abnormal blood flow will be underestimated due to compression of vessels. For example, the patellar tendon should ideally

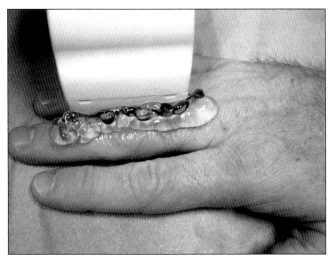

Fig. 14.2 Jelly stand-off. The use of copious amounts of ultrasound gel ensures that excessive pressure is not exerted, whilst maintaining good contact.

be scanned with the knee extended rather than flexed.

Angle of insonation

The angle of insonation is of particular importance when examining in colour Doppler. Ideally, to ensure an accurate representation of blood flow, the angle of insonation should be less than 60°. This may be achieved by angling the probe or the sample box. If it is not possible to obtain an appropriate angle, power Doppler should be employed.

> **Practical tip**
>
> Ideally, to ensure an accurate representation of blood flow with Doppler ultrasound, the angle of insonation should be less than 60°.

Dynamic localisation

Doppler sonography is extremely sensitive to motion artefact. This may be used to one's advantage in the dynamic localisation of certain structures, such as the median nerve. Flexing and extending the fingers results in motion artefact in the flexor tendons but not the median nerve, which may help in differentiating the structures (Figs 14.3a and 14.3b).

Ambient temperature

There is evidence that the ambient temperature may affect regional blood flow (6). Therefore, particular care should be taken to ensure that ambient temperatures remain relatively constant if serial investigations are planned. If the area to be scanned is an extremity, such as the hand, it may help to use a temperature-controlled water bath.

Comparison with normal

Often it is difficult to be certain whether blood flow demonstrated on Doppler sonography is pathological. If the contralateral limb is asymptomatic, then a direct comparison is invaluable.

Spectral Doppler trace

The use of a spectral Doppler trace may allow confirmation that the colour or power Doppler

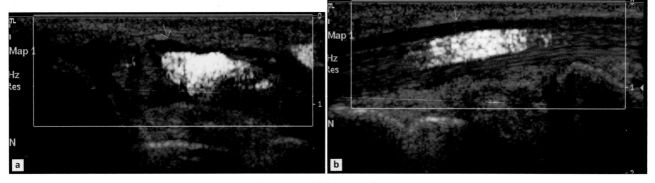

Fig. 14.3 Dynamic localisation of the median nerve. (a) Axial and (b) longitudinal images at the wrist. Flexion and extension of the fingers results in motion artefact in the flexor tendons, but not in the median nerve, allowing localisation of the median nerve at the wrist.

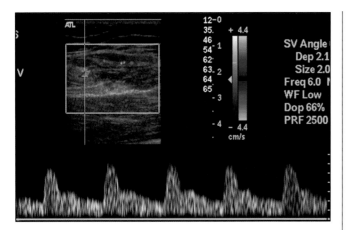

Fig. 14.4 Spectral Doppler trace. The spectral Doppler trace confirms that the power Doppler signal obtained in this vascular soft-tissue mass (biopsy proven haemangioma) has a phasic waveform, and therefore represents true flow.

signal is not artefactual, as a phasic waveform should be obtained (Fig. 14.4). The routine acquisition of spectral Doppler traces, however, adds little further information in most circumstances.

CLINICAL APPLICATIONS

Distinguishing solid from fluid-containing structures

Cysts or fluid-containing structures or lesions typically appear anechoic, with posterior acoustic enhancement. On dynamic assessment, compressibility may be a feature. However, the differentiation between a low-echogenicity solid mass and an echogenic fluid collection may be difficult using only greyscale

sonography. In these situations, the presence of internal blood flow on Doppler imaging may allow rapid confirmation of a solid lesion (7). Similarly, synovial hypertrophy may demonstrate a blood flow on Doppler interrogation, allowing differentiation from synovial fluid (8).

Assessment of increased blood flow in musculoskeletal disorders

Greyscale ultrasound with high-resolution linear array transducers provide excellent structural detail of musculoskeletal structures such as tendons and muscles, but despite this, there are limitations in evaluating inflammatory conditions, tendinopathy and tumours. The use of Doppler adds a more functional and dynamic assessment of disease activity often confirming the diagnosis, and allowing assessment of therapeutic response.

Interpretation of increased blood flow

Increased local blood flow may be depicted by power Doppler sonography in a variety of musculoskeletal conditions (9). This increased flow has been variously attributed to increased vascularity, increased perfusion or hyperaemia (9, 10). These phenomena are undoubtedly related—increased vascularity (i.e. more vessels) may lead to increased perfusion of a structure and thus to hyperaemia. There may, however, be situations in which there is increased blood flow coursing through the same number of vessels—in which case there may be increased perfusion and hyperaemia without increased vascularity. Strictly speaking, therefore, these terms are not directly interchangeable.

Injured soft tissues undergo repair through a complex series of events that involve both physical and chemical processes. These processes are currently undergoing extensive investigation as efforts are directed towards achieving accelerated wound healing (11). There are three main phases of wound healing (12). The *inflammatory* phase is characterised by platelet accumulation, coagulation and leucocyte migration. The *proliferative* phase comprises re-epithelialisation, angiogenesis, fibrous proliferation and wound contraction. Finally, the *remodelling* phase occurs over several months, during which the dermis responds to injury with the production of collagen and matrix proteins and then returns to its preinjury phenotype. Increased blood flow on Doppler sonography following acute muscle or tendon injury should therefore be recognised as a normal healing response (Figs 14.5a and 14.5b).

Tendon pathology

In patents with tendinosis, the thickened abnormal tendon has been shown to correspond to tenocyte hyperplasia and prominent angiogenesis with endothelial hyperplasia (13). There is associated loss of the normal collagen architecture with microtears and separation of the collagen fibres. These degenerative, angiofibroblastic changes are the result of chronic repetitive microtrauma and may be exquisitely demonstrated by ultrasound as ill-defined areas of low echogenicity. Doppler interrogation has a useful role in the ultrasound examination as it has been suggested that neovascularisation may help distinguish acute from chronic tendinosis (14) and may be related to the pathogenesis of pain (15) (Figs 14.6a and 14.6b). In support of this latter hypothesis, it has been shown that sclerosing the neovessels in painful Achilles tendinosis may result in significant alleviation of symptoms (16). Furthermore, increased blood flow seen on Doppler sonography in calcific tendinopathy affecting the rotator cuff has been shown to correlate well with the painful resorptive phase of the calcification (17).

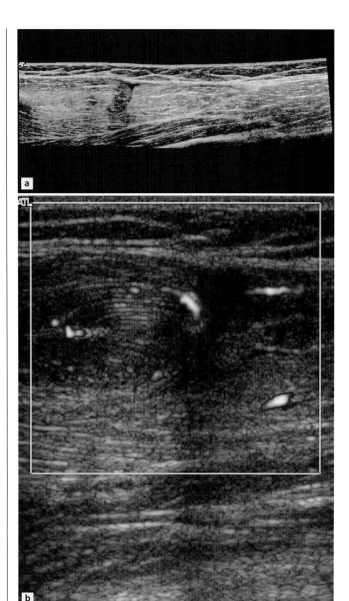

Fig. 14.5 Rectus femoris rupture. (a) Longitudinal extended field-of-view image of the rectus femoris demonstrating a full thickness rupture. (b) Power Doppler demonstrates increased local blood flow as part of the reparative process.

Key point

Doppler interrogation has a useful role in the ultrasound examination as it has been suggested that neovascularisation may help distinguish acute from chronic tendinosis and may be related to the pathogenesis of pain.

Tenosynovitis is characterised by low-echogenicity thickening of the synovial sheath, which may either be due to synovial hypertrophy or fluid. The tendon itself may demonstrate normal morphology or appear thickened or hypoechoic. For patients with symptomatic

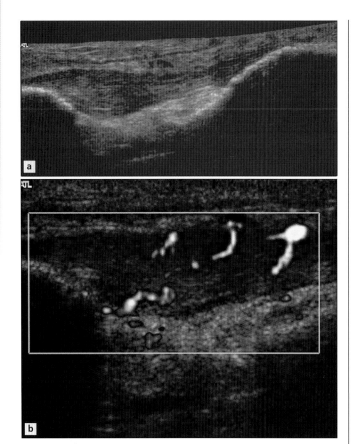

Fig. 14.6 Patellar tendinopathy. (a) Longitudinal extended field-of-view image demonstrating proximal thickening of the patellar tendon. (b) Power Doppler demonstrates florid neovascularity, indicating a chronic process.

tenosynovitis, it has been shown that a significant proportion of the hypoechoic rim represents vascularised synovium rather than complex fluid, using power Doppler (8) (Figs 14.7a and 14.7b).

Cellulitis

On ultrasound, cellulitis is characterised by thickening and induration of the skin and subcutaneous tissues (18). There may be loss of architecture of the subcutaneous fat, with oedema leading to increased echogenicity and poor ultrasound penetration of the tissues. Associated abscess formation may occur. Doppler interrogation may reveal increased blood flow in the affected areas, and thus allow differentiation of inflammatory (i.e. infective) from other noninflammatory causes of oedema such as fluid overload (Figs 14.8a and 14.8b).

Reflex sympathetic dystrophy is a potentially disabling syndrome of pain, hyperaesthesia and vasomotor disturbance, usually occurring in the lower limb following trauma. Eventually it may lead to muscle atrophy, trophic skin changes and bone and joint abnormalities. Skin thickening or thinning and soft-tissue oedema has been described on MRI (19). Using power Doppler, increased flow in the skin and subcutaneous

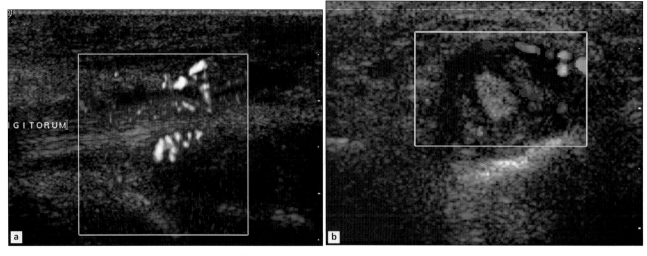

Fig. 14.7 Tenosynovitis. (a) Longitudinal image of flexor digitorum longus demonstrating synovial thickening and increased power Doppler signal indicating tenosynovitis. (b) Axial image with colour Doppler demonstrates that a significant portion of the low-echogenicity rim surrounding the tendon is vascularised synovium.

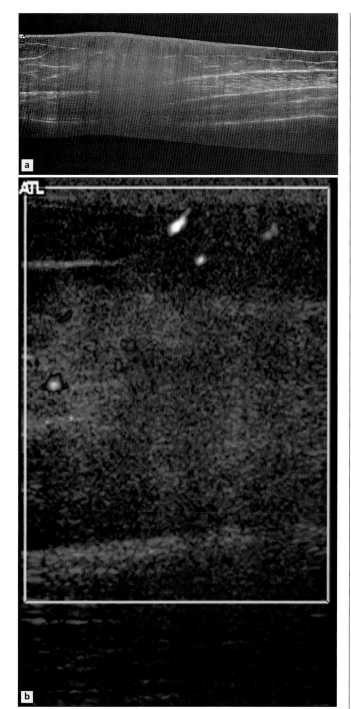

Fig. 14.8 Cellulitis. (a) Longitudinal extended field-of-view image of the anterior thigh demonstrating cellulitis, with oedema and loss of normal architecture of the subcutaneous fat. (b) Power Doppler demonstrates increased local blood flow, indicating an inflammatory process.

tissues of patients with reflex sympathetic dystrophy has been described (20).

Muscle inflammation

There are many conditions that may lead to myositis, including autoimmune diseases, infections, vasculitidies, trauma and paraneoplastic disease. The inflammatory changes result in diffuse swelling and oedema, with loss of the normal pennate structure of the muscle fibres with increased blood flow on Doppler imaging (Figs 14.9a–14.9c). The ultrasound appearances, however, are usually nonspecific and biopsy is usually required for diagnosis. In these circumstances, Doppler imaging may be useful for guiding biopsy to areas of active inflammation.

Traumatic myositis ossificans occurs following muscle contusion (21). There is usually a well-defined sequence of events: initially, in the first week following trauma, periosteal new bone formation occurs in association with a soft-tissue mass. Over the next 2–6 weeks, there is progressive calcification starting in the periphery, which eventually matures into ossification over the following 6 months or so. Eventually, rather bizarre new bone formation may develop. The lesion may diminish in size and occasionally resorb. The ultrasound features of myositis ossificans depend on the stage at which imaging has occurred. Often ultrasound is performed in the initial inflammatory phase, when calcification and early ossification is developing. During this period, there is muscle oedema in association with echogenic foci, indicating ossification, with evidence of neovascularity on Doppler ultrasound (22) (Figs 14.10a–14.10c). When the lesion is mature, there is usually no increased Doppler flow.

Distinguishing inflammatory from noninflammatory collections

Greyscale sonography is neither sensitive nor specific for characterising inflammatory collections. Doppler sonography, however, may allow demonstration of increased blood flow to

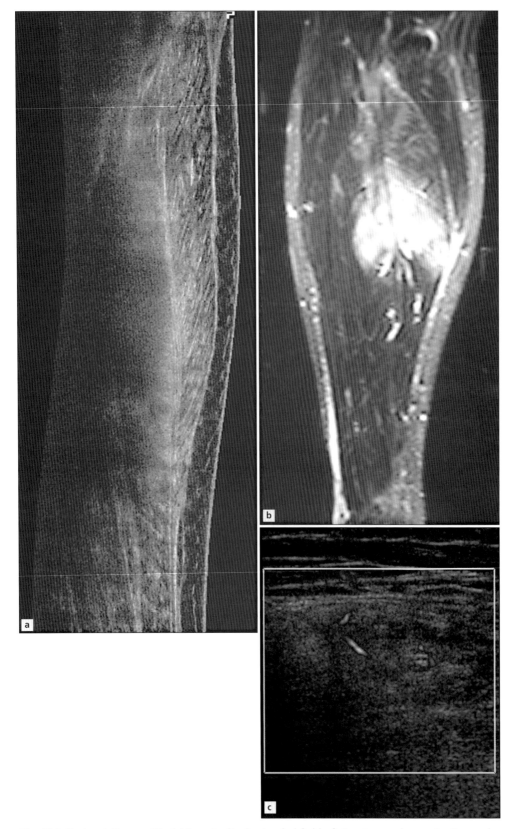

Fig. 14.9 Eosinophilic myositis. (a) Longitudinal extended field-of-view image demonstrating oedema and loss of normal architecture in the soleus muscle. (b) Corresponding STIR sequence on MRI showing oedema in the soleus. (c) Axial scan of the soleus demonstrates increased flow on power Doppler, indicating an inflammatory process.

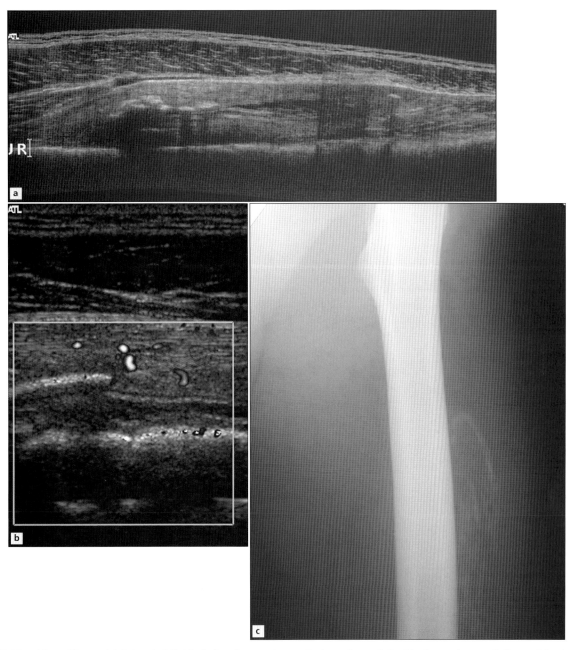

Fig. 14.10 Myositis ossificans. (a) Extended field-of-view image demonstrates echogenic foci in the vastus medialis consistent with ossification. (b) Adjacent to the ossification there is increased flow on power Doppler indicating the inflammatory phase of the process. (c) Plain radiograph confirms the presence of ossification in the soft tissues.

the inflammatory tissue surrounding collections (Fig. 14.11). Chronic, walled-off abscesses and tuberculous cold abscesses, however, may not demonstrate increased flow in the adjacent soft tissues (Figs 14.12a and 14.12b). Breidhal *et al.* (21) examined 39 patients with joint effusions or collections and found that power Doppler sonography could help distinguish inflammatory fluid collections from those that are non-inflammatory. All inflammatory collections were graded as either having moderate or marked hyperaemia in the adjacent soft tissues, whereas all noninflammatory conditions had no evidence of hyperaemia. Power Doppler was unable to differentiate between inflammatory collections of infective and noninfective origin.

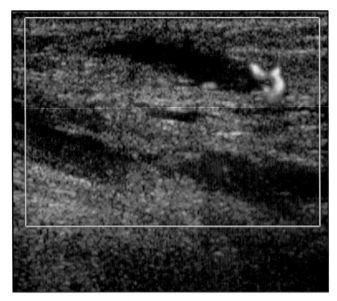

Fig. 14.11 Infected collection. There is increased blood flow on power Doppler in the adjacent tissues surrounding this infected collection in the forearm, indicating adjacent cellulitis.

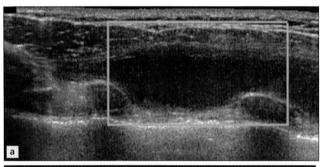

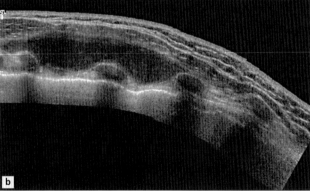

Fig. 14.12 Tuberculous cold abscess. (a) A low-echogenicity collection in the chest wall with no demonstrable flow in the surrounding tissues, in a patient who subsequently had thick pus aspirated. (b) Extended field-of-view image demonstrating the extent of the chest wall collection.

Synovitis

Synovitis may be encountered in patients with infective or inflammatory arthropathies. On greyscale sonography there is low-echogenicity material within the joint, which may indicate fluid or synovial thickening, or components of both of these. Although Doppler imaging is useful for confirmation of inflammatory change, it is unhelpful in differentiating between infective and noninfective conditions (22), as the appearances may be identical. Furthermore, when a joint effusion is present, the lack of increased periarticular flow on power Doppler does not exclude septic arthritis, and should not therefore preclude aspiration (Figs 14.13 and 14.14).

Early detection of inflammatory athropathy

For patients with inflammatory arthropathy, assessment of disease activity and therapeutic response has predominantly relied on clinical assessment and serum markers of inflammation. Plain radiography, although sensitive for established erosions, gives little information on synovial inflammation and early erosions. Greyscale sonography allows demonstration of effusions, synovial hypertrophy and erosions before any abnormal plain radiographic features are manifest. Combined with greyscale sonography, power Doppler imaging now plays an important role in the detection of early synovitis (23–25). In rheumatoid arthritis (RA), angiogenesis is recognised as the key event in the production of pannus, which is associated with the erosive phase of the disease (26). The detection of vascular pannus therefore has an important role in determining whether disease-modifying drugs should be introduced (Fig. 14.15a).

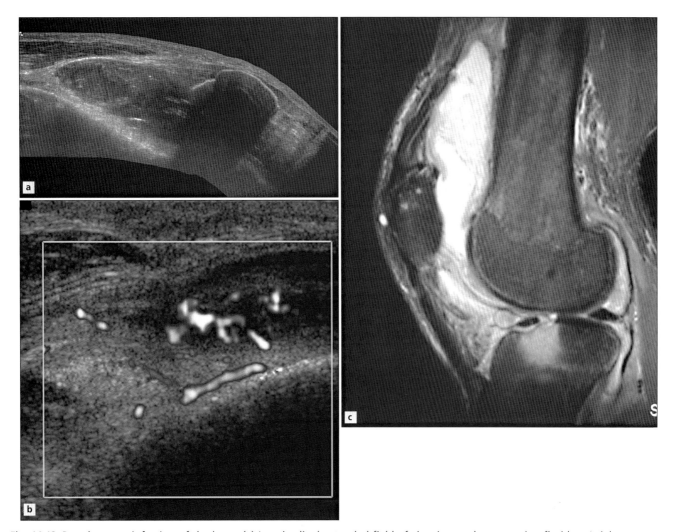

Fig. 14.13 Pseudomonas infection of the knee. (a) Longitudinal extended field-of-view image demonstrating florid synovial hypertrophy in the suprapatellar pouch. (b) Marked increased flow on power Doppler, confriming the inflammatory nature of the infected synovitis. There is no significant joint effusion. (c) Sagittal STIR image confirming the presence of florid synovitis.

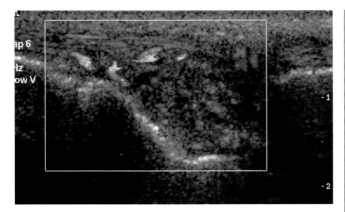

Fig. 14.14 Inflammatory synovitis of the wrist in rheumatoid arthritis. There is marked synovial hypertrophy at the carpus with increased flow on colour Doppler.

Backhaus *et al.* (23) prospectively examined 60 patients with inflammatory arthropathy and found that clinical evaluation, scintigraphy, MRI and ultrasound were each more sensitive than conventional radiography in detecting inflammatory soft-tissue lesions, as well as destructive joint processes in arthritis. In this study, ultrasound was found to be even more sensitive than MRI in the detection of synovitis.

The degree of blood flow demonstrated in pannus or synovial hypertrophy in established disease may allow some indication of activity (25), with active disease showing greater flow than inactive disease.

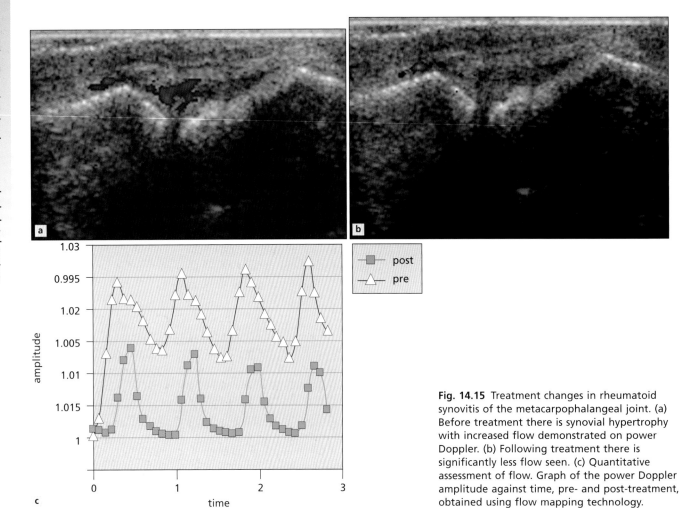

Fig. 14.15 Treatment changes in rheumatoid synovitis of the metacarpophalangeal joint. (a) Before treatment there is synovial hypertrophy with increased flow demonstrated on power Doppler. (b) Following treatment there is significantly less flow seen. (c) Quantitative assessment of flow. Graph of the power Doppler amplitude against time, pre- and post-treatment, obtained using flow mapping technology.

Several investigators (27–29) have used contrast agents to assess synovial blood flow in patients with inflammatory athropathy. For patients with rheumatoid arthritis it has been found that the use of a microbubble ultrasound contrast agent significantly improved the detection of intra-articular blood flow to finger joints, allowing earlier detection of synovitis (29). Further research, however, is required to determine whether this improved detection of microvascular flow in these patients is of clinical importance.

There are potential advantages of MRI over ultrasound for evaluating early synovitis, in that it may cover a wider area in a single field of view and thus cover several joints in the hands relatively quickly in a single examination. Assessment of disease activity using MRI, however, relies on measurement of synovial volume and rates of synovial enhancement, rather than direct assessment of blood flow. Nevertheless, a close relationship exists between presence of vascular flow seen on power Doppler and the rate of early synovial enhancement on dynamic contrast-

enhanced MRI (30). There is also good concordance between contrast-enhanced power Doppler sonography and contrast-enhanced MRI in demonstrating synovitis (27). Ultimately, the technique chosen should reflect local expertise.

Monitoring therapeutic response

The ability to monitor therapeutic response is crucial in evaluating the effectiveness of different treatment regimens. Traditionally, clinicians have relied on clinical examination, self-assessment questionnaires and serological markers of inflammation such as the C-reactive protein. Newman *et al.* (10) used power Doppler sonography to examine symptomatic knees in patients with inflammatory arthritis, before and after joint aspiration, and intra-articular steroid administration. A qualitative decrease in synovial perfusion was observed in all knees, corresponding to symptomatic improvement. Other workers (31) have shown a subjective reduction in power Doppler signal in the metacarpophalangeal joints of patients with rheumatoid arthritis who were treated by systemic steroid therapy.

Software that allows colour pixels representing power Doppler signal to be separated from the background grey pixels—a process termed "flow mapping" has now been developed allowing objective quantification of Doppler signal. By pixel counting and equating the intensity of each color pixel to a value the quantity of Doppler signal can be measured. The value of this technique is that it may allow simple longitudinal studies on regional blood flow to be performed, as long as all the imaging parameters remain constant (Figs 14.15b and 14.15c). Using this method, a therapeutic response to systemic steroid therapy has been shown in patients with rheomatoid arthritis (33). Various flow mapping techniques have been described using both intrinsic software supplied with the ultrasound equipment, or exporting the captured colour images to desktop imaging software with pixel count and histogram facilities. The particular disadvantage of these methods, is that the are dependent not only on the particulat ultrasound machine used, but also on the version of software currently supplied with that machine. Comparisons between different ultrasound machines is difficult which makes it difficult to compare results from different centres. Software upgrades can affect colour sensitivity and alter colour maps which makes longitudinal studies challenging. The search for a more sustainable and comparable reading has focussed on the resistive index (RI) as a more reliable measurement. This has the advantage of being more robust, reproducible and less machine-dependent but requires a good strong spectral trace to measure from, and this is not always apparent in very small synovial vessels, particularly in older machines.

Tumour assessment

Ultrasound is often the first imaging modality used in the investigation of musculoskeletal soft-tissue masses. It provides a rapid and inexpensive means of confirming the presence of a lesion, and provides information on the site, size and morphology. Despite this numerous studies have shown that greyscale ultrasound is unable to distinguish between benign and malignant lesions (34–36). Magnetic resonance imaging can provide useful information on morphology, signal characteristics, pattern of contrast enhancement and local staging, but is also unable to differentiate between benign and malignant lesions with high accuracy (37).

Certain benign lesions may have characteristic appearances on combined greyscale and Doppler sonography. Superficial lipomas are readily recognised (35) and usually do not require further investigations. Glomus tumours are typically located in a subungual position or in the pulp of the finger (40). These are small, exquisitely tender lesions that arise from the neuromyoarterial glomus, an organ that controls temperature, and are classically highly vascular on Doppler interrogation (Figs 14.16a and 14.16b).

Soft-tissue vascular anomalies may broadly be classified into two distinct categories, benign neoplasms and vascular malformations (38). These lesions have different biologic and clinical behaviour and therapeutic requirements but they are often confused (39). Haemangiomas are benign neoplasms that proliferate rapidly in infancy only to involute in early childhood. Capillary and cavernous haemangiomas have been the terms classically used for the most common variants of benign vascular neoplasms, but they may not be the most appropriate

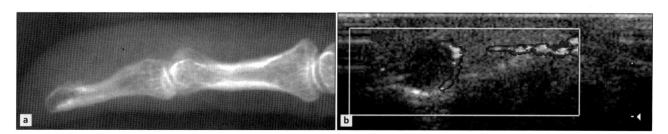

Fig. 14.16 Glomus tumour. (a) Plain radiograph of the index finger demonstrating bony erosion of the volar aspect of the distal phalanx. (b) A small rounded mass in the pulp of the finger with erosion of the underlying bone is demonstrated. Colour Doppler reveals a vascular lesion.

descriptions for these lesions (40). Many so-called cavernous haemangiomas are in fact not true neoplasms but represent vascular malformations. Haemangiomas may have a variable appearance both macroscopically and microscopically, and may demonstrate no flow on Doppler sonography (41). Typically, the cavernous type (Figs 14.17a and 14.17b) is composed of large, thin-walled, dilated vessels lined by flattened endothelial cells, whereas the capillary type is nonvascular and spongy in appearance (Fig. 14.18).

Vascular malformations are always present at birth, and their growth is commensurate with the patient's, never involute and are not tumours. They instead represent vessel anomalies due to errors of vascular morphogenesis. They are derived from embryonal capillary, venous, arterial or lymphatic channels, or combinations

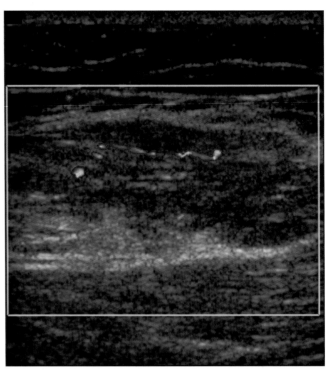

Fig. 14.18 Capillary haemangioma. An intramuscular heterogeneous mass in the upper thigh with minor flow on Doppler interrogation, shown on biopsy to be a capillary haemangioma.

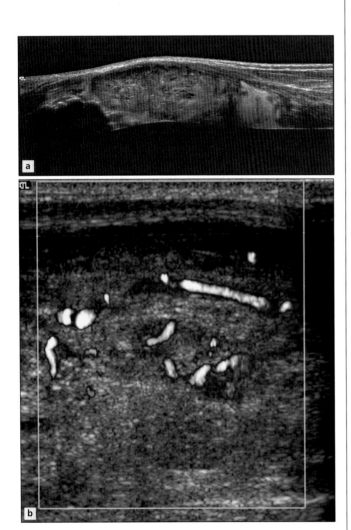

Fig. 14.17 Cavernous haemangioma. (a) Extended field-of-view image of the forearm demonstrating a predominantly solid heterogeneous mass. (b) On power Doppler the lesion is shown to be highly vascular, indicating a cavernous haemangioma.

of these (42). Paltiel *et al*. found that the most significant distinguishing feature between haemangiomas and vascular malformations is the presence of a solid soft-tissue mass (41). In this study vessel density and mean arterial peak velocity were comparable for haemangiomas and arteriovenous malformations (AVMs). Mean venous peak velocity was significantly higher for AVMs than for other vascular malformations and haemangiomas.

Benign versus malignant lesions

Histologically, the vessels in malignant lesions are characterised by a lack of a muscle layer and an irregular margin. The vessels often demonstrate an "anarchic pattern" with calibre changes, occlusions, stenoses and arteriovenous shunts and loops (43). These appearances may be visualised by angiography and sonography. Not all malignant soft-tissue tumours have an anarchic pattern, however (Figs 14.19a–14.19c).

Several researchers have attempted to define ultrasound criteria for malignant neovascularity with varying success. The morphologic analysis of tumour vessels appears to be more reliable

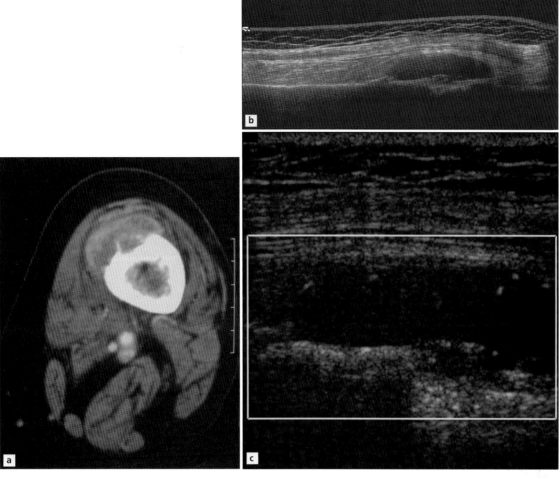

Fig. 14.19 Periosteal metastasis from adenocarcinoma. (a) Axial CT scan demonstrating a "cookie-bite" lesion of the lower femur. (b) Extended field-of-view image demonstrates a low-echogenicity mass involving the periosteum. (c) Power Doppler reveals homogeneous neovascularity throughout the lesion.

than quantitative parameters such as flow velocities or resistive indices (44, 45). Recent research suggests that by using a combination of colour and power Doppler and spectral wave analysis, evaluation of tumour vascular architecture may enable differentiation of benign from malignant lesions (46). This study, however, only included lesions that exhibited at least five vessels. The major characteristics for malignancy were found to be a combination of occlusions, stenoses, vascular pattern and trifurcations. Trifurcations were defined when three vessels branched out from the same point of the original vessel. Loops and shunts, leading to abnormal resistive indices were described as minor characteristics, and were thought to be less accurate for malignancy as these features are also present in arteriovenous malformations. Combining any two of the major characteristics struck the best compromise with respect to

achieving the highest sensitivity and specificity (Figs 14.20a and 14.20b).

> **Key point**
>
> A combination of colour and power Doppler and spectral wave analysis in the evaluation of tumour vascular architecture may enable differentiation between benign and malignant lesions. The major characteristics for malignancy are a combination of occlusions, stenoses and trifurcations.

Although there is a growing body of evidence that meticulous Doppler examination may help differentiate benign from malignant lesions, in practice, a cautious approach to ultrasound diagnosis should be taken. It should be recognised that necrotic lesions and low-grade

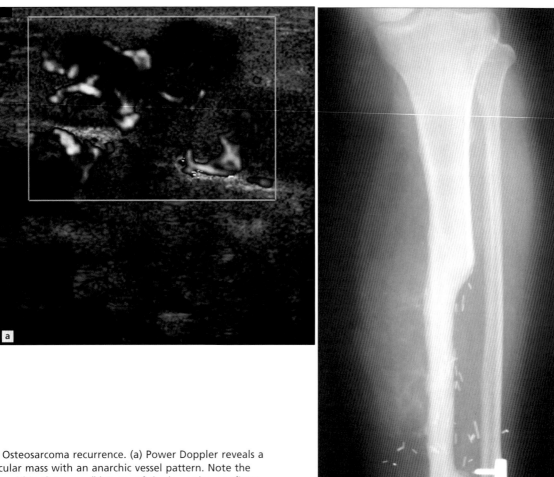

Fig. 14.20 Osteosarcoma recurrence. (a) Power Doppler reveals a highly vascular mass with an anarchic vessel pattern. Note the ossification within the mass. (b) X-ray of the lower leg confirms the presence of a recurrent osteosarcoma.

neoplasms may not demonstrate neovascularity, and therefore, the absence of flow does not necessarily indicate benignity. Ultimately, ultrasound is unable to provide a histological diagnosis, which can only be obtained by biopsy.

Monitoring tumour regression

For patients with osteosarcoma or Ewing's sarcoma, the clinical outcome can be predicted by the histological response to adjuvant chemotherapy, as determined at the time of surgery. Those patients that respond poorly may benefit from a change of chemotherapy regimen, or early surgery to reduce the risk of metastasis. Van der Woude et al. (47) used colour Doppler sonography to assess intratumoural blood flow in the extraosseous component of patients with either osteosarcoma or Ewing's sarcoma, before, during and after chemotherapy. They found that the resistive indices in arteries that fed tumours

were significantly lower than in the contralateral normal arteries. After chemotherapy, persistent intratumoural flow corresponded to poor histological response. In practical terms, if after chemotherapy there is less vascularity in a lesion, and the resistive index of the feeding vessel decreases, tumour necrosis can be assumed. It may be difficult to ensure exact probe repositioning for follow-up studies, but if examinations are performed by a single operator, and landmarks are used scrupulously, this may be overcome.

MISCELLANEOUS APPLICATIONS OF DOPPLER SONOGRAPHY

Neonatal femoral head blood flow

Avascular necrosis is an iatrogenic complication of placing a child in a hip spika for treatment of developmental dysplasia of the hip. This is thought to arise from vascular compromise of the femoral head when the hip is abducted. Intrinsic blood flow to the unossified neonatal femoral head has been demonstrated by power Doppler (48). At between 60° to 85° of abduction, flow became undetectable in 11 of 13 neonates, and reappeared during adduction. Power Doppler may therefore help to identify neonates at risk of avascular necrosis from abduction hip restraints.

Muscle blood flow changes with exercise

Power Doppler sonography has been used to evaluate exercise-induced changes in muscle blood flow, by comparing ultrasound scans of the biceps muscle performed before and after a standardised exercise protocol (49). With exercise there was a marked increase in intramuscular vessel conspicuity, in addition to increases in fractional blood volume estimates. The effectiveness of an exercise regimen might therefore be evaluated using this method. There are implications that Doppler sonography may be useful for assessing exercise-induced compartment syndrome.

Digital arteries in Raynaud's phenomenon

Doppler sonography has been used to assess the digital arteries in Raynaud's phenomenon, a disorder characterised by vasospasm of the arteries. During an attack of Raynaud's, the skin first turns white then blue. As the arteries relax the skin then turns red. Primary Raynaud's is of unknown aetiology, whereas secondary Raynaud's occurs as a result of an underlying factor such as smoking or connective tissue disease. The diagnosis of Raynaud's is essentially clinical, and the use of ultrasound is reserved for cases where there is uncertainty. Compared to healthy subjects, patients with Raynaud's have been found to have significantly higher resistive and pulsatility indices, but lower peak systolic and end-diastolic velocities, indicating stenoses (50). Nail bed vascularity at ambient temperature has been shown to differ between healthy subjects and patients with Raynaud's (6).

REFERENCES

1. Rubin JM. Musculoskeletal power Doppler. Eur Radiol 1999;9(Suppl 3):S403–6.
2. Rubin JM, Bude RO, Carson PL, Bree RL, Adler RS. Power Doppler US: A potentially useful alternative to mean frequency-based color Doppler US. Radiology 1994;190(3): 853–6.
3. Ophir J, Parker KJ. Contrast agents in diagnostic ultrasound. Ultrasound Med Biol 1989;15(4):319–33.
4. Harvey CJ, Blomley MJ, Eckersley RJ, Cosgrove DO. Developments in ultrasound contrast media. Eur Radiol 2001;11(4):675–89.
5. Rubin JM. Spectral Doppler US. Radiographics 1994;14(1):139–50.
6. Keberle M, Tony HP, Jahns R, Hau M, Haerten R, Jenett M. Assessment of microvascular changes in Raynaud's phenomenon and connective tissue disease using colour Doppler ultrasound. Rheumatology 2000;39(11):1206–13.
7. Fornage BD. Role of color Doppler imaging in differentiating between pseudocystic malignant tumors and fluid collections. J Ultrasound Med 1995;14(2):125–8.
8. Breidahl WH, Stafford Johnson DB, Newman JS, Adler RS. Power Doppler sonography in tenosynovitis: significance of the peritendinous hypoechoic rim. J Ultrasound Med 1998;17(2): 103–7.
9. Newman JS, Adler RS, Bude RO, Rubin JM. Detection of soft-tissue hyperemia: Value of power Doppler sonography. Am J Roentgenol 1994;163(2):385–9.
10. Newman JS, Laing TJ, McCarthy CJ, Adler RS. Power Doppler sonography of synovitis: Assessment of therapeutic response—preliminary observations. Radiology 1996;198(2):582–4.
11. Suh DY. Understanding angiogenesis and its clinical applications. Ann Clin Lab Sci 2000;30(3):227–38.
12. Kirsner RS, Eaglstein WH. The wound healing process. Dermatol Clin 1993;11(4):629–40.
13. Yu JS, Popp JE, Kaeding CC, Lucas J. Correlation of MR imaging and pathologic findings in athletes undergoing surgery for chronic patellar tendinitis. Am J Roentgenol 1995;165(1):115–8.
14. Weinberg EP, Adams MJ, Hollenberg GM. Color Doppler sonography of patellar tendinosis. Am J Roentgenol 1998; 171(3):743–4.
15. Ohberg L, Lorentzon R, Alfredson H. Neovascularisation in Achilles tendons with painful tendinosis but not in normal tendons: An ultrasonographic investigation. Knee Surg Sports Traumatol Arthrosc 2001;9(4):233–8.
16. Ohberg L, Alfredson H. Ultrasound guided sclerosis of neovessels in painful chronic Achilles tendinosis: Pilot study of a new treatment. Br J Sports Med 2002;36(3):173–5; discussion 176–7.
17. Chiou HJ, Chou YH, Wu JJ, Hsu CC, Huang DY, Chang CY. Evaluation of calcific tendonitis of the rotator cuff: Role of color Doppler ultrasonography. J Ultrasound Med 2002;21(3):289–95; quiz 296–7.
18. Chao HC, Lin SJ, Huang YC, Lin TY. Sonographic evaluation of cellulitis in children. J Ultrasound Med 2000;19(11):743–9.
19. Schweitzer ME, Mandel S, Schwartzman RJ, Knobler RL, Tahmoush AJ. Reflex sympathetic dystrophy revisited: MR imaging findings before and after infusion of contrast material. Radiology 1995;195(1):211–4.
20. Nazarian LN, Schweitzer ME, Mandel S, Rawool NM, Parker L, Fisher AM, et al. Increased soft-tissue blood flow in patients with reflex sympathetic dystrophy of the lower extremity revealed by power Doppler sonography. Am J Roentgenol 1998;171(5):1245–50.
21. Breidahl WH, Newman JS, Taljanovic MS, Adler RS. Power Doppler sonography in the assessment of musculoskeletal fluid collections. Am J Roentgenol 1996;166(6):1443–6.

22. Strouse PJ, DiPietro MA, Adler RS. Pediatric hip effusions: Evaluation with power Doppler sonography. Radiology 1998; 206(3):731–5.

23. Backhaus M, Kamradt T, Sandrock D, Loreck D, Fritz J, Wolf KJ, et al. Arthritis of the finger joints: A comprehensive approach comparing conventional radiography, scintigraphy, ultrasound, and contrast-enhanced magnetic resonance imaging. Arthritis Rheum 1999;42(6):1232–45.

24. Giovagnoni A, Valeri G, Burroni E, Amici F. Rheumatoid arthritis: Follow-up and response to treatment. Eur J Radiol 1998;27(Suppl 1):S25–30.

25. Hau M, Schultz H, Tony HP, Keberle M, Jahns R, Haerten R, et al. Evaluation of pannus and vascularization of the metacarpophalangeal and proximal interphalangeal joints in rheumatoid arthritis by high-resolution ultrasound (multidimensional linear array). Arthritis Rheum 1999;42(11): 2303–8.

26. Taylor PC. VEGF and imaging of vessels in rheumatoid arthritis. Arthritis Res 2002;4(Suppl 3):S99–107.

27. Magarelli N, Guglielmi G, Di Matteo L, Tartaro A, Mattei PA, Bonomo L. Diagnostic utility of an echo-contrast agent in patients with synovitis using power Doppler ultrasound: A preliminary study with comparison to contrast-enhanced MRI. Eur Radiol 2001;11(6):1039–46.

28. Carotti M, Salaffi F, Manganelli P, Salera D, Simonetti B, Grassi W. Power Doppler sonography in the assessment of synovial tissue of the knee joint in rheumatoid arthritis: A preliminary experience. Ann Rheum Dis 2002;61(10):877–82.

29. Klauser A, Frauscher F, Schirmer M, Halpern E, Pallwein L, Herold M, et al. The value of contrast-enhanced color Doppler ultrasound in the detection of vascularization of finger joints in patients with rheumatoid arthritis. Arthritis Rheum 2002; 46(3):647–53.

30. Szkudlarek M, Court-Payen M, Strandberg C, Klarlund M, Klausen T, Ostergaard M. Power Doppler ultrasonography for assessment of synovitis in the metacarpophalangeal joints of patients with rheumatoid arthritis: A comparison with dynamic magnetic resonance imaging. Arthritis Rheum 2001;44(9): 2018–23.

31. Stone M, Bergin D, Whelan B, Maher M, Murray J, McCarthy C. Power Doppler ultrasound assessment of rheumatoid hand synovitis. J Rheumatol 2001;28(9):1979–82.

32. Cosgrove D, Eckersley R, Blomley M, Harvey C. Quantification of blood flow. Eur Radiol 2001;11(8):1338–44.

33. Teh J, Stevens K, Williamson L, Leung J, McNally EG. Power Doppler ultrasound of rheumatoid synovitis: quantification of therapeutic response. Br J Radiol. 2003 Dec;76(912):875–879.

34. Alexander AA, Nazarian LN, Feld RI. Superficial soft-tissue masses suggestive of recurrent malignancy: Sonographic localization and biopsy. Am J Roentgenol 1997;169(5): 1449–51.

35. Belli P, Costantini M, Mirk P, Maresca G, Priolo F, Marano P. Role of color Doppler sonography in the assessment of musculoskeletal soft tissue masses. J Ultrasound Med 2000; 19(12):823–30.

36. Lagalla R, Iovane A, Caruso G, Lo Bello M, Derchi LE. Color Doppler ultrasonography of soft-tissue masses. Acta Radiol 1998;39(4):421–6.

37. Kransdorf MJ, Murphey MD. Radiologic evaluation of soft-tissue masses: A current perspective. Am J Roentgenol 2000;175(3):575–87.

38. Mulliken JB, Glowacki J. Classification of pediatric vascular lesions. Plast Reconstr Surg 1982;70(1):120–1.

39. Gampper TJ, Morgan RF. Vascular anomalies: Hemangiomas. Plast Reconstr Surg 2002;110(2):572–85; quiz 586; discussion 587–8.

40. Requena L, Sangueza OP. Cutaneous vascular proliferation. Part II. Hyperplasias and benign neoplasms. J Am Acad Dermatol 1997;37(6):887–919; quiz 920–2.

41. Paltiel HJ, Burrows PE, Kozakewich HP, Zurakowski D, Mulliken JB. Soft-tissue vascular anomalies: Utility of US for diagnosis. Radiology 2000;214(3):747–54.

42. Fishman SJ, Mulliken JB. Hemangiomas and vascular malformations of infancy and childhood. Pediatr Clin North Am 1993;40(6):1177–200.

43. Less JR, Skalak TC, Sevick EM, Jain RK. Microvascular architecture in a mammary carcinoma: Branching patterns and vessel dimensions. Cancer Res 1991;51(1):265–73.

44. Schroeder RJ, Maeurer J, Gath HJ, Willam C, Hidajat N. Vascularization of reactively enlarged lymph nodes analyzed by color duplex sonography. J Oral Maxillofac Surg 1999; 57(9):1090–5.

45. Schroeder RJ, Maeurer J, Vogl TJ, Hidajat N, Hadijuana J, Venz S, et al. D-Galactose-based signal-enhanced color Doppler sonography of breast tumors and tumorlike lesions. Invest Radiol 1999;34(2):109–15.

46. Bodner G, Schocke MF, Rachbauer F, Seppi K, Peer S, Fierlinger A, et al. Differentiation of malignant and benign musculoskeletal tumors: combined color and power Doppler US and spectral wave analysis. Radiology 2002;223(2): 410–6.

47. van der Woude HJ, Bloem JL, van Oostayen JA, Nooy MA, Taminiau AH, Hermans J, et al. Treatment of high-grade bone sarcomas with neoadjuvant chemotherapy: The utility of sequential color Doppler sonography in predicting histopathologic response. Am J Roentgenol 1995;165(1): 125–33.

48. Bearcroft PW, Berman LH, Robinson AH, Butler GJ. Vascularity of the neonatal femoral head: In vivo demonstration with power Doppler US. Radiology 1996;200(1):209–11.

49. Newman JS, Adler RS, Rubin JM. Power Doppler sonography: Use in measuring alterations in muscle blood volume after exercise. Am J Roentgenol 1997;168(6):1525–30.

50. Chikui T, Izumi M, Eguchi K, Kawabe Y, Nakamura T. Doppler spectral waveform analysis of arteries of the hand in patients with Raynaud's phenomenon as compared with healthy subjects. Am J Roentgenol 1999;172(6):1605–9.

Musculoskeletal interventional ultrasound

15

Eugene G McNally

GENERAL

Ultrasound is an ideal method for guiding interventional musculoskeletal procedures. The purpose of this chapter is to describe the most commonly performed procedures. In most cases a 21-G needle is all that is necessary to puncture the majority of relatively superficial musculoskeletal structures. Complex preparation is not required and with sensible attention to sterility, extra-articular soft-tissue injections have a remarkably low complication profile when placed in their intended locations. Preliminary examination locates the intended target structure and approach route. For very superficial structures, a small footprint probe approximates the puncture point and target and is ideal for guiding the injection of small joints of the hand or foot. The puncture point can be marked in variety of ways. Traditionally skin-marking pens are used but have the slight disadvantage of either being wiped clear during skin sterilisation if they are water soluble or smearing and staining the probe if not. Pressure with the blunt end of a needle or needle cover avoids this. The author prefers to use a marking line rather than a point as this not only gives a puncture point but an initial needle direction. With practice, this means that the needle can be inserted close to its destination blind; then once the probe is in position, the needle can be advanced the final distance to its intended target. A line can be created either with a skin-marking pen, or by pressure from an extended paperclip. Pressing for 10 sec produces an impression that lasts about 5 min, plenty of time for scrubbing and skin preparation. Combining skin pressure and a marker pen is another alternative. In some cases, it is not even necessary to remove the probe during skin preparation. For SASD bursal injections, for example, the shoulder examination sequence can end with the probe in the correct position for injection. A quick wipe with a sterile swab is followed by the bursal injection. In this way a diagnostic procedure can be combined with a guided injection with little prolongation of the examination time. In children, the use of a topical local anaesthetic cream or ethyl chloride spray or both helps to reduce even the small initial discomfort of the initial injection. These can also be used in adults in areas that are more uncomfortable such as the sole of the foot. Whether they provide any more than placebo effect in adults is questionable. The sting from some anaesthetic preparations can also be reduced by the addition of a 1% bicarbonate solution.

The patient experience can also be improved by careful attention to a number of small but thoughtful details. The injection trolley should be prepared in advance if possible and be kept out of view until needed. It is unnecessary to draw up drugs in full view of the patient. Ideally the patient should not see a needle until the moment it is to be inserted into the skin. Adequate time should be given for local anaesthesia to work. When more complex preparations are necessary, such as application of a sterile probe cover, it is suggested that skin preparation and local anaesthesia injection are carried out first. Any minor distraction at the precise moment of needle insertion, such as asking the patient to take a breath or directing a question can help. Particular attention to the needs of children with familiar personnel, parents, nurses and play therapist as necessary can improve the experience and reduce the future development of needle phobia.

The injection cocktail most frequently used is a combination of a corticosteroid mixed with a local anaesthetic. Either long- or short-acting local anaesthetics can be used. The author's preference is for a combination of triamcinolone 40 mg mixed with 0.5% bupivacaine. For more superficial injections where there is significant risk of subcutaneous leak, Depo-Medrone® replaces triamcinolone as the corticosteroid of choice. There is some evidence to suggest that this preparation is less prone to cause subcutaneous fat necrosis.

In all cases care should be taken not to inject corticosteroid directly into tendons as an area of focal necrosis may lead to tendon rupture. With practice there is little difficulty but for those less certain about correct needle placement, a preliminary injection of a small quantity of local anaesthetic on its own can be helpful to distend the tendon sheath and confirm correct needle placement. Local anaesthetics are less damaging to tendons than corticosteroid but in all cases it is unwise to continue with injection when undue or unexpected resistance is encountered.

The degree of sterility required will vary with the target, personal practice and local guidelines.

A minimalist approach can be justified for the majority of soft-tissue injections, using rigorous skin antisepsis and sterile contact jelly. For guided injections into joints, and in particular to implanted joints, a higher level of sterility is warranted with gloved hands, skin preparation and sterile probe covers.

SUBACROMIAL SUBDELTOID BURSAL INJECTION

Patient position

Most shoulders are examined with the patient seated and there is no need to change position prior to injection. The commonest approach to the blind subacromial subdeltoid (SASD) bursa injection carried out without ultrasound guidance surgically is via a posterior approach. The most lateral and posterior margin of the acromium is palpated and the needle inserted approximately 1 cm below this, directed upwards. This blind technique is reported to have good success and the needle is said to be in the subacromial subdeltoid bursa if free lateral side-to-side movement of its tip is possible. During injection, a finger placed anteriorly should feel the contrast injection if it is free flowing within the bursa. Postinjection ultrasound can be used to confirm correct placement of the injected material; however, if a small volume injection is used, it may be difficult to detect this underneath the bony acromium.

Ultrasound-guided injections are generally from a lateral or anterior approach. The author's preference is to use a guided injection using direct ultrasound screening of the needle during its entry into the bursa. For this approach an anterior or an anterolateral puncture site provides the best visualisation of the route of the needle to the correct location.

Needle and drugs

In the majority of cases a 21-G needle suffices for all but the deepest bursae. The subacromial subdeltoid bursa is a large structure and can accommodate quite considerable volumes of fluid although a total injection dose of more than 5 ml is usually not necessary. The author uses a combination of 40 mg triamcinolone mixed with 0.5% bupivacaine.

Approach and puncture point

The simplest approach is to place the probe in the same position as used to generate a coronal image of the cuff (Fig. 15.1). From this position, the needle can approach either from above the probe as shown in Fig. 15.1 or from below (Fig. 15.2). Either method is valid. A common approach for a right-handed operator, for a left shoulder injection, is to hold the needle in the right hand and the probe in the left hand whilst the operator stands behind the seated patient. The reverse is true for the right shoulder. With

practice, the degree of dexterity required to manipulate the needle becomes less and the author prefers to approach both sides with the needle above the probe (Fig. 15.1). An approach from above has the advantage of not having the probe cable interfere with the needle. An alternative is to place the probe axially in an anterior position until clear visualisation of the supraspinatus tendon and subacromial subdeltoid bursa is obtained (Fig. 15.3). The skin is punctured just medial to the probe and the needle directed towards the bursa.

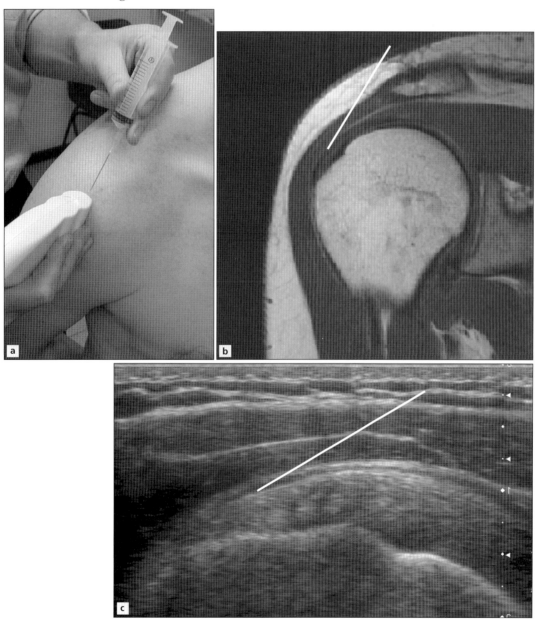

Fig. 15.1 (a) Position of probe and needle for preferred approach to subacromial subdeltoid bursa. As the bursa is large the on position is less critical but the author tends to complete the examination with an injection and hence the patient is asked to leave their arm in the final position with shoulder abducted and internally rotated. (b) Sagittal T1-weighted MRI showing schematically the approach of the needle lateral to the tip of the acromion paralleling the bursa, close to the lateral margin of the supraspinatus. (c) Comparative coronal ultrasound examination with direction of needle approach as indicated.

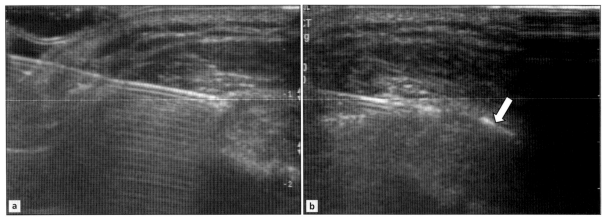

Fig. 15.2 Coronal image during SASD bursal injection via lateral approach. (a) The needle bevel is in the SASD bursa. (b) This is only reliably confirmed as the subsequent injection quickly disperses (reflective material) (arrow). Focal conglomeration indicates incorrect positioning.

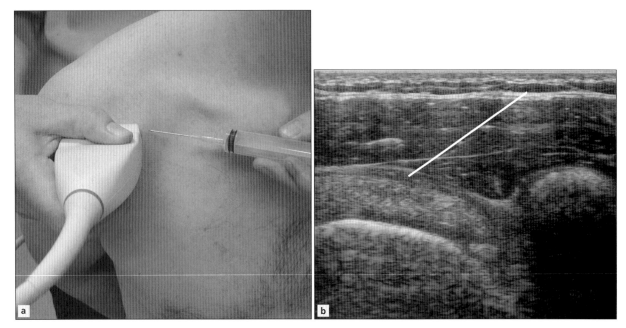

Fig. 15.3 Alternative anterior approach to subacromial subdeltoid bursa. (a) The probe is in the position to demonstrate the anterior free edge. The skin can be punctured either medial or lateral to the probe but access is easier for the medial puncture. (b) Ultrasound at the same position showing needle approach.

Target area

As long as the needle is kept in the same axial plane as the probe it can be followed accurately until it reaches the superficial surface of the supraspinatus tendon. A preliminary injection in this location may confirm the correct positioning in the bursa as evident by rapid flow of injected material away from the needle tip. More commonly, a local injection is observed, indicating that the needle tip still lies on the deltoid side of the bursa. A gentle manoeuvre of the needle with a slight hooking action to direct the needle under the reflective bursa is usually sufficient to ensure firm placement within the bursa and the injection can be completed.

Postprocedure

Following the injection it is often useful to manipulate the shoulder gently and then determine whether the patient's range of movement within the painful arch has improved. A diminution of symptoms with increased range of motion is termed a positive impingement test.

SUPRASPINATUS CALCIFICATION BARBOTAGE

Calcific tendinopathy is a relatively common disorder and ultrasound detects calcification relatively early when compared with plain films and more accurately in many cases than MRI (Fig. 15.4). Not all supraspinatus calcification causes symptoms and barbotage is generally reserved for patients who suffer severe and acute pain as a consequence of crystal shedding into the subacromial subdeltoid bursa. Symptoms in many cases are so acute that a diagnosis of septic arthritis is often considered. Although ultrasound is more sensitive to the detection of calcification, it is difficult to determine on ultrasound criteria which lesions are most likely to respond to treatment. Inflammatory changes in the surrounding tendon and a more poorly demarcated calcification are clues. The author prefers to use plain films to make this assessment. Well-defined, hard, often-ossified lesions are probably of long-standing, are unlikely to be contributing to acute calcific tendinopathy and are less likely to respond to barbotage. More poorly defined homogeneous and milky appearances on the plain X-ray are more optimistic findings.

Patient position

The technique for aspiration is similar to subacromial subdeltoid bursa injection described previously. The patient should be warned that calcium aspiration can be painful and in some cases the examination should be carried out with the patient recumbent.

Needle and drugs

A single- or double needle-technique may be used. Some authors argue that calcium is easier to flush out by using one needle to inject saline and a second to drain the area.

Approach and puncture point

The principle difference between SASD bursal injection and barbotage is that the coronal approach may not provide the best aspect on the calcification, although it frequently does. Once the calcification and the best approach to it have been identified, the skin is punctured at the midpoint of the lateral short axis of the probe.

Target area

The needle is first advanced to the subacromial subdeltoid bursa, which is injected with local anaesthetic. The author prefers to carry this out before the barbotage procedure as the procedure itself can release calcium pyrophosphate crystals into the bursa, which can be excruciatingly painful. Once the bursa has been infiltrated, the needle is advanced into the calcium and an aspirate is attempted. If the appearances are rather homogeneous and cloudy on the X-ray then milk of calcium can often be aspirated into the syringe. If the lesion is too hard and does not appear to aspirate then, agitation of the needle on the surface and within the lesion can help to promote calcium dispersion. Following this a small quantity of local anaesthetic and hydrocortisone is injected into the calcium.

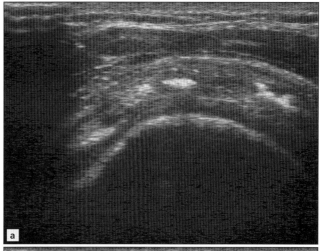

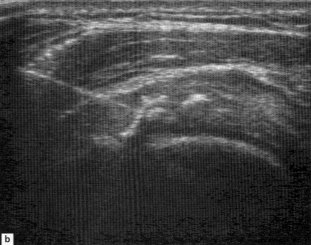

Fig. 15.4 a) Supraspinatus calcification. b) needle in situ prior to aspiration.

ACROMIOCLAVICULAR JOINT INJECTION

Patient position

Most shoulders are examined with the patient seated and there is no need to change position prior to injection.

Needle and drugs

A 21-G green needle with 30 mg Depo-Medrone® mixed with 0.5% bupivacaine is suggested. The joint is generally a rather tight structure and it is unlikely that much more than 0.5 to 1 ml will be accepted by it.

Approach and puncture point

The AC joint is easily identified in the coronal plane but is best injected in the sagittal plane. Standing beside the seated patient during the examination (Fig. 15.5) gives good access to the AC joint, which is most easily identified in the sagittal plane by placing the probe initially medial to it and identifying the bony reflective margin of the clavicle. The probe is then slid laterally until the bony reflection disappears, indicating that it is now positioned directly over the joint. Further lateral movement brings up the bony acromion, which is a useful confirmatory procedure. The needle and probe are inserted at 90° to one another with the probe in the sagittal plane on the anterior aspect of the joint and the

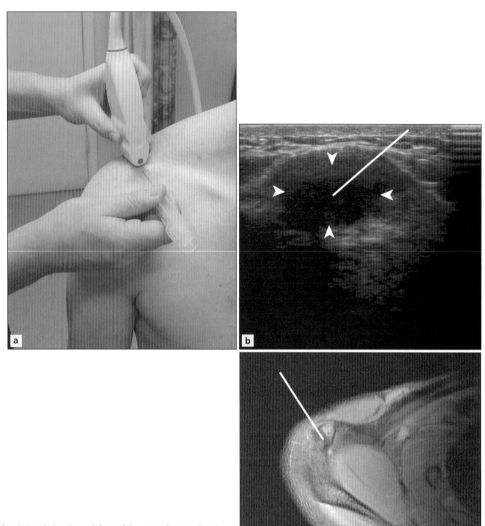

Fig. 15.5 Position for acromioclavicular joint injection. (a) In this case the probe is on the posterosuperior aspect of the joint and the puncture side anterosuperior. Reversing needle and probe is equally effective. (b) Rounded poorly reflective joint is identified (arrowheads) and the needle's approach shown schematically. (c) Axial fat-saturated T1-weighted MR image showing schematically the direction of the needle.

needle inserted from posterior. In this position it is easily seen entering into the joint (Fig. 15.5).

SHOULDER ARTHROGRAPHY/INJECTION

Patient position

Direct MR arthrography is a common procedure used to determine the intra-articular components contributing to an unstable shoulder. As most shoulder dislocations are anterior and, as a consequence, the structures of interest also lie anteriorly (the anterior labrum and capsule), a posterior approach provides the best means of reducing artefacts that may subsequently impede interpretation of the study. Ultrasound or fluoroscopic guidance is helpful and reduces the small risk of failure associated with a blind approach. Ultrasound equipment is more portable than fluoroscopic equipment and is therefore often more readily available in more remote MR units. Guided injections are also used for therapeutic purposes.

Needle and drugs

Depending on the depth of the joint, a 21-G spinal needle is recommended in most cases. The injectate depends on the indication for the procedure.

Approach and puncture point

Once again the probe is best positioned in the axial plane and is manipulated until the posterior glenoid margin with its attached labrum can be identified (Fig. 15.6). The puncture site is lateral to the probe.

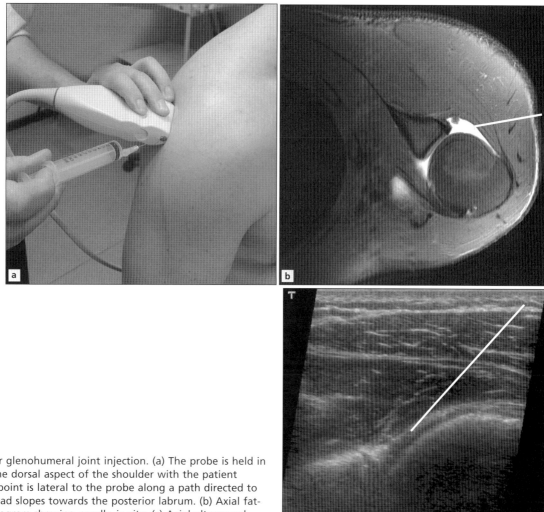

Fig. 15.6 Approach for glenohumeral joint injection. (a) The probe is held in the axial plane over the dorsal aspect of the shoulder with the patient seated. The puncture point is lateral to the probe along a path directed to where the humeral head slopes towards the posterior labrum. (b) Axial fat-saturated T1 MR arthrogram showing needle *in situ*. (c) Axial ultrasound image correlating with (a) and (b) showing direction of approach to the joint.

Target area

The needle is advanced in the axial plane under ultrasound screening, aiming for a point approximately halfway between the most posterior point of the humeral head and the labrum or glenoid margin. Care should be taken not to aim for the glenoid margin itself as a large labrum can displace the needle posteriorly and prevent accurate placement in the joint. Once again a small injection of local anaesthetic will confirm intra-articular location, following which arthrographic material or an anti-inflammatory cocktail can be injected.

COMMON EXTENSOR ORIGIN

Patient position

The principal indication for injecting the common extensor origin is recalcitrant tennis elbow that has failed to respond to physiotherapy and blind injection treatment. The probe is positioned in the coronal plane, with the arm in the same "praying" position as is used for diagnosis (see Chapter 1).

Needle and drugs

A 21-G green needle is used to approach both the common flexor and extensor origins. For a corticosteroid infiltration, Depo-Medrone 30 mg mixed with 0.5% bupivacaine is suggested. The area is generally infiltrated with 2–3 ml. An alternative procedure that does not involve corticosteroids is to make multiple punctures with the needle, termed dry needling. The aim of this procedure is to addess a maladaptive repair by combining re-injury with a rehabilitation program to induce corrective repair. Dry needling can be combined with autologous blood injection to achieve the same result.

Approach and puncture point

The skin is punctured proximal to the probe with the needle advanced medially and distally to the surface of the extensor origin (Fig. 15.7).

Target area

A line of approach should be taken that will allow the needle to be advanced further, directed towards the deeper portion of the common extensor origin. The radiocapitellar joint makes a useful landmark for this purpose. If a small footprint probe is not available then care should be taken to ensure that the probe is advanced a little more distally so that the proximal puncture point will be in the correct location to allow the needle to pass towards the radiocapitellar joint.

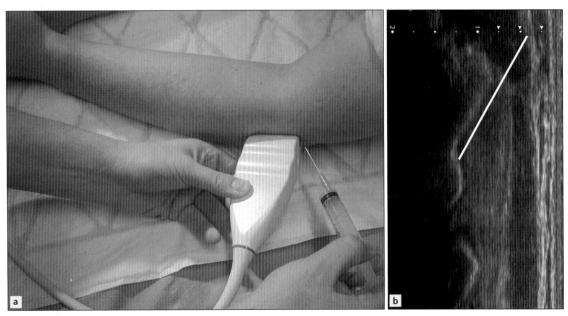

Fig. 15.7 (a) Position of probe giving coronal view of common extensor origin. The puncture point is proximal to the probe with a line of approach towards the radiocapitellar joint as shown in (b).

INTRA-ARTICULAR INJECTION ELBOW

Patient position

The patient can be seated or lying with their arm held across their chests (Fig. 15.8). In children where septic arthritis of the elbow is not uncommon, the child sits facing mother on her lap, with their arms wrapped around the mother's side. A nurse or assistant can stand behind the mother and hold the child's hands to prevent excessive movement. This presents the posterior aspect of the elbow in a good position for both examination and aspiration.

Approach and puncture point

A posterior approach is simplest particularly when there is an effusion. A path adjacent to the triceps tendon rather than through it is recommended. An alternative approach in adults is through the radiocapitellar joint or just lateral to the olecranon process where a small groove can be palpated between the olecranon and the humerus. This is similar to the ulnar notch but

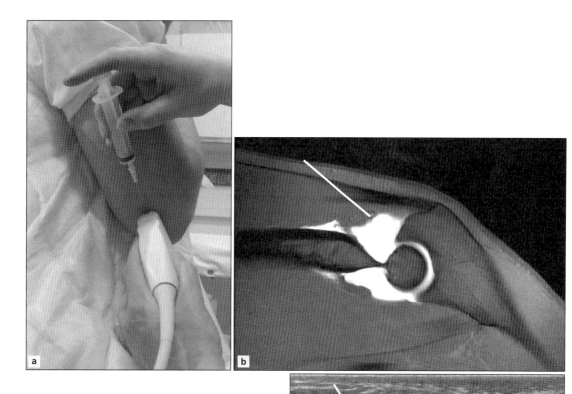

Fig. 15.8 Dorsal approach to the elbow joint. (a) The patient is seated with his/her back to the operator. The probe position demonstrates a sagittal view of the dorsal aspect of the joint as in (b) the fat-saturated T1-weighted MR arthrogram and (c) correlating ultrasound in a different patient. The puncture point is proximal and directed as shown.

lies on the radial aspect rather than the ulnar aspect of the olecranon.

Needle and drugs

A 21-G green needle and 40 mg triamcinolone mixed with 0.5% bupivacaine is a common combination. The joint will generally accept 10 ml. The technique of ultrasound arthrography can be used in the detection of loose bodies within a joint and also as guidance for joint distension and gadolinium injection prior to MR arthrography.

Target area

The joint is easily identified by any of the approaches already described. Depending on the approach used, once cannulation has been achieved, it is often helpful to move the probe to visualise the olecranon fossa prior to injecting the joint. This allows easy confirmation of joint filling and allows the movement of suspected loose bodies to be observed.

TENDON SHEATH INJECTION

The basic principles that have been described already can be readily applied to the injection of tendon sheaths. In many respects tendon sheath injection is relatively easy due to the proximity of tendon sheath to the surface and their elongated nature providing a large target zone.

Approach and puncture point

The probe is orientated along the long axis of the tendon and a small mark is made on the skin to indicate the central point of the tendon (Fig. 15.9). The author prefers to use a line rather than a point mark as this provides both the puncture point and the direction of further advancement. If local anaesthetic is to be used, the skin can be punctured and infiltrated along the direction indicated by the mark and when the probe is placed in position, with experience, the needle tip will be found to lie in close approximation to its target area.

Needle and drugs

A 21-G green needle and 40 mg triamcinolone mixed with 0.5% bupivacaine. A large sheath joint will generally accept 5–8 ml.

Target area

Under ultrasound guidance the needle can be advanced with further infiltration of local anaesthetic, to help with anaesthesia but also to distend the tendon sheath once the needle is in the correct location. Rotating the needles so that the bevel points towards the tendon is a simple technique that will further reduce the unlikely possibility of tendon puncture. Once the tendon sheath has been cannulated and preliminary injection is confirmed with the free flow of material within the sheath and away from the needle, the full injection can be administered. It should be noted that the injection should result in distension of the tendon sheath with filling on both sides of the tendon. If filling is limited to one side alone it is probable that the needle lies outside the tendon sheath. This general

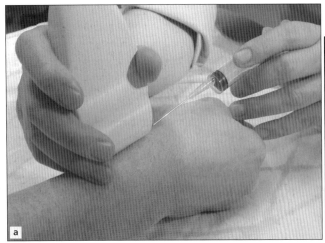
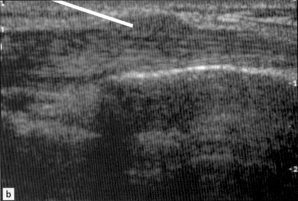

Fig. 15.9 Cannulation of extensor tendon. The probe parallels the tendon to be injected. In this case the puncture point is proximal with the needle directed at a shallow angle towards the tendon sheath as shown in (b).

technique can be applied to all tendon sheath injections. However, it should be noted that in de Quervain's tenosynovitis, the sclerosing nature of this process does not result in a large amount of tendon sheath fluid and that cannulation is not only a little more difficult but is also painful, presumably reflecting the underlying nature of this disease.

CARPAL TUNNEL INJECTION

The standard injection point for carpal tunnel injection is between the flexor carpi radialis tendon and the median nerve. The skin is marked proximal to the flexor retinaculum. The puncture point can be identified by placing the probe first in the transverse plane to identify the flexor carpi radialis and the median nerve. The probe can then be rotated until its midpoint is centred over the space between these two structures. The puncture point is then proximal to the midpoint of the probe and directed into this space. The tip of the needle can be confirmed under ultrasound control prior to the injection. The small size of the target space means that a combination of sagittal and axial views with the probe are most helpful in confirming accurate placement.

INJECTION OF SMALL JOINT OF THE HAND

Patient position

Seating the patient opposite the seated operator allows good access to the small joints of the hand. A small footprint ultrasound probe is best.

Needle and drugs

A 21-G green needle and 30 mg Depo-Medrone® mixed with 0.5% bupivacaine. The joint generally accepts 1–2 ml.

Approach and puncture point

An approach from the sagittal plane, either dorsally or ventrally, allows easy access to the joint (Figs 15.10 and 15.11). Ultrasound guidance can also be used to sample periarticular erosions whereby a 21-G needle is used to aspirate a small

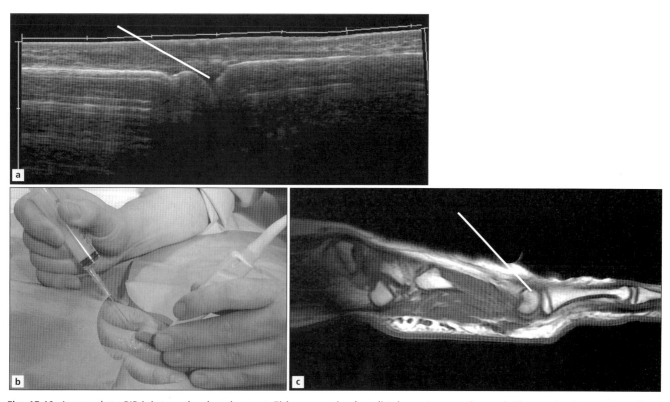

Fig. 15.10 Approach to PIP joint on the dorsal aspect. Either a proximal or distal puncture can be used. The proximal puncture point allows the needle to parallel the curved head of the proximal phalanx as shown on the sagittal T1-weighted MRC. Note the use of a small footprint probe that allows the puncture point to be closer to the centre of the image.

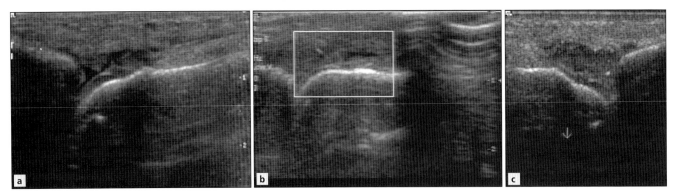

Fig. 15.11 (a) Sagittal image of MTPJ synovitis with (b) synovial Doppler study. (c) Postinjection image.

quantity of histological material. Cytological analysis helps to differentiate between seropositive, seronegative, crystal and other causes of arthropathy.

Target area

Directing the needle tip distally, aiming to place it under the "roof" of the more distal bone, is suggested. The anatomy of these superficial joints is well demonstrated and is usually sufficiently clear to allow access from distal to proximal if necessary.

ASPIRATION OF THE INFANT HIP

Patient position

The child is supine with hips extended in a position of comfort. Some authors recommend that toes be approximated and loosely strapped together. The author does not do this as it might increase the child's apprehension of what is to follow.

Needle and drugs

Local anaesthetic cream is applied to the skin anterior to the affected hip as soon as the patient presents to hospital. See Chapter 8 for method and timeframe.

Approach and puncture point

This is one of a few ultrasound techniques where the actual aspiration is carried out without real-time guidance. Accurate placement of the needle tip is confirmed by withdrawing joint fluid. Successful aspiration in an accurate and quick

fashion depends on accurate identification of the point of maximal anterior capsular distension. Localisation depends on keeping the probe held vertically over the hip with an angle of 90° to the skin. The puncture point is determined by marking the skin, creating a blanched area with the probe and/or using an extended paperclip to triangulate (Fig. 15.12b).

The first method involves marking the central point of each side of the probe when the point of maximal distension has been identified (Fig. 15.12a). The intersection of lines joining opposite points identifies the puncture point. A modification of this method is to mark the central points of the narrow ends of the probe. The puncture point will lie somewhere along this line. The exact point is determined by moving a small wire, such as a straightened paper clip, and noting where the acoustic shadows cross the point of maximal joint distension (L. Berman: personal communication). Another useful technique is to apply a little pressure to the probe once the point of maximal joint distension has been identified. If the probe is quickly removed from the skin, the blanched foot plate can be identified and a mark placed at its centre. Combining these techniques means that the aspiration point can be identified with great confidence. The probe should not be removed until the operator is 100% confident that the effusion lies directly underneath the marked puncture point.

Target area

Once removed, following a sterile technique, direct puncture with the needle directed at 90° to the skin and without ultrasound guidance will result in aspiration in almost every case.

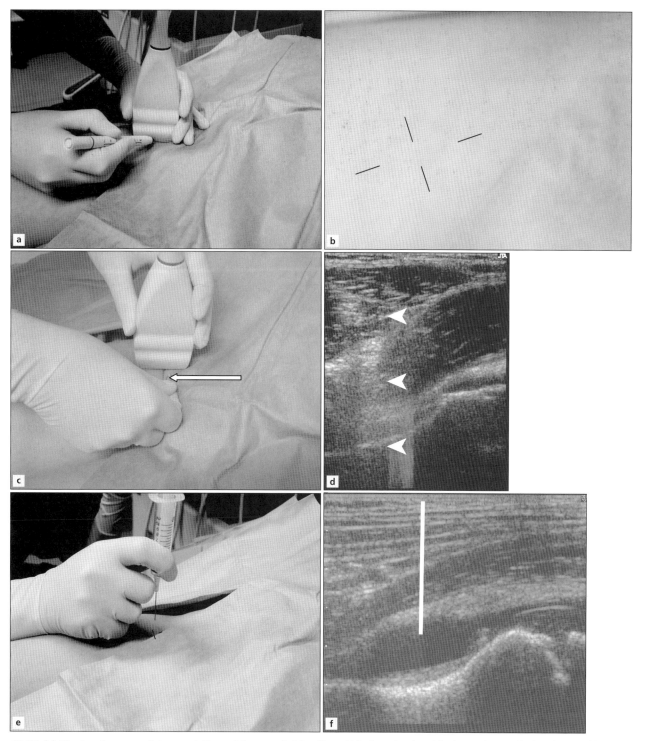

Fig. 15.12 (a) The key to successful cannulation of the paediatric effused hip is to begin with the probe vertical and centrally positioned over the point of maximal joint distension. If the subsequent aspiration is also with a vertical needle, then aspiration is markedly simplified. With the probe in the correct position, several techniques can be used to locate the puncture point. These are often best used in combination. The central point of all four sides of the probe can be marked. When the probe is removed the intersection of opposite lines gives the central puncture point. (b) A small amount of pressure has been applied to the probe, then the probe has been removed to review an area of blanched skin. The central point of the blanched area is easy to determine and provides useful confirmation of the marking technique. (c) An extended paper clip (long arrow) is placed underneath the probe and moved so that the acoustic shadow it casts (d, arrowheads) passes over the point of maximal distension. This can be used either on its own or in conjunction with a small mark placed at the midpoint at the narrow ends of the probe. The intersection between the marker points and the position determined by the paper clip gives the puncture point. Again this method can be used in conjunction with the methods described in (a) and (b) with each additional method providing firmer reassurance on the correct puncture point. Note that the figure shown in (d) with the paper clip shadow does not have an effusion. (e) Once the puncture point is determined with complete confidence the probe is removed and the joint punctured with a vertical needle. (f) The line of approach is shown.

ASPIRATION AND INJECTION OF THE ADULT HIP

Patient position

The approach to the adult hip joint is similar to that in children although due to the depth of this joint the anatomy is rarely as clearly demarcated as it is in the child.

Needle and drugs

A reflective spinal needle or similar and 40 mg triamcinolone mixed with 0.5% bupivacaine are used. A large sheath joint will generally accept 5–8 ml.

Approach and puncture point

Two approaches can be used, depending on preference, the patient's body habitus and the presence of effusion. If the joint is distended, it is usually easily seen with the probe aligned along the femoral neck (Fig. 15.13). In thin patients and noneffused joints, a good view of the anterior joint can be gained using an anterior approach with the probe turned into an axial position (Fig. 15.14). The anterior approach is lateral to the femoral vessels, remembering that the nerve is also lateral to the artery and not as conspicuous. This is the same approach as for injecting an iliopsoas bursa.

Target area

With the sagittal approach, the rounded contour to the anterior aspect of the femoral head contrasts sharply with the triangular-shaped acetabulum and the joint is relatively easy to identify particularly in the presence of an effusion. The target for the axial approach is just lateral to the anterior labrum.

In obese individuals the bony landmarks and soft-tissue distension that follows hip injection can be more difficult to identify with certainty. Although the confidence with which intra-articular injection can be confirmed is higher for fluoroscopic procedures using iodinated contrast media, ultrasound has the advantage of being superior in guiding synovial biopsy, which makes up for some of its deficiencies with regard to intra-articular confirmation. Having said this, in the majority of patients, intra-articular

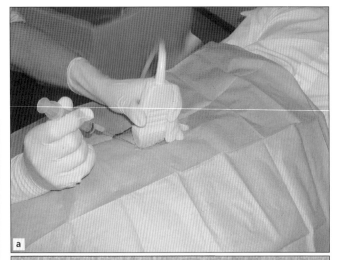
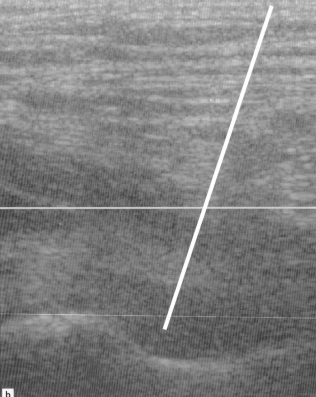

Fig. 15.13 Standard, sagittal approach to the hip. (a) The patient is recumbent. The probe is positioned to give a sagittal view of the anterior joint space. (b) The puncture point is proximal with the needle directed towards the joint.

confirmation of the needle position is relatively easy to achieve and confirm.

Synovial biopsy is a useful adjunct for the investigation of complications following hip replacement and the resulting microbiological specimens are more likely to reflect the true microbiology within the infected implant. Where possible, three separate specimens should be obtained, ideally using a different needle each time. This reduces the possibility of a false

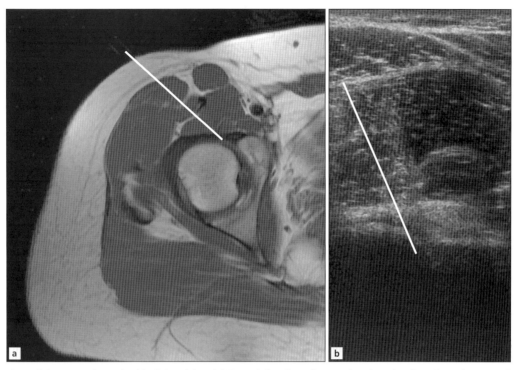

Fig. 15.14 Alternative axial approach to the hip joint. (a) Axial T1-weighted MR image showing the direction of approach. (b) Corresponding axially orientated ultrasound image. Note that the needle is lateral to the neurovascular bundle and directed to a point lateral to the anterior labrum.

positive result from instrument contamination. Restrained use of lidocaine (lignocaine) local anaesthetic is also recommended, as it is bacterostatic.

HIP BURSAL INJECTION

Trochanteric bursitis is a common disorder causing pain in the lateral aspect of the hip. Symptoms can be mimicked by gluteal bursitis although this is less common. A precise anatomical knowledge is necessary to distinguish the different bursae. The trochanteric bursa is the largest of these and lies posterior to the greater trochanter. The ultrasound features of trochanteric bursitis are quite variable but in many cases the bursa is not particularly distended with fluid but is seen more as a thickened rind of tissue when compared with the contralateral side. The gluteal bursae, of which there are two main structures, lie more anterior and deep to the tendons of gluteus minimis and medius.

Patient position

All these bursa are best approached with the patient lying in a ducibutus position with the affected side upwards. The probe is placed in the coronal position so that the greater trochanter can be visualised. It is then moved slightly posteriorly if the trochanteric bursa is to be injected and left in this location if the gluteal bursae are to be injected. Axial scanning during the procedure helps to confirm placement in the correct bursa.

Needle and drugs

A reflective spinal needle or similar and 40 mg triamcinolone mixed with 0.5% bupivacaine are used. The bursa will generally accept 5–8 ml.

Approach and puncture point

The puncture point is on the proximal aspect of the probe (Fig. 15.15).

Target area

The trochanteric bursa lies deep to gluteus maximus insertion. The subgluteus medius bursa is reached by passing the needle deep to the tendons of gluteus medius. The needle should lie anterolateral to the greater trochanter rather than posterolateral as for the trochanteric bursa.

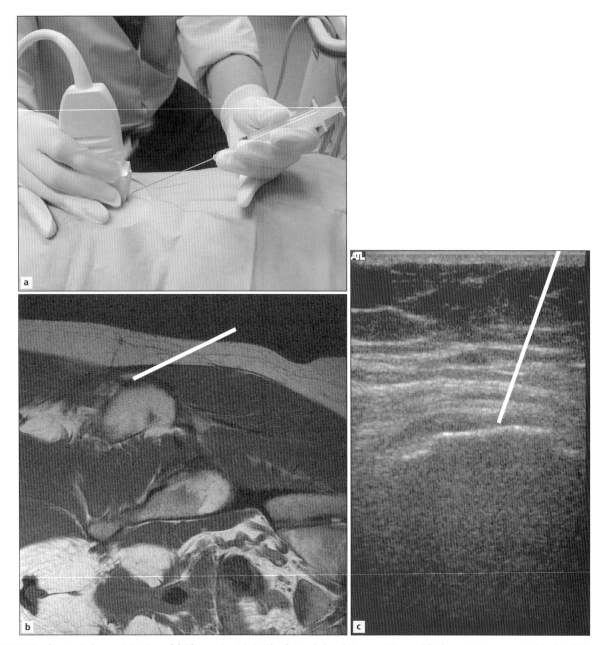

Fig. 15.15 Trochanteric bursa injection. (a) The patient is in the lateral decubitus position with the examiner seated behind them. The probe is positioned over the greater trochanter then moved slightly posteriorly to identify the trochanteric bursa. The puncture point is proximal using a narrow gauge spinal needle. (b) Corresponding T1-weighted coronal MR image showing direction of needle approach. (c) Corresponding coronally orientated ultrasound image with needle directed towards trochanteric bursa.

Psoas bursitis is a less common cause of bursal symptoms around the hip. The bursa can be identified lying lateral to the neurovascular bundle, which is easily seen, particularly if colour flow is used. The close proximity of the bursa to the femoral artery means that cannulation is best achieved by an oblique approach. The probe is placed in axial orientation overlying the femoral artery. The puncture site is lateral to this and the needle passes deep and medially until it reaches a point posterior to the femoral artery itself.

ADDUCTOR ORIGIN AND SYMPHYSEAL INJECTION

Groin strain in the athlete is multifactorial and often due to a combination of lesions. If due to adductor origin sprain this area can be injected under ultrasound control. Like trochanteric bursitis, on some occasions the ultrasound findings are not prominent and correlation with the area of inflammation on enhanced MR images is helpful. It should be remembered that, particularly in the case of symphyseal changes, that abnormal signal changes on MRI can be detected in the asymptomatic athlete.

Patient position

Injection to the adductor origin is best achieved with the patient supine. The area is exposed better if the leg is abducted and externally rotated.

Needle and drugs

A reflective spinal needle or similar and 40 mg triamcinolone mixed with 0.5% bupivacaine are used.

Approach and puncture point

For an adductor origin injection, the probe is oriented along the adductor tendon. The bony landmark of the inferior pubic ramus is easily identified with the adductor arising from it.

Target area

The puncture point should be chosen so that the needle can be inserted close to and paralleling the adductor origin so that the greatest area of infiltration can be achieved (Fig. 15.16).

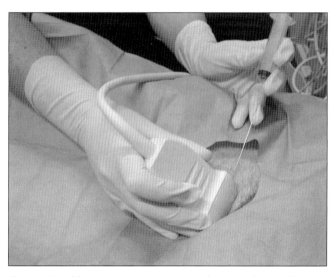

Fig. 15.16 Adductor origin injection can be carried out either from a transverse approach (shown here) or by aligning the probe along the tendon origin and puncturing from above. The axial approach allows the symphysis to be located and provides more recognisable anatomy if there is uncertainty.

The symphysis can be injected axially but a sagittal approach is easier. The puncture point is above the probe. Moving the probe from side to side helps to identify the surrounding bony landmarks and it becomes obvious when the probe is positioned directly above the symphysis. This technique is similar to that used to isolate the acromioclavicular joint. The patient should be warned that symphyseal injection can be painful.

KNEE JOINT ASPIRATION AND SYNOVIAL BIOPSY

Patient position

Injection or aspiration of the knee is best achieved with the patient supine and the knee slightly flexed to a position of comfort.

Needle and drugs

A reflective 21-G, spinal needle or similar, depending on the depth of the joint, and 40 mg triamcinolone mixed with 0.5% bupivacaine are used as a therapeutic injection. The knee joint can hold large amounts of fluid and over 50 ml can be injected with ease but this is rarely necessary.

Approach and puncture point

The suprapatellar pouch is the easiest area to access the distended knee joint. A sagitally orientated probe allows cannulation of the superolateral portion of the suprapatellar bursa. The puncture point is proximal (Fig. 15.17).

Target area

The area between the patella and the bony distal femur provides an excellent target area for small effusions. Larger effusions are straightforward.

As in the hips, synovial biopsy is a better means of determining the microbiological content of the septic implant when compared with simple fluid aspiration. In view of the relative thinness of the synovium, biopsy is best achieved by inserting the needle parallel to the area of

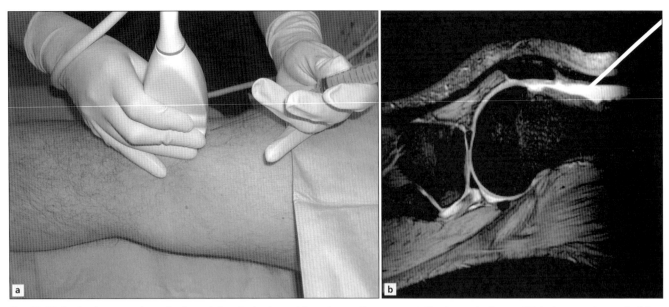

Fig. 15.17 Sagittal approach to the knee joint. Probe is positioned over the suprapatellar bursa in the sagittal plane as shown in (a). The puncture point is proximal and directed towards the distended bursa. (b) Corresponding sagittally orientated gradient echo image.

synovium to be biopsied. A slight vibration on the needle allows the specimen to imbed in the biopsy port prior to closure.

Other intra-articular lesions include ganglion cysts, including Hoffa's ganglion and cruciate ganglia. Hoffa's ganglia are aspirated from anterior with the needle inserted adjacent to the patellar tendon. A probe orientated in the axial plane overlying the patellar tendon provides good visualisation of Hoffa's fat pad. The needle can then be inserted medially or laterally, depending on the position of the ganglion. Cruciate ganglia are much more difficult to deal with. They require a posterior approach and, in view of their depth, visualisation in all but the slimmest individuals is difficult and it is difficult to be certain that aspiration has been completed. The outcome following cruciate ganglion aspiration/injection is variable as, in keeping with ganglia elsewhere, the fluid is often somewhat gelatinous and difficult to aspirate and even if aspiration is successful, they may recur.

Outside the joint interventional indications include peripatellar tendon injection for patellar tendinopathy and aspiration injection of the proximal tibiofibula joint.

PROXIMAL TIBIOFIBULAR JOINT

Patient position

Injection is best achieved with the patient in lateral decubitus with the affected knee upwards.

Needle and drugs

A 21-G green needle and 40 mg triamcinolone mixed with 0.5% bupivacaine are best used. The joint will generally accept 2–3 ml.

Approach and puncture point

An axial or parasagittal orientation to the probe posterolaterally identifies the superolateral aspect of the proximal tibiofibular joint. The puncture point is proximal to the probe (Fig. 15.18).

Target area

The needle is directed distally and into the soft-tissue triangle that directs the needle towards the upper aspect of the joint.

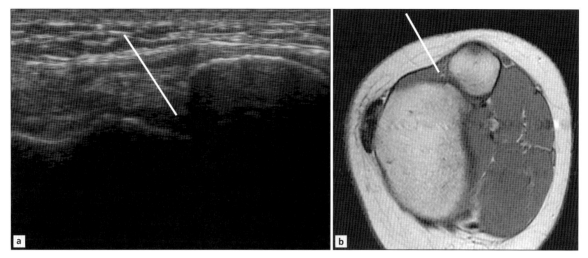

Fig. 15.18 (a) Axially orientated ultrasound image showing approach to proximal tibiofibular joint. (b) Corresponding axial T1-weighted image with needle direction *in situ*.

HINDFOOT INJECTIONS

The principle indications for interventional procedures in the hindfoot are for Achilles bursa injection, treatment of plantar fasciitis and occasionally distension of the Achilles paratenon. Peroneal and tibialis posterior tendon injections are technically similar to the tendon sheath injection described above.

Achilles bursa

Patient position

Injection is best achieved with the patient prone with feet extended over the end of the examination couch as per the Achilles examination.

Needle and drugs

A 21-G green needle and 30 mg Depo-Medrone® mixed with 0.5% bupivacaine. The bursa will easily accept 5 ml, but a large volume injection is not usually necessary.

Approach and puncture point

The Achilles bursa is best approached by a lateral puncture. The ultrasound probe is held in the axial plane placed directly over the Achilles tendon.

Target area

In this position an excellent view can be obtained of the needle approaching from the lateral side (Fig. 15.19). The puncture point should be kept low, particularly if the degree of bursal distension is relatively minor. Preliminary injection of a small quantity of local anaesthetic may be necessary to distend small bursa and confirm intrabursal positioning.

Paratenon injection

Patient position

The patient is best positioned prone as per examination of the Achilles tendon itself.

Needle and drugs

A 21-G green needle is suggested. Injection of the paratenon is somewhat controversial. Some authors advocate the use of relatively large volumes of either normal saline or local anaesthetic in order to disrupt adhesions that may have formed between the paratenon and the tendon itself. The inclusion of a corticosteroid preparation is thought to increase the risk of tendon rupture.

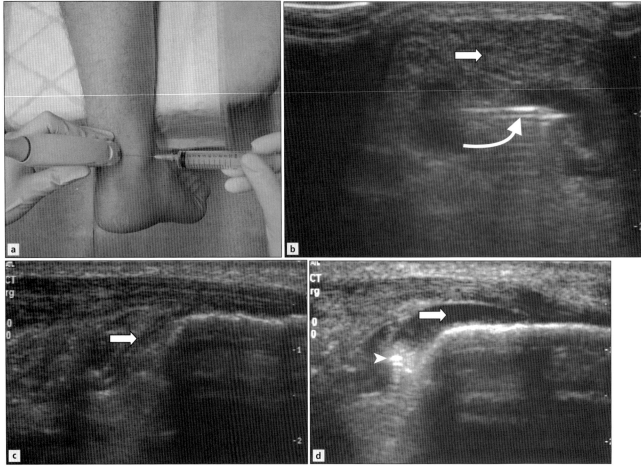

Fig. 15.19 Pre-Achilles bursa injection. (a) The probe is held axially with the lateral puncture. The puncture point should be sufficiently anterior to the tendon to avoid striking it. (b) Corresponding axial image showing transverse section through the Achilles tendon (arrow) with needle *in situ* in pre-Achilles bursa (curved arrow). (c) Long-axis view through tendon insertion showing a somewhat difficult to see pre-Achilles bursitis (arrow). (d) Corresponding image to (c) following injection. The needle is seen in transverse section (arrowhead) and the pre-Achilles bursa is now distended with poorly reflective fluid.

Approach and puncture point

A sagittally oriented probe is best. The puncture point is proximal.

Target area

The needle can be positioned on the dorsal aspect of the tendon sheath. Axial scanning can help to confirm that the tendon itself has not been breached.

Plantar fascia

Patient position

Injecting the plantar fascia is most commonly carried out with the patient prone with feet extended over the end of the couch as per the standard examination technique. A sagittal or axial approach is used in this position.

Needle and drugs

A 21-G green needle and 40 mg triamcinolone mixed with 0.5% bupivacaine. As much as 5 ml is ample to infiltrate the fascia.

Approach and puncture point

The probe is placed initially in a sagittal location overlying the abnormal fascia. Three injection techniques are possible. The most commonly described approach is to puncture the skin above the probe followed by a sagittal approach with

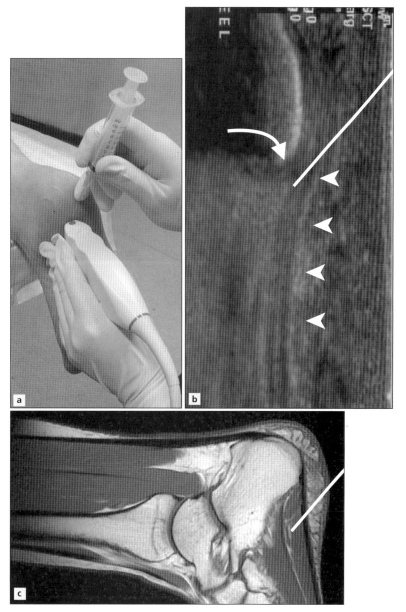

Fig. 15.20 (a) Standard position for plantar fascia injection. The probe is in sagittal plane with the patient prone as per standard fascia examination. The puncture point is proximal and directed towards the area lying between the fascia (arrowheads) and the os calcis (curved arrow). Note that this image is for demonstration purposes, as the fascia is normal. (c) Corresponding sagittal T1-weighted MRI image showing the needle approach.

the needle directed towards the fascial origin (Fig. 15.20). A puncture point should be chosen so that the needle can traverse the plantar fascia as it leaves its origin from os calcis and inject on its deep surface. The second approach is to puncture below the probe (Fig. 15.21). This has the advantage of allowing easier access to the deep aspect of the fascia and punctures through thinner and potentially less painful skin. Its main disadvantage is that needle and syringe manipulation is a little more awkward though with practice this is a very useful approach. A third method, and the authors preference, is to rotate the probe 90° to show the plantar fascia in axial section (Figs 15.22 and 15.23). A medial puncture point is chosen, the proximal distance of this point is dependent on heel pad thickness. Ideally, the puncture is at the same level as the plantar fascia. This allows easy access to both superficial and deep surfaces of the fascia.

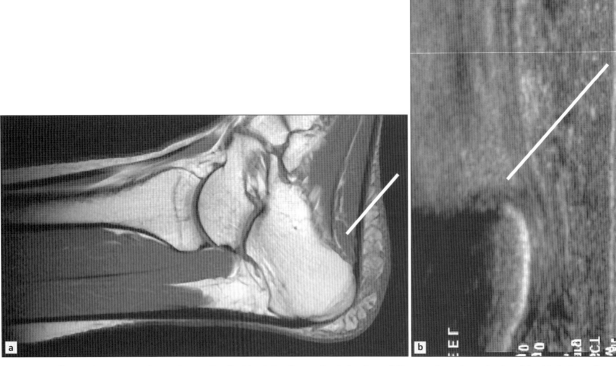

Fig. 15.21 Alternative approach to plantar fascia. The injection point is in the midfoot rather than the heel (a, b). It is easier to direct the needle towards the angle between the fascia and os calcis from this position. Its disadvantage is that the patient often must be turned from the prone examining position to supine in order to achieve access. This position can be used with the patient prone but it is a little more cumbersome.

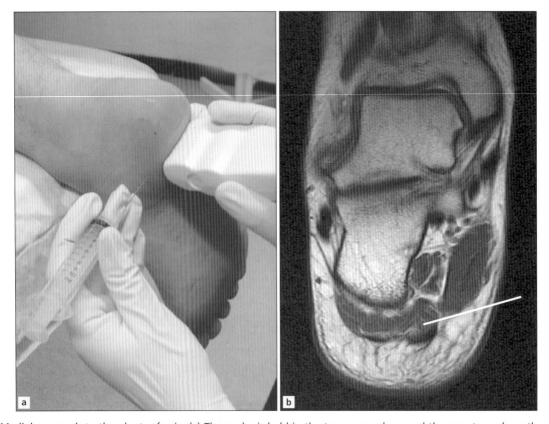

Fig. 15.22 Medial approach to the plantar fascia. (a) The probe is held in the transverse plane and the puncture along the medial aspect of the sole. Advantages are said to include a less painful injection but anatomical localisation is less familiar.

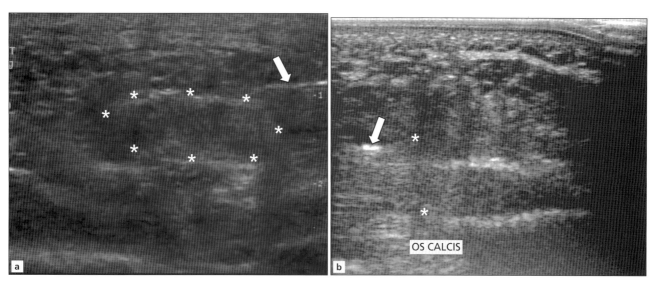

Fig. 15.23 (a) Axial image of thickened planatar fascia (between asterisks). A needle has been inserted on the medial aspect of the foot and advanced towards the fascia (arrow), aiming for its superficial surface as in sagittal image (b, arrow). Following superficial surface injection, the needle is withdrawn and manipulated to the deep surface where the injection is augmented.

Target area

The author prefers to inject both superficial and deep to the plantar fascia so the angle of approach should be carefully chosen as to allow this. Once the skin has been penetrated, passage to the plantar fascia is straightforward. The inferior surface (i.e. that first encounter) is infiltrated first before passing the needle distally to the fascia to infiltrate the deep surface.

MORTON'S NEUROMA INJECTION

Patient position

The patient is placed supine and the interdigital spaces are examined in the usual way.

Needle and drugs

A 21-G green needle and 40 mg triamcinolone mixed with 0.5% bupivacaine are best used. Only 1 ml is required to infiltrate the neuroma and bursa.

Approach and puncture point

Once the neuroma has been identified, several approaches to injection are possible. To approach from the plantar surface, a small mark is placed at the centre of the distal end of the probe between the toes on the involved interspace (Fig. 15.24) with the probe in the sagittal plane and clearly over the neuroma. To approach from the dorsal surface, pressure between the toes dorsally with the blunt end of a needle will indent the skin and show the optimal puncture point over the neuroma. The route chosen is a matter of personal preference. The dorsal route is through less thickened skin and may therefore be more comfortable for the patient. Needle visualisation is less good that the plantar approach, as the needle tip is perpendicular rather than parallel to the probe. The 2nd and 3rd toes may also lie very close together and may indeed overlap in some patients, making the dorsal approach difficult.

Target area

The needle is inserted firmly at the puncture point and along the line of the mark prior to anaesthetic being infiltrated. Following this, when the probe is placed in the sagittal position, it is usually seen that the needle lies close to the neuroma. It is then a straightforward matter to advance into the neuroma and inject it. Rotating 90° to show the needle within the interspace prior to injection is a useful confirmatory manoeuvre (Fig. 15.25).

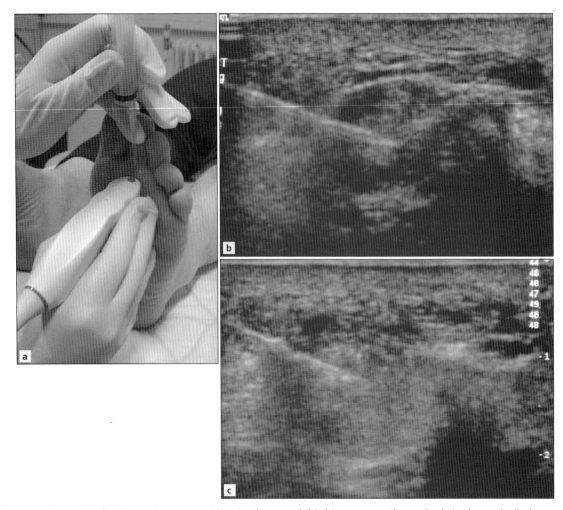

Fig. 15.24 (a) Puncture point for Morton's neuroma injection in second/third interspace. The probe is in the sagittal plane with the neuroma located within the interspace. The puncture point is on the plantar aspect of the foot distal to the probe as shown (b) schematically by the sagittal T1-weighted image. (c) Corresponding ultrasound image showing needle approaching neuroma.

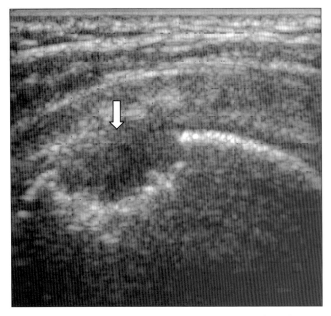

Fig. 15.25 "Cookie bite" in bone (arrow). Ultrasound can be used to guide bone biopsy if the surface is involved.

FOREIGN BODY LOCALISATION

Most superficial foreign bodies are easily located close to the entry point. Thorns, wood splinters and glass are readily seen on high-resolution ultrasound even if quite small. Unless there is a fibrous reaction around the foreign material (Fig. 15.26), ultrasound localisation can be followed by removal either by aspiration through a large bore needle or following a limited incision. For deeper or fibrosed FBs a mark can be placed on the skin overlying the lesion to guide surgical removal. Occasionally a sensation of foreign body implantation can persist following removal of the material. This may relate to haematoma or scar tissue formation along the track. In some patients, this sensation can lead to the firm belief that some material remains and ultrasound can provide reassurance on this. The author has found that placing a small-bore plastic

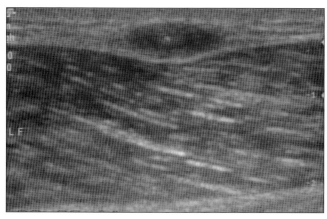

Fig. 15.26 Sagittal sonogram of thigh with implanted wood splinter that has formed a fibrous reaction.

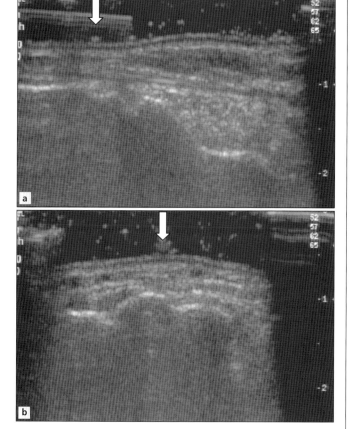

Fig. 15.27 (a) Sagittal and (b) axial of patient convinced of the presence of retained foreign material. A small plastic canula has been placed over the puncture point (arrows) to reassure that the underlying tissues are normal.

cannula embedded in a pool of coupling gel can provide the additional reassurance needed as the patient can see the tiny cannula over the skin clearly, yet no material within the soft tissues (Fig. 15.27).

SOFT-TISSUE AND BONE BIOPSY

The techniques for the ultrasound-guided biopsy of soft-tissue masses is well described in the radiological literature. The most important aspect from the perspective of musculoskeletal soft-tissue tumours is to ensure that the biopsy track is in a position that can be excised during the subsequent surgical treatment of the soft-tissue tumour. Equally important is to ensure that the track chosen does not traverse another limb compartment as this would adversely alter the staging and potentially the prognosis of a malignant lesion. Using ultrasound to guide a soft-tissue biopsy allows the core to be taken from the more solid or aggressive elements of a soft-tissue tumour and away from the more liquid or necrotic areas, which may be less likely to yield diagnostic material.

Biopsy of bone tumours has traditionally been the remit of fluoroscopic or CT control; however, for lesions that disrupt the cortex, ultrasound offers some advantages. In particular, it can demonstrate where cortical breach is maximal and hence transcortical biopsy will be easiest (Fig. 15.25). This can sometimes be difficult to determine on fluoroscopy. In the author's experience ultrasound-guided bone biopsies also tend to be quicker than fluoroscopic procedures although they cannot be applied in all cases. Bone lesions without cortical breach or those where the biopsy is directed at a more aggressive portion of the interosseous lesion, which cannot be visualised on ultrasound, are less successful.

Ultrasound of groin injury

16

Philip Robinson

INTRODUCTION

The clinical role of ultrasound in the assessment of patients with groin pain has yet to be fully established. This technique has great potential in a number of conditions; however, as with other areas of the body, the examiner must be aware of its strengths and limitations especially in the assessment of athletes.

Commoner causes of groin discomfort in the general population include inguinal hernias and muscle strains in the lower abdominal wall and upper thigh. Muscular strains in this group of patients often do not present to a primary care physician and certainly further management in the form of imaging is not necessary. The majority of symptomatic inguinal hernias can also be diagnosed clinically but there is a potential role for imaging in equivocal cases as there are well-recognised limitations to clinical assessment (1, 2).

The situation in the professional athlete is more controversial with a number of aetiologies for chronic groin pain described (2–10). Especially in the case of osteitis pubis, adductor dysfunction and the prehernia complex (or sportsman's hernia) research has been relatively anecdotal, describing a number of differing pathologies and treatments (2–12). Review of this literature and its relative strengths and weaknesses is not within the remit of this book. The following chapter will concentrate on the use of ultrasound for assessing patients with groin pain.

Although there are a large number of pathologies that can cause groin pain, including infection, neuralgia or tumour (2, 4, 5, 13, 14), the following discussion will focus on inguinofemoral hernias and muscular strain.

ANATOMICAL BOUNDARIES

For descriptive purposes the groin will be defined as the soft tissues of the inguinofemoral region between the anterior superior iliac spine and symphysis pubis, involving the upper thigh and inferior abdominal wall. Soft-tissue structures include the skin, superficial fat and fascia, musculature, extra peritoneal (preperitoneal) fat and the peritoneum (15, 16).

INGUINAL CANAL

Normal anatomy

The inguinal canal allows the passage of vessels, nerves, lymphatics and the spermatic cord (round ligament in females) from within the abdomen to the external genitalia (15, 16). The posterior wall of the canal is formed by the muscle, aponeurosis and fascia of transversus abdominis and also part of the internal oblique. The anterior wall is formed from the fascia of the external oblique muscle (Fig. 16.1) (15, 16). The deep (internal) inguinal ring is a defect within the transversus abdominis fascia that allows the contents of the inguinal canal to leave the abdomen and enter the canal proper (15, 16). The canal then extends obliquely, medially and inferiorly towards the

pubic crest where the superficial (external) inguinal ring, a defect in the external oblique fascia, allows the contents to leave the canal (Fig. 16.2) (15, 16). Superficial to the canal is subcutaneous fat and skin, whereas deep to the canal passes the iliopsoas muscle on its medial aspect and the external iliac vessels pass on the lateral aspect (as they enter the thigh) (15, 16). The peritoneum and small bowel lie posterosuperiorly (Fig. 16.1).

Important landmarks include the inferior epigastric vessels, which arise from the external iliac vessels and course superiorly to lie deep to the rectus abdominis (Fig. 16.3) (15, 16). Just after their origin from the external iliac vessels they lie

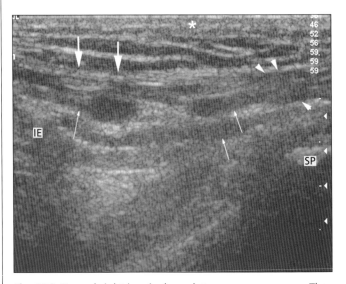

Fig. 16.2 Normal right inguinal canal, transverse sonogram. The inferior epigastric vessels (IE) lie medial to the internal ring. The thick echogenic inguinal ligament (large arrows) lies anteriorly, deep to the subcutaneous fat (*). Multiple tubular structures are seen (small arrows) passing medially towards the symphysis pubis (SP) and passing through the external ring where a defect (arrowheads) in the inguinal ligament can be visualised.

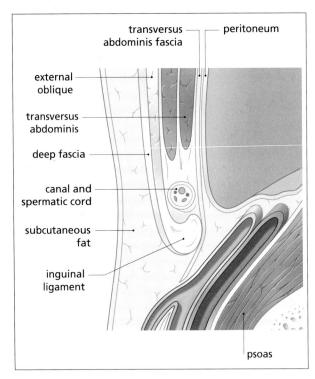

Fig. 16.1 Line drawing of a sagittal section through the lower oblique muscles and inguinal canal. The oblique muscles with external oblique anteriorly and transversus abdominis posteriorly lie superior to the canal and spermatic cord (*). The subcutaneous fat and deep fascia lie anterior and blend with the external oblique fascia, which inferiorly forms the inguinal ligament. The psoas muscle and femoral vessels run deep to the canal with the transversus abdominis fascia and peritoneum lying posteriorly and superiorly.

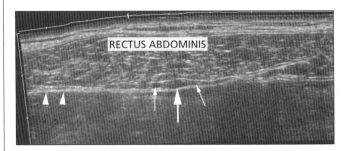

Fig. 16.3 Normal inferior epigastric vessels, transverse sonogram, lower abdomen. Normal appearances of rectus abdominis with its thick investing fascia (arrowheads). The inferior epigastric artery (large arrow) and veins (small arrows) can be seen deep to the muscle but still within the investing fascia.

immediately medial to the deep inguinal ring. Therefore if a hernia arises lateral to these vessels, it is indirect (passing through the internal ring) but if it arises medial to the vessels it is a direct hernia (bulging through the posterior wall) (17).

Examination technique and normal ultrasound appearances

It is important to identify the deep inguinal ring when assessing for inguinal hernias. The author has two main methods of visualising the epigastric vessels and thus obtaining his landmark for assessing the deep ring on dynamic examination. The first method is to scan the rectus abdominis muscle transversely and identify the inferior epigastric vessels within the rectus sheath on its deep aspect (Fig. 16.3). By continuous scanning in the transverse plane the vessels can be followed inferiorly as they sweep to join the external iliac vessels. However, in obese patients with lax musculature, although it is relatively easy to identify the vessels deep to the rectus abdominis, it is difficult to continuously follow them because of the patient's body habitus. Therefore another technique is to scan the femoral vessels in the transverse plane and move cranially until the epigastric vessels are seen at their origin and are beginning to pass medially. However, at this point, because the

actual course of the inguinal canal is in the transverse oblique plane the transducer should also be obliqued by rotating the medial aspect of the transducer inferiorly.

In this position a longitudinal image of the canal is obtained, which includes the epigastric vessels, femoral vessels and proximal inguinal canal. The inguinal ligament is seen as an echogenic line deep to the subcutaneous fat blending with the deep fascia (Figs 16.2 and 16.4) (15, 16, 18). Deep to the ligament are multiple hyperechoic and hypoechoic linear structures (representing vessels, nerves and cords) within the canal. Their prominence is variable and they pass medially to exit the canal through the external ring (seen as a defect of the inguinal ligament) (Figs 16.2 and 16.4). Deep to the canal lies the psoas muscle but echogenic peritoneum and hypoechoic bowel (and a varying amount of preperitoneal fat) lie posterosuperiorly (Figs 16.1 and 16.5).

Assessment of this area with the patient at rest and straining (performing a slow Valsalva manoeuvre) is now performed. Normally mild bulging of the posterior wall and peritoneum can be found but it should not occlude the canal (please see later) (Fig. 16.4). Occasionally the venous structures within the canal can also distend but again this is quite variable. It is important to instruct the patient to perform the Valsalva manoeuvre slowly (i.e. not cough) and to ensure that transducer pressure is not applied too firmly; otherwise, any potential hernia will be maintained in reduction.

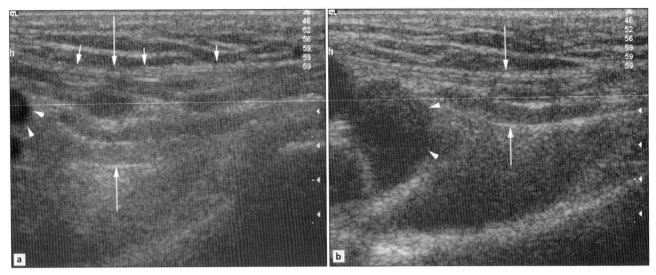

Fig. 16.4 Normal right inguinal canal, transverse sonograms. (a) At rest the femoral and inferior epigastric vessels can be seen (arrowheads) at the medial aspect of the canal. Multiple tubular structures are seen traversing the canal deep to the inguinal ligament (short arrows). Note the anteroposterior dimension of the canal (long arrows). (b) On straining there is marked distension of the vessels (arrowheads) at the medial aspect of the canal, a narrowing of the canal anteroposteriorly (long arrows) but no alteration in the contents of the canal itself.

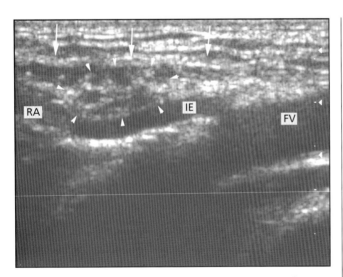

Fig. 16.5 Normal left inguinal canal, sagittal sonogram. This image was obtained at the level of the inferior epigastric vein (IE) as it arises from the femoral vein (FV). The inguinal canal can be seen as an oval-shaped soft-tissue area containing multiple tubular structures (arrowheads). The inguinal ligament and muscular fascia (arrows) can be seen anterior to the canal with rectus abdominis (RA) lying superiorly.

The canal should then be assessed in its short axis, which is the anatomical sagittal plane (Fig. 16.1) (15, 16, 19). To obtain this view scan the external iliac/femoral vessels longitudinally and move the transducer medially to view the inferior epigastric vessels as they arise and begin to pass superiorly towards rectus abdominis (Fig. 16.5). At this point the transducer should be moved slightly more medially to come off the epigastric vessels. The short axis of the inguinal canal with its hypoechoic tubular contents can now be visualised with peritoneum and bowel posterosuperiorly (Fig. 16.6). On straining in a normal subject, there may be slight dilatation of the vessels within the canal and bowel should move towards the canal but should not completely efface or enter the canal (Fig. 16.6).

Practical tip

To assess the inguinal canal along its short axis, identify the origin of the inferior epigastric vessels in long axis and move the probe slightly more medially.

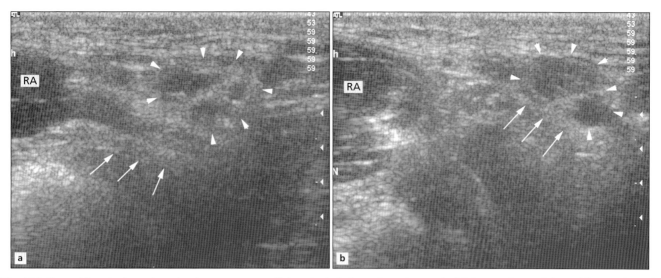

Fig. 16.6 Normal inguinal canal, sagittal sonograms medial to the inferior epigastric vessels. (a) At rest the oval-shaped inguinal canal can be seen (arrowheads) with rectus abdominis (RA) lying superiorly. Posterosuperiorly lies the echogenic peritoneum and bowel (small arrows). (b) On straining the echogenic peritoneum and hypoechoic bowel push inferiorly and anteriorly (arrows) approaching the inguinal canal. The overall canal shape is maintained with distension of the vessels within it (arrowheads). Note also the contraction of rectus abdominis (RA) on straining.

Ultrasound appearance of inguinal hernias

> **Key point**
>
> Indirect hernias protrude through the internal inguinal ring and extend along the inguinal canal parallel to its long axis.

Indirect hernias protrude through the internal inguinal ring and extend along the inguinal canal parallel to its long axis (1, 17). The hernia usually consists of peritoneum, fat and bowel. Occasionally the hernia can be congenital due to a persistent processus vaginalis; however, it should be noted that this can be an incidental finding with the condition persisting in 29% of adults (20, 21).

Direct inguinal hernias occur due to a weakness in the posterior inguinal wall within the transversus abdominis fascia, allowing protrusion of peritoneum and bowel through the wall into the inguinal canal (1, 22, 23). Because of this the hernia rarely continues distally along the inguinal canal itself and is more localised in comparison to indirect hernias (1, 22, 23).

On ultrasound the appearance of the normal inguinal contents can be variable and, unless there is a large irreducible hernia present, it is difficult to determine a small hernia within the canal on static imaging. It is during the dynamic component of the examination that the hernia sac and its contents can be observed moving into the canal and reducing (partially or completely) on rest with transducer pressure.

> **Key point**
>
> During the dynamic component of the examination the hernia sac and its contents can be observed moving into the canal and reducing (partially or completely) on rest with transducer pressure.

In the transverse plane an indirect hernia arises lateral to the epigastric vessels and extends through the long axis of the canal (Fig. 16.7). When scanning sagittally (short axis of the canal) the indirect hernia can be seen distending the canal and effacing its contents (Fig. 16.8).

In the transverse plane a direct hernia will protrude through the posterior canal wall medial to the epigastric vessels (Fig. 16.9). In the sagittal plane (short axis of the canal) the direct hernia will push into the canal from the posterior and superior aspects and efface its contents (Fig. 16.10).

The contents of any hernia have a similar appearance on ultrasound with a relatively hyperechoic margin of the peritoneum and hypoechoic bowel contents (predominantly fluid and gas) (Fig. 16.10). If the hernia is a persistent processus vaginalis it will appear similar to peritoneum with two opposing echogenic layers

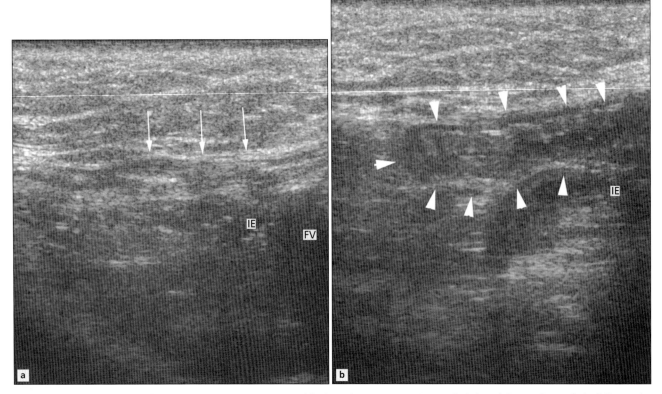

Fig. 16.7 Left indirect inguinal hernia, transverse sonograms. (a) The inferior epigastric vessels (IE) and femoral vessels (FV) lie on the medial aspect of the canal, marking the internal inguinal ring. The inguinal ligament is seen as a condensation of the echogenic fascia (arrows), but it is difficult to clearly visualise the tubular structures within the canal in this particular patient. (b) On straining there is marked distension of the canal by hypoechoic bowel and echogenic peritoneum (arrowheads) arising lateral to the inferior epigastric vessels (IE) and pushing along the canal.

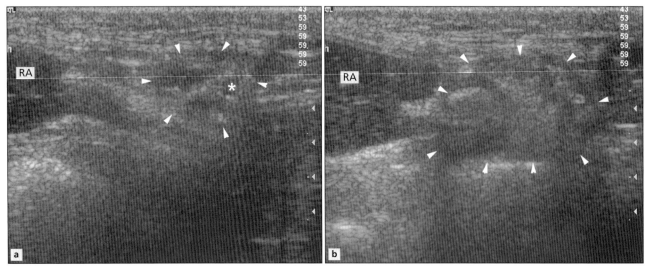

Fig. 16.8 Right indirect inguinal hernia, sagittal sonograms. (a) At rest the normal inguinal canal is visualised (arrowheads) containing tubular structures (*). (b) On straining there is marked distension of the canal with obliteration of the normal contents by bowel (arrowheads).

seen sliding over each other on straining (20, 24). Occasionally preperitoneal fat will also herniate into the canal, appearing more homogenous and hyperechoic than bowel and sometimes moving with the bowel and peritoneum (Fig. 16.11) (25).

Careful note should also be made on scanning in either plane for other less-common inguinal abnormalities, e.g. lipoma, haematoma, lymph node or undescended testicle (25, 26) (Figs 16.11 and 16.12).

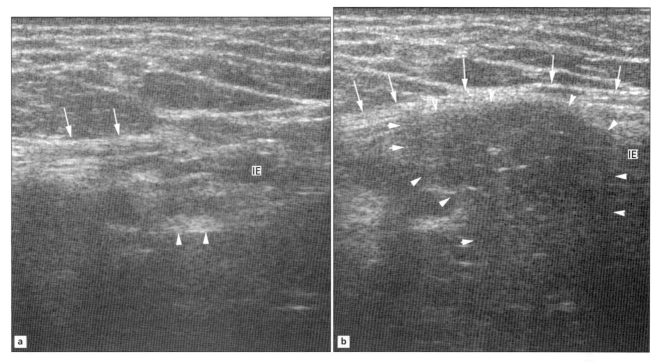

Fig. 16.9 Left direct hernia, transverse sonograms. (a) At rest the inferior epigastric vessels (IE) are seen on the medial aspect of the canal with the echogenic inguinal ligament (arrows) lying anteriorly and echogenic peritoneum lying posteriorly (arrowheads). (b) On straining there is anterior displacement of the inguinal ligament (arrows) by a predominantly hypoechoic loop of bowel (arrowheads) pushing through the posterior wall medial to the epigastric vessels (IE).

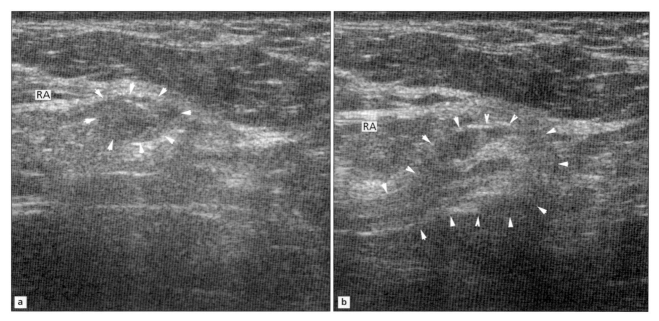

Fig. 16.10 Left direct hernia, sagittal sonograms. (a) At rest the normal inguinal canal can be seen (arrowheads). Note fatty atrophy of rectus abdominis (RA). (b) On straining, bowel can be seen entering and effacing the canal (arrowheads) from the posterosuperior aspect, consistent with a direct hernia.

A diagnostic problem arises in cases where the posterior inguinal wall almost occludes the canal on straining but no actual herniation occurs. Some authors have advocated this may represent the prehernia complex or sportsman's hernia.

One study has described this feature in nine athletes with groin pain who subsequently underwent posterior wall strengthening surgery (19). However, postsurgery six of the nine patients were rescanned and four still had similar

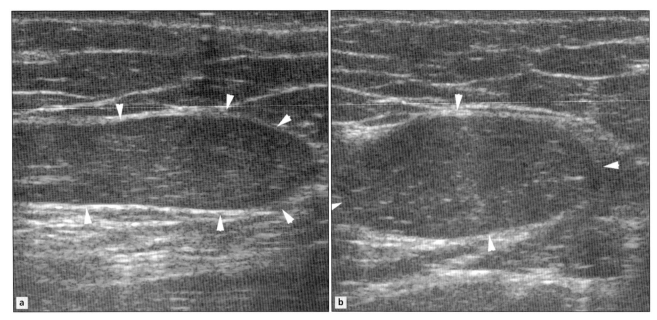

Fig. 16.11 Indirect hernia due to a preperitoneal lipoma. (a) Transverse sonogram shows a well-defined homogenous hyperechoic mass extending along the inguinal canal (arrowheads), consistent with a lipoma. (b) Sagittal sonogram confirms the homogenous hyperechoic mass filling the inguinal canal and effacing its contents (arrowheads).

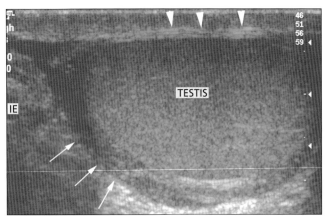

Fig. 16.12 Right inguinal mass, transverse sonogram. A well-defined oval homogenous soft-tissue mass lies medial to the inferior epigastric vessels (IE) and is surrounded by hypoechoic fluid. The inguinal ligament can be seen anteriorly (large arrowheads). The features on ultrasound were consistent with an undescended testicle and this was confirmed at surgery.

marked posterior wall bulging despite being asymptomatic. The three other patients (who were not rescanned) were still symptomatic after posterior wall surgery and underwent further adductor surgery or nerve block (19). Obviously this area requires further evaluation, but it is best only to comment on wall bulging when it occurs on the symptomatic side and is asymmetrical with the asymptomatic side.

Postoperative evaluation

There are a number of surgical procedures described for hernia repair but all involve reduction of the hernia and then correction of the defect by oversewing or mesh insertion (17, 27, 28). When a mass recurs after surgical repair ultrasound can help differentiate between recurrent hernia and a static haematoma or seroma (Fig. 16.13) (24). If a mesh is used to repair the hernia, it is usually situated around the internal inguinal ring or posterior wall, depending on the type of hernia repaired. The metallic mesh can be visualised as a hyperechoic linear structure just adjacent to the epigastric vessels (Fig. 16.14) (24). Occasionally after operative repair of indirect hernias the peritoneum can still be seen herniating into the canal although the repair is sufficient to prevent bowel herniation. This is because the peritoneal sac is often left intact to reduce any trauma to the spermatic vessels during surgery (17, 24, 27, 28). Patients can also develop a preperitoneal lipoma within the canal, which does show some movement on straining but is usually differentiated from a recurrent hernia by the fact that it is more homogeneous with increased echotexture (Fig. 16.15) (24, 25). Neuralgia is another relatively common postoperative complication (2%) but in this instance ultrasound

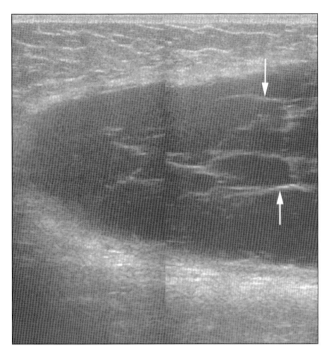

Fig. 16.13 Increasing right iliac fossa soft-tissue mass 14 days after hernia repair, transverse sonogram. A well-defined mass with a hyperechoic margin, complex hypoechoic contents and septa (arrows), consistent with a complex seroma.

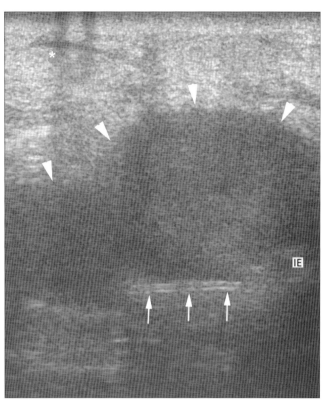

Fig. 16.14 Left inguinal mass after direct hernia repair, transverse sonogram. A well-defined hyperechoic linear structure (arrows) lies medial to the inferior epigastric vessels (IE). This has the typical appearance of a mesh and is placed over the posterior inguinal wall. However, filling the canal is a lobulated, predominantly hypoechoic soft-tissue mass consistent with a postoperative haematoma. Oedema of the subcutaneous fat is also noted (*).

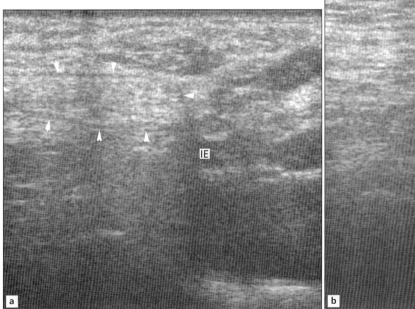

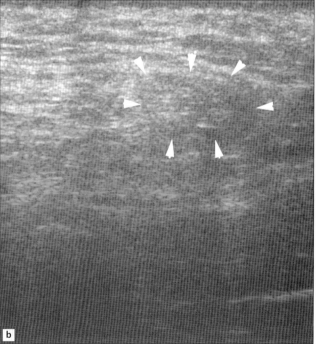

Fig. 16.15 Palpable mass after left indirect hernia repair. (a) Transverse sonogram shows a well-defined and homogeneous hyperechoic soft-tissue mass within the canal medial to the inferior epigastric vessels (IE). Features are consistent with a lipoma. (b) Sagittal sonogram confirms the hyperechoic lipoma filling the inguinal canal.

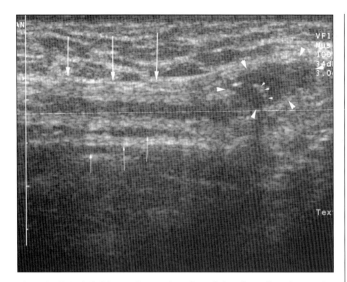

Fig. 16.16 Painful lump 8 months after right direct hernia repair, transverse sonogram. The tubular contents of the inguinal canal can be seen (small arrows) with the inguinal ligament anteriorly (large arrows). The medial aspect of the ligament is displaced anteriorly by a hypoechoic mass (large arrowheads) containing a small linear hyperechoic structure (small arrowheads). This small linear structure had the appearance of a foreign body and was confirmed to be a stitch granuloma at surgery.

is usually normal; however, postsurgical neuromas and stitch granulomas have been described (Fig. 16.16) (17, 24).

Evaluation by other imaging techniques

Although ultrasound has been found to be an accurate technique for detecting hernias already evident on clinical examination (18, 20, 29–31), there has been no evaluation in equivocal cases, which potentially is where its clinical role lies.

Herniography has been extensively evaluated in patients with equivocal clinical features and has been shown to be a very sensitive but relatively nonspecific technique demonstrating a large number of asymptomatic hernias (22, 23, 32–41). Although herniography has been shown to have a low complication rate the procedure is still invasive and requires ionising radiation (23, 42, 43).

The use of MR imaging in evaluating inguinal hernias has only been described in a limited number of studies (31, 44) with one series comparing the accuracy of MR imaging with ultrasound and clinical examination (31). The MR imaging technique described involved rapid acquisition of coronal images while the patient performed a Valsalva manoeuvre. Although accurate (sensitivity 94% and specificity 96%), the majority of the hernias were clinically evident and differentiation between direct and indirect hernias was not always possible. In this study ultrasound was found to be equally sensitive to MR imaging (94%) (both greater than clinical examination, 74%) but the significance of the additional subclinical hernias detected was not discussed. Ultrasound was found to be less specific (81%) than clinical examination (96%) or MR imaging (96%); however, the authors erroneously recorded posterior wall bulging as actual herniation. Further research is necessary to evaluate these techniques in patients with equivocal clinical features.

FEMORAL HERNIA

The femoral canal is a largely potential space containing fat and lymph nodes that lies medial to the femoral vein just distal to the inguinal ligament (15, 16).

Femoral hernias are relatively infrequent in male patients and are commoner in middle-aged female patients (45). Pathologically the hernia sac passes from the abdomen deep to the inguinal canal and into the femoral canal. Quite commonly bowel does not completely enter the canal but pushes preperitoneal fat into it.

The femoral canal is located by scanning the femoral vessels in the transverse plane. Just below the inguinal canal the femoral canal lies immediately medial to the femoral vein (Fig. 16.17) (46, 47). The patient is then asked to perform a Valsalva manoeuvre and the femoral vein and canal assessed. Normally the femoral vein should distend with no distortion of the adjacent tissues (Fig. 16.17). This expansion of the vein into the potential space of the adjacent femoral canal implies there is no mass effect from within the canal itself (46).

A femoral hernia expands the canal, compressing or preventing the normal expansion of the femoral vein (Fig. 16.18). When this appearance is noted, the hernia should be confirmed by scanning over the canal in the longitudinal plane. This can be achieved by obtaining a longitudinal image of the femoral vein and then moving the transducer medially. When the Valsalva manoeuvre is performed,

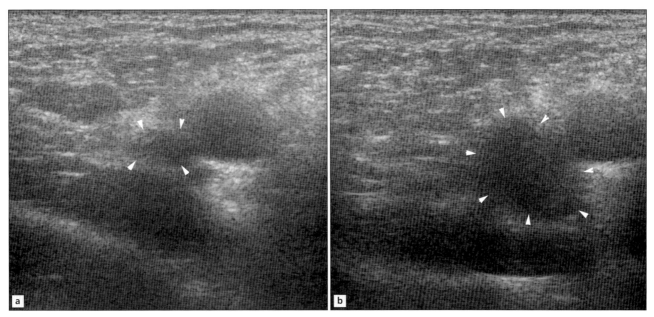

Fig. 16.17 Normal left femoral canal, transverse sonograms. (a) At rest the femoral vein is not distended (arrowheads). (b) On straining there is marked distension of the vein (arrowheads) with no hernia evident in the femoral canal.

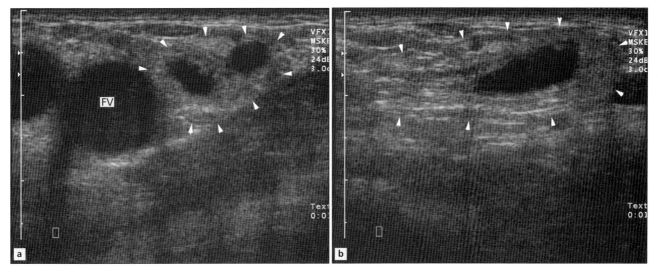

Fig. 16.18 Right femoral hernia. (a) Transverse sonogram on straining. A hernia of fat, bowel and fluid is present (arrowheads) within the femoral canal medial to the femoral vein (FV). (b) Longitudinal sonogram medial to the femoral vein. The femoral hernia (arrowheads) can be seen extending from the abdomen into the canal.

bowel and peritoneum can be seen extending inferiorly into the canal (Fig. 16.18).

Practical tip

Failure of the femoral vein to distend during valsalva is a sign of a femoral hernia or other local space occupying lesion.

ABDOMINAL MUSCLES

The musculature of the lower abdominal wall includes the external oblique, internal oblique, transversus abdominis and rectus abdominis muscles (15, 16). As previously discussed, these muscles have a postural function with a linear configuration that predominantly consists of type T1 fibres (see Chapter 12). The rectus abdominis lies either side of the midline raphe, running inferiorly to blend with the superior aspect of the symphysis pubis and the adductor musculature. The other abdominal muscles form three layers at the lateral margin of the rectus abdominis with external oblique outermost, internal oblique and then transversus abdominis lying innermost (Fig. 16.19) (15, 16). Tears of these muscles are relatively rare except in athletes where rectus abdominis is the most commonly affected (especially in weightlifters and gymnasts) (48). Haematomas can form after trauma, surgery or spontaneously in patients taking anticoagulants. However, abdominal wall hernias are not uncommon (see next section).

The easiest way to examine this group of muscles is to scan transversely in the midline, locating rectus abdominis and then moving laterally to the oblique abdominal muscles (Fig. 16.19). On ultrasound this muscle group has the appearance of any other skeletal muscle (please see Chapter 12). The rectus sheath is visualised as thick echogenic fascia, which blends with the investing fascia of the oblique muscles (Figs 16.3 and 16.19). Once the anatomy of these muscles has been defined, the position of any pathology can be identified.

Abdominal wall hernias

Apart from inguinofemoral hernias there are three other types of abdominal wall hernia: Spigelian, incisional and umbilical (45, 49–51). All three types of hernia involve protrusion of at least peritoneum and preperitoneal fat through a defect in the abdominal wall musculature and fascia (45).

Spigelian hernias occur through a weakness of the lateral rectus abdominis sheath at its margin with the oblique muscles (linea semilunaris) at the point where the inferior epigastric vessels penetrate the rectus sheath. Incisional hernias arise from muscular weakness due to previous surgery and resulting scar tissue (Fig. 16.20). This is a common clinical problem with an estimated 10% of all hernia operations being for repair of this type of hernia (45). Umbilical hernias present in the midline and can be congenital but usually occur in patients who are overweight or have marked abdominal distension due to ascites (45).

For all these conditions the area to be evaluated can be confirmed on taking a history. The role of ultrasound is to confirm the contents of the hernia (fat and/or bowel) and determine the size of the fascial defect (Fig. 16.20).

SYMPHYSIS PUBIS

The symphysis pubis is a fibrocartilaginous joint of the anterior pelvis and is also the confluence for the thigh adductors, rectus abdominis and the medial aspect of the inguinal ligament (15, 16, 25).

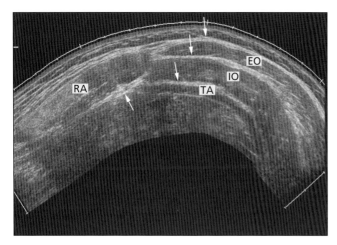

Fig. 16.19 Normal abdominal muscles, extended field-of-view (SieScape) transverse sonogram. Rectus abdominis (RA) can be seen medially with the oblique muscles lying laterally (external oblique (EO), internal oblique (IO) and transversus abdominis (TA)). Note the thick continuous investing fascia (arrows).

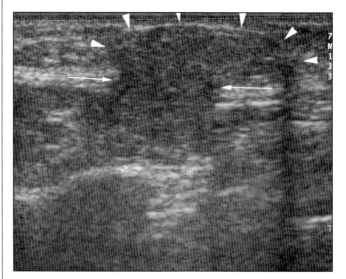

Fig. 16.20 Incisional hernia, sagittal sonogram. Cholecystectomy performed 8 months previously. A defect in the deep fascia (arrows) can be seen with a homogenous protrusion of soft tissue (arrowheads) extending into the subcutaneous fat. Although hypoechoic compared to the subcutaneous fat, no bowel could be demonstrated during scanning and features were consistent with a protrusion of preperitoneal fat.

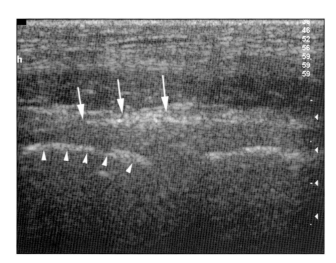

Fig. 16.21 Normal symphysis pubis, transverse sonogram. The echogenic cortical margin of the pubic body (arrowheads) can be seen. The overlying capsule with its echogenic margin (arrows) is also identified.

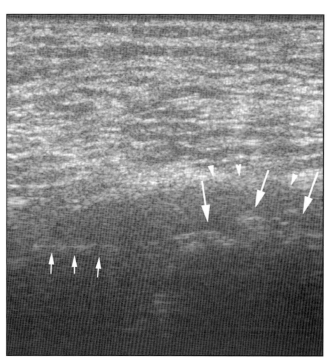

Fig. 16.22 Chronic degeneration of the left pubic body, transverse sonogram. The articular irregularity of the left pubic cortex can be seen (large arrows) compared to the relatively normal right side (small arrows). There is some displacement of the capsular tissues (arrowheads).

The symphysis pubis can be visualised on ultrasound by placing the transducer over the joint after direct palpation or by scanning the rectus abdominis transversally and moving inferiorly to the joint. Only the superior and anterior aspect of the joint can be visualised by ultrasound (52). The joint margin is seen as the echogenic pubic cortex with the echo-poor joint space in between (Fig. 16.21). A faint echogenic line representing the capsular margin and superior pubic ligament spans the joint with the fibrocartilaginous disc occasionally seen within the joint as an echogenic stripe (16).

Chronic degeneration and irregularity of the symphysis pubis is commonly seen in the elderly population, postpartum women and professional athletes (Fig. 16.22) (2, 8, 13, 53, 54). Joint margin irregularity can also occur secondary to chronic enthesopathic change of the adductor tendons or with more acute inflammatory joint conditions (e.g. fracture or osteomyelitis) (13, 14). Osteitis pubis is an acute noninfectious inflammatory condition of the joint characterised by joint and enthesopathic inflammation, which are presumed to be mechanical in origin (2, 55). It is most commonly seen in athletes and is usually self-limiting (over 3–6 months) with active rehabilitation (2, 13, 55, 56).

Symphyseal articular irregularity is seen on ultrasound as an irregular echogenic pubic cortex with, if a joint effusion is present, hypoechoic fluid displacing the capsular margin (Fig. 16.22).

Unfortunately, as mentioned previously, this appearance is nonspecific and these findings must always be correlated with the clinical examination and history. If osteitis pubis, stress fracture or infection is suspected clinically MR imaging is usually more sensitive and specific than ultrasound. However, ultrasound-guided needle placement is valuable in performing joint aspiration in infection or therapeutic injection in osteitis pubis (54, 55, 57).

ADDUCTOR MUSCLES

Normal anatomy and examination technique

The thigh adductor muscle group consists of adductor longus, brevis and magnus as well as gracilis. These muscles originate from the pubic body and inferior pubic ramus and pass distally to the femur and tibia (Fig. 16.23) (15, 16). Their main action is thigh adduction with some hip flexion and are functionally important in sports where frequent changes of direction are required (e.g. soccer, ice hockey, fencing, Australian-rules football) (2, 5, 58–60).

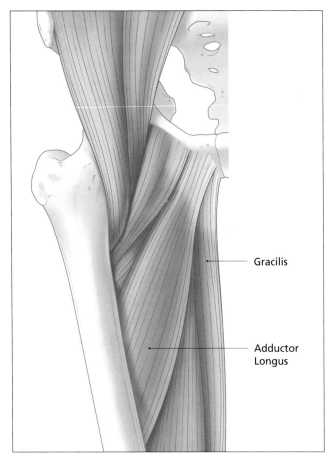

Fig. 16.23 Line drawing of the normal thigh musculature. Adductor longus (AL) is the most superficial muscle extending from the pubic body towards the femur. Gracilis (Gr) can be seen to originate posterior and medial to the adductor longus.

Gracilis

Adductor Longus

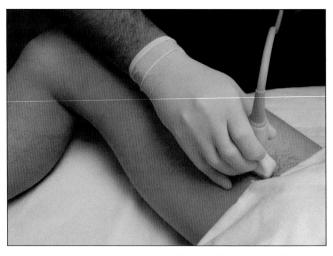

Fig. 16.24 Examination technique for visualising the adductor longus. The optimal position to examine the adductor longus is with the thigh flexed and externally rotated and the knee flexed. The transducer is then placed on the most prominent muscle (adductor longus).

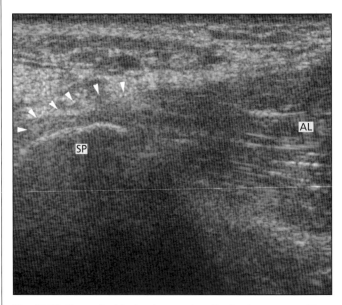

Fig. 16.25 Normal adductor longus, longitudinal sonogram. The normal muscle (AL) and tendon (arrowheads) can be seen originating from the symphysis pubis (SP).

Practical tip

The adductor muscles are best visualised as they originate from the pubis and inferior pubic ramus with the thigh in abduction and external rotation and the knee flexed.

The adductor muscles are best visualised as they originate from the pubis and inferior pubic ramus with the thigh in abduction and external rotation and the knee flexed (Fig. 16.24). In this position adductor longus is the most prominent muscle and is easily palpable. On palpating the muscle the transducer can be placed on its longitudinal axis and moved obliquely along this plane towards the symphysis pubis, following the muscle through the myotendinous junction to its tendon and origin at the body of the pubis (Figs 16.23 and 16.25) (61). Moving medially and posteriorly the other adductor

muscles (brevis and magnus) and gracilis can be visualised. It should be noted that adductor brevis usually has a limited proximal tendon and the muscle appears to originate directly from the bone. The normal ultrasound appearances of muscle and tendon have already been described (see Chapters 2 and 15).

Adductor muscle injury

In the general population serious adductor muscle injuries or chronic symptoms are relatively rare. Acute injuries usually occur in the younger population and athletes when the leg undergoes forced abduction (2). The adductor longus is the most commonly injured muscle in the adductor group (2, 13, 61–63). Acute injury in a normal muscle results in a muscle strain or tear at the distal myotendinous junction although proximal rupture is more common in mature athletes due to proximal tendinopathy further weakening the myotendinous junction (48) (Fig. 16.26).

This group of muscles are a common chronic problem especially in soccer where there is repetitive kicking and frequent forceful changes of direction (2, 13, 62). Chronic tendinopathy especially of the proximal adductor longus is common in many athletes (professional and recreational) and is often relatively asymptomatic (Fig. 16.27) (2, 13). Acute injuries in this group of patients can result in avulsion or disruption of the prematurely degenerate proximal tendon rather than a purely muscular tear (Fig. 16.28). However, the main clinical difficulty is defining whether chronic groin pain in athletes is due to adductor tendinopathy/dysfunction, osteitis pubis or a prehernia complex. All these

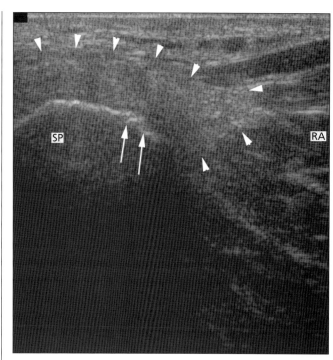

Fig. 16.27 Chronic adductor longus tendinopathy, longitudinal sonogram. The adductor longus tendon (AL) is homogenously hyperechoic with loss of definition of its tissue planes extending towards the myotendinous junction (arrowheads). There is some mild underlying irregularity of the pubis (small arrows). In comparison to Fig. 16.30, the tendon is less swollen and was asymptomatic. SP = symphysis pubis.

conditions can present with diffuse groin pain and multiple tender areas on examination (2, 8, 13). A number of professional soccer players will also have previously undergone partial or complete avulsions with subsequent haematoma and scarring; therefore identifying abnormal tendon architecture does not necessarily explain the patient's current symptoms (Figs 16.27 and 16.29).

> **Key point**
>
> The main clinical difficulty with adductor muscle injury is defining whether chronic groin pain in athletes is due to adductor tendinopathy/ dysfunction, osteitis pubis or a prehernia complex.

Ultrasound examination should fully evaluate the tendons, looking for any specific area of focal tenderness that reproduces the patient's symptoms. Additionally the rest of the myotendinous area and muscle should be assessed (including dynamic evaluation) for strains or tears (Fig. 16.26). Ultrasound evaluation

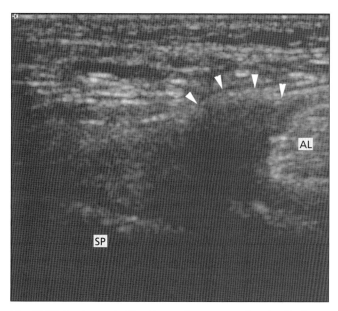

Fig. 16.26 Acute grade III adductor longus tear, longitudinal sonogram. The adductor longus (AL) can be seen retracted from the symphysis pubis (SP). In the intervening space there is hypoechoic fluid displacing overlying fascia (arrowheads), consistent with haematoma.

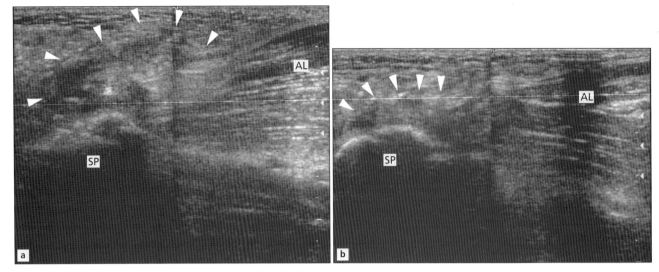

Fig. 16.28 Professional soccer player with acute on chronic right groin pain, longitudinal sonograms (dual screen to extend field of view). (a) On the symptomatic right side, there is marked distortion of the adductor longus tendon, which is swollen and replaced by a mixed hypo- and hyperechoic mass (arrowheads). The adductor longus (AL) muscle appears normal. Features are consistent with an acute tendinous rupture from the symphysis pubis (SP) and haematoma. (b) On the asymptomatic side the tendon is predominantly hyperechoic with loss of its normal tissue planes but is homogeneous and not swollen. Features are consistent with chronic tendinopathy.

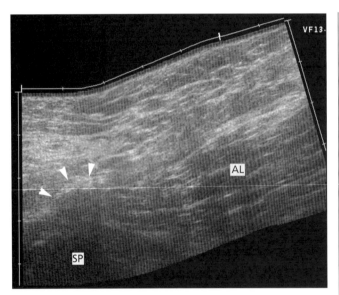

Fig. 16.29 Previous adductor longus avulsion, longitudinal sonogram (dual screen to extend field of view). The adductor longus muscle (AL) appears normal; however, at its insertion into the symphysis pubis (SP), there is a displaced hyperechoic avulsion fragment (arrowheads). The patient was a professional soccer player and was currently asymptomatic in this region.

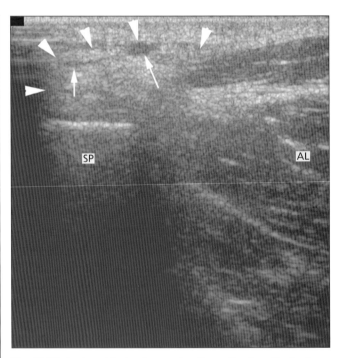

Fig. 16.30 Acute adductor longus tendinopathy, longitudinal sonogram. The adductor longus (AL) muscle has normal echotexture; however, the tendon is markedly swollen (arrowheads) and heterogeneous with loss of normal definition and hypoechoic areas present (small arrows).

of acute muscle and tendon abnormalities has already been described and the same basic principles apply to this muscle group (Figs 16.26 and 16.30) (see Chapter 12). Features that suggest that an area of chronic tendinopathy may be the origin of the player's symptoms are marked focal tenderness on transducer pressure and evidence of superimposed acute changes within the tendon, including haematoma or oedema, causing convex swelling of the soft-tissue planes with hypoechoic intrasubstance fluid (Figs 16.26 and 16.28) (61).

Other imaging techniques

There have been relatively few studies evaluating pelvic MR imaging in athletes with chronic groin pain (64–66). These studies admit to problems in obtaining a homogenous subject group due to difficultly in clinically defining the initial diagnosis and a measurable endpoint (6, 64, 66). Symphyseal bone marrow oedema, adductor longus oedema and rectus abdominis asymmetry on MR imaging have been described in differing proportions among symptomatic athletes (64, 66). There was a trend for these features to be present on the symptomatic side but abnormality did exist on the opposite side and was also described in asymptomatic patients. A small proportion of symptomatic athletes also had normal MR imaging appearances (66).

It is this author's belief that in athletes with groin pain ultrasound is effective in detecting inguinofemoral hernias and acute or chronic pathology in the adductor muscles and tendons, whereas MR imaging is better at defining bone marrow oedema associated with osteitis pubis or adductor dysfunction in this patient group where ultrasound examination is normal or shows only chronic changes (67). However, the sensitivity and specificity of these MR imaging features has yet to be fully established.

In the sportsman's hernia there have been various pathologies described, mainly involving microtears of the conjoint tendon or external oblique with subsequent neuropathy (2, 65). From an imaging point of view it is not possible to positively diagnose this condition and, at present, it remains a clinical diagnosis.

CONCLUSION

Ultrasound has the potential to become an integral tool in the imaging of patients with groin pain. Ultrasound is noninvasive and allows real-time evaluation of the groin, giving this technique a great potential advantage over other modalities in the examination of hernias and inguinal pathology. Postoperatively ultrasound can also play an important role in differentiating recurrent hernias from other complications.

In muscle and tendon injuries ultrasound is already established as an accurate and effective technique in diagnosing and grading injuries; however, in the assessment of athletes with chronic groin pain interpretation should be more cautious. In this patient group the underlying disease mechanisms are not clearly understood at present and there is often asymptomatic chronic tendon and symphyseal disease already present. Therefore identifying an imaging abnormality does not necessarily imply that this is the source of the athlete's current problem. In this troublesome clinical area, a multidisciplinary approach is necessary, for diagnosis and treatment, and different imaging modalities may be necessary to assess all aspects of the injury process.

REFERENCES

1. Kark A, Kurzer M, Waters KJ. Accuracy of clinical diagnosis of direct and indirect inguinal hernia. Br J Surg 1994;81(7):1081–2.
2. Renstrom P, Peterson L. Groin injuries in athletes. Br J Sports Med 1980;14(1):30–6.
3. Ashby EC. Chronic obscure groin pain is commonly caused by enthesopathy: "Tennis elbow" of the groin. Br J Surg 1994;81(11):1632–4.
4. Fredberg U, Kissmeyer-Nielsen P. The sportsman's hernia—Fact or fiction? Scand J Med Sci Sports 1996;6(4):201–4.
5. Lovell G. The diagnosis of chronic groin pain in athletes: A review of 189 cases. Aust J Sci Med Sport 1995;27(3):76–9.
6. Martens MA, Hansen L, Mulier JC. Adductor tendinitis and musculus rectus abdominis tendopathy. Am J Sports Med 1987;15(4):353–6.
7. Taylor DC, Meyers WC, Moylan JA, Lohnes J, Bassett FH, Garrett WE, Jr. Abdominal musculature abnormalities as a cause of groin pain in athletes. Inguinal hernias and pubalgia. Am J Sports Med 1991;19(3):239–42.
8. Thomas JM. Groin strain versus occult hernia: Uncomfortable alternatives or incompatible rivals? Lancet 1995;345(8964):1522–3.
9. Williams P, Foster ME. "Gilmore's groin"—Or is it? Br J Sports Med 1995;29(3):206–8.
10. Ziprin P, Williams P, Foster ME. External oblique aponeurosis nerve entrapment as a cause of groin pain in the athlete. Br J Surg 1999;86(4):566–8.
11. Ekberg O, Persson NH, Abrahamsson PA, Westlin NE, Lilja B. Longstanding groin pain in athletes. A multidisciplinary approach. Sports Med 1988;6(1):56–61.
12. Akermark C, Johansson C. Tenotomy of the adductor longus tendon in the treatment of chronic groin pain in athletes. Am J Sports Med 1992;20(6):640–3.
13. Fricker PA. Management of groin pain in athletes. Br J Sports Med 1997;31(2):97–101.
14. Lynch SA, Renstrom PA. Groin injuries in sport: Treatment strategies. Sports Med 1999;28(2):137–44.
15. Agur A. Grant's atlas of anatomy, 9th ed. Baltimore, MD: Williams and Wilkins; 1991.
16. Clemente C. Gray's anatomy. Philadelphia: Lea & Febiger; 1985.
17. Tetik C, Arregui ME, Dulucq JL, Fitzgibbons RJ, Franklin ME, McKernan JB, et al. Complications and recurrences associated with laparoscopic repair of groin hernias. A multi-institutional retrospective analysis. Surg Endosc 1994;8(11):1316–22; discussion 1322–3.

18. Deitch EA, Soncrant MC. Ultrasonic diagnosis of surgical disease of the inguinal-femoral region. Surg Gynecol Obstet 1981;152(3):319–22.

19. Orchard JW, Read JW, Neophyton J, Garlick D. Groin pain associated with ultrasound finding of inguinal canal posterior wall deficiency in Australian Rules footballers. Br J Sports Med 1998;32(2):134–9.

20. Lawrenz K, Hollman AS, Carachi R, Cacciaguerra S. Ultrasound assessment of the contralateral groin in infants with unilateral inguinal hernia. Clin Radiol 1994;49(8): 546–8.

21. Erez I, Schneider N, Glaser E, Kovalivker M. Prompt diagnosis of "acute groin" conditions in infants. Eur J Radiol 1992;15(3): 185–9.

22. Ekberg O. The herniographic appearance of direct inguinal hernias in adults. Br J Radiol 1981;54(642):496–9.

23. Ekberg O. Inguinal herniography in adults: Technique, normal anatomy, and diagnostic criteria for hernias. Radiology 1981;138(1):31–6.

24. Furtschegger A, Sandbichler P, Judmaier W, Gstir H, Steiner E, Egender G. Sonography in the postoperative evaluation of laparoscopic inguinal hernia repair. J Ultrasound Med 1995; 14(9):679–84.

25. van den Berg JC, Rutten MJ, de Valois JC, Jansen JB, Rosenbusch G. Masses and pain in the groin: A review of imaging findings. Eur Radiol 1998;8(6):911–21.

26. Sandler MA, Alpern MB, Madrazo BL, Gitschlag KF. Inflammatory lesions of the groin: Ultrasonic evaluation. Radiology 1984;151(3):747–50.

27. Sandbichler P, Draxl H, Gstir H, Fuchs H, Furtschegger A, Egender G, et al. Laparoscopic repair of recurrent inguinal hernias. Am J Surg 1996;171(3):366–8.

28. Smedberg SG, Broome AE, Gullmo A. Ligation of the hernial sac? Surg Clin North Am 1984;64(2):299–306.

29. Lilly MC, Arregui ME. Ultrasound of the inguinal floor for evaluation of hernias. Surg Endosc 2002;16(4):659–62.

30. Zhang GQ, Sugiyama M, Hagi H, Urata T, Shimamori N, Atomi Y. Groin hernias in adults: Value of color Doppler sonography in their classification. J Clin Ultrasound 2001;29(8): 429–34.

31. van den Berg JC, de Valois JC, Go PM, Rosenbusch G. Detection of groin hernia with physical examination, ultrasound, and MRI compared with laparoscopic findings. Invest Radiol 1999;34(12):739–43.

32. Ekberg O, Blomquist P, Fritzdorf J. Herniography in patients with clinically suggested recurrence of inguinal hernia. Acta Radiol Diagn (Stockh) 1984;25(3):225–9.

33. Ekberg O, Blomquist P, Olsson S. Positive contrast herniography in adult patients with obscure groin pain. Surgery 1981;89(5):532–5.

34. Ekberg O, Fork FT, Fritzdorf J. Herniography in atypical inguinal hernia. Br J Radiol 1984;57(684):1077–82.

35. Ekberg O, Fritzdorf J, Blomquist P. Herniographic appearance of contralateral inguinal hernia. Acta Radiol Diagn (Stockh) 1984;25(2):125–8.

36. Gullmo A. Herniography. The diagnosis of hernia in the groin and incompetence of the pouch of Douglas and pelvic floor. Acta Radiol Suppl 1980;361:1–76.

37. Jones RL, Wingate JP. Herniography in the investigation of groin pain in adults. Clin Radiol 1998;53(11):805–8.

38. Smedberg SG, Broome AE, Elmer O, Gullmo A. Herniography: A diagnostic tool in groin symptoms following hernial surgery. Acta Chir Scand 1986;152:273–7.

39. Smedberg SG, Broome AE, Elmer O, Gullmo A. Herniography in the diagnosis of obscure groin pain. Acta Chir Scand 1985;151(8):663–7.

40. Smedberg SG, Broome AE, Gullmo A, Roos H. Herniography in athletes with groin pain. Am J Surg 1985;149(3):378–82.

41. van den Berg JC, Strijk SP. Groin hernia: Role of herniography. Radiology 1992;184(1):191–4.

42. Ekberg O. Complications after herniography in adults. Am J Roentgenol 1983;140(3):491–5.

43. Sutcliffe JR, Taylor OM, Ambrose NS, Chapman AH. The use, value and safety of herniography. Clin Radiol 1999;54(7): 468–72.

44. van den Berg JC, de Valois JC, Go PM, Rosenbusch G. Groin hernia: Can dynamic magnetic resonance imaging be of help? Eur Radiol 1998;8(2):270–3.

45. Zarvan NP, Lee FT, Jr., Yandow DR, Unger JS. Abdominal hernias: CT findings. Am J Roentgenol 1995;164(6):1391–5.

46. Deitch EA, Soncrant MC. The value of ultrasound in the diagnosis of nonpalpable femoral hernias. Arch Surg 1981;116(2):185–7.

47. Gitschlag KF, Sandler MA, Madrazo BL, Hricak H, Eyler WR. Disease in the femoral triangle: sonographic appearance. Am J Roentgenol 1982;139(3):515–9.

48. Peterson L, Renstrom P. Sports injuries. Chicago: Year Book Medical; 1986.

49. Harrison LA, Keesling CA, Martin NL, Lee KR, Wetzel LH. Abdominal wall hernias: Review of herniography and correlation with cross-sectional imaging. Radiographics 1995; 15(2):315–32.

50. Shadbolt CL, Heinze SB, Dietrich RB. Imaging of groin masses: Inguinal anatomy and pathologic conditions revisited. Radiographics 2001;21 Spec No:S261–71.

51. Yeh HC, Lehr-Janus C, Cohen BA, Rabinowitz JG. Ultrasonography and CT of abdominal and inguinal hernias. J Clin Ultrasound 1984;12(8):479–86.

52. Gibbon WW. Diagnostic ultrasound in sports medicine. Br J Sports Med 1998;32(1):3.

53. Holmich P, Uhrskou P, Ulnits L, Kanstrup IL, Nielsen MB, Bjerg AM, et al. Effectiveness of active physical training as treatment for long-standing adductor-related groin pain in athletes: Randomised trial. Lancet 1999;353(9151): 439–43.

54. Karlsson J, Sward L, Kalebo P, Thomee R. Chronic groin injuries in athletes. Recommendations for treatment and rehabilitation. Sports Med 1994;17(2):141–8.

55. Fricker PA, Taunton JE, Ammann W. Osteitis pubis in athletes. Infection, inflammation or injury? Sports Med 1991;12(4): 266–79.

56. Harris NH, Murray RO. Lesions of the symphysis in athletes. Br Med J 1974;4(5938):211–4.

57. Holt MA, Keene JS, Graf BK, Helwig DC. Treatment of osteitis pubis in athletes. Results of corticosteroid injections. Am J Sports Med 1995;23(5):601–6.

58. Hawkins RD, Hulse MA, Wilkinson C, Hodson A, Gibson M. The association football medical research programme: An audit of injuries in professional football. Br J Sports Med 2001;35(1): 43–7.

59. Holmich P, Darre E, Jahnsen F, Hartvig-Jensen T. The elite marathon runner: Problems during and after competition. Br J Sports Med 1988;22(1):19–21.

60. Tyler TF, Nicholas SJ, Campbell RJ, McHugh MP. The association of hip strength and flexibility with the incidence of adductor muscle strains in professional ice hockey players. Am J Sports Med 2001;29(2):124–8.

61. Kalebo P, Karlsson J, Sward L, Peterson L. Ultrasonography of chronic tendon injuries in the groin. Am J Sports Med 1992; 20(6):634–9.

62. Ekstrand J, Hilding J. The incidence and differential diagnosis of acute groin injuries in male soccer players. Scand J Med Sci Sports 1999;9(2):98–103.

63. Andreasson G, Lindenberger U, Renstrom P, Peterson L. Torque developed at simulated sliding between sport shoes and an artificial turf. Am J Sports Med 1986;14(3): 225–30.

64. Albers SL, Spritzer CE, Garrett WE, Jr., Meyers WC. MR findings in athletes with pubalgia. Skeletal Radiol 2001; 30(5):270–7.

65. Meyers WC, Foley DP, Garrett WE, Lohnes JH, Mandlebaum BR. Management of severe lower abdominal or inguinal pain in high-performance athletes. PAIN (Performing Athletes with Abdominal or Inguinal Neuromuscular Pain Study Group). Am J Sports Med 2000;28(1):2–8.

66. Verrall GM, Slavotinek JP, Fon GT. Incidence of pubic bone marrow oedema in Australian rules football players: Relation to groin pain. Br J Sports Med 2001;35(1):28–33.

67. Robinson P, Barron DA, Parsons W et al. Adductor-related groin pain in athletes: correlation of MR imaging with clinical findings. Skeltal Radiol. 2004 Aug 33(8):451–7.

Index